Improving
Your Skills in
12-Lead ECG
Interpretation

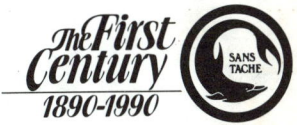

Improving Your Skills in 12-Lead ECG Interpretation

Gerry C. Mulholland

RN, MSN, CCRN

Manager, Cardiac Cath Lab
Cardiology Services
Lawrence & Memorial Hospital
New London, Connecticut

Barbara B. Brewer

MSN, RNC, CCRN, MALS

Administrative Director, Cardiology Services
Lawrence & Memorial Hospital
New London, Connecticut

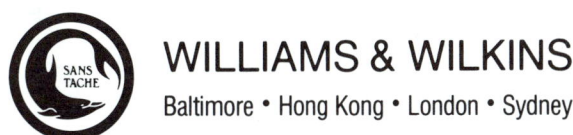

WILLIAMS & WILKINS

Baltimore • Hong Kong • London • Sydney

Editor: Susan M. Glover
Associate Editor: Marjorie Kidd Keating
Copy Editor: Susan S. Vaupel
Designer: JoAnne Jonowiak
Illustration Planner: Lorraine Wrzosek
Production Coordinator: Adèle Boyd
Cover Designer: Dan Pfisterer

Copyright © 1990
Williams & Wilkins
428 East Preston Street
Baltimore, Maryland 21202, USA

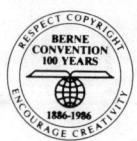

Printed in the United States of America

Library of Congress Cataloging in Publication Data

Mulholland, Gerry.
    Improving your skills in 12-lead ECG interpretation / Gerry Mulholland, Barbara Brewer.
        p.   cm.
    Includes bibliographical references.
    ISBN 0-683-06152-6
    1. Electrocardiography.   I. Brewer, Barbara,   II. Title.
RC683.5.E5M85   1990
616.1′207547—dc20   89-77622
                                                                  CIP

90 91 92 93 94
1 2 3 4 5 6 7 8 9 10

PREFACE

Suppose you are working in the coronary care unit or in the cardiac step-down unit. It is 12 midnight and your patient's call light goes on. You answer the light and discover your patient is having new onset chest pain. After assessing the patient and recording a 12-lead ECG, you call the physician to inform him or her of the change in the patient's condition. The physician asks if the ECG shows signs of ischemia or infarction and asks you to compare it with the patient's most recent ECG. Will you be able to interpret the 12-lead ECG? Will you immediately understand the significance of the ECG changes and modify the patient's plan of care?

Now suppose your patient has a diagnosis of an anterior wall myocardial infarction (MI). The rhythm strip shows normal sinus rhythm (NSR) with right bundle branch block (RBBB). Will you be able to determine whether the patient has extended the block? What monitoring lead would be more helpful to use?

If you cannot answer or need to research the answers to the above questions, *Improving Your Skills in 12-Lead ECG Interpretation* is for you! It will assist you in learning how to interpret a 12-lead ECG using a *systematic* approach and will assist you in applying the information in your clinical practice.

Improving Your Skills in 12-Lead ECG Interpretation is a text-workbook designed for nurses, medical students, paramedics and allied health professionals who have a background in basic dysrhythmia interpretation and who work in a hospital, ambulatory or office setting where 12-lead ECGs are done on a regular basis. The purpose of the book is to provide the learner with a *systematic* approach to interpreting both normal and abnormal 12-lead ECGs and to understand the clinical significance of the interpretation. This book is patterned after the approach used in basic dysrhythmia textbooks and courses. It is designed to show the learner where to begin and what information is essential.

In meeting the objectives of this book the learner will:

1. Develop a *systematic* and consistent approach to 12-lead ECG Interpretation.
   Each chapter addresses one aspect of the *systematic* process in detail and reinforces the material learned in previous chapters.
2. Improve his/her skill in 12-lead ECG interpretation.
   The book provides sufficient self assessment exercises for the learner to practice. The final chapter allows the learner to apply the completed *systematic* pro-

cess. Drill and practice will strengthen and improve one's skill.
3. Understand the significance of the interpretation in terms of the patient's plan of care.
   The ECG changes presented are related to their clinical significance. Patient care interventions are provided.
4. Learn a method that will simplify 12-lead ECG interpretation.

How can this text-workbook be utilized? It can be used as the primary text in a formal 12-lead ECG course. The text will provide the essential content needed to analyze 12-lead ECGs and provide sufficient practice exercises. It will free the coordinator or instructor of the course from the time consuming task of collecting practice ECG examples. The text can also be used by an individual for self-study and as a means of maintaining competence in this skill.

The book is unique in the way the chapters are written and organized. Each chapter builds upon the lessons learned in the previous one. The first chapter outlines the features of the normal 12-lead ECG and describes a step by step approach for use in its analysis. Chapters 2 through 8 each cover, in detail, *one* step of the *systematic* approach. In Chapter 8 *all* the steps of the process are reviewed and integrated to arrive at a final ECG interpretation. Six clinical situations and ECG exercises are included in Chapters 1 to 7 and 25 exercises are included in Chapter 8 for the learner's practice. The suggested answers to the ECG exercises are provided at the end of each chapter and in Appendix A, and are based on the clinical situations described.

How does the text-workbook differ from other textbooks on the market? This text-workbook picks up where others fail by providing a *systematic* approach for the learner. Content is integrated with application by asking the reader to complete six practice exercises at the end of each chapter. It focuses on everyday information a practicing nurse or health care worker needs to know. The book's primary concentration is on *how to* interpret a 12-lead ECG and *how to* apply the interpretation to the clinical situation. The book is sequenced in the order of a recommended systematic process. This will assist one in applying what is learned to the clinical area. There are many excellent content specific textbooks on the subject of interpreting the 12-lead ECG, but most lack practical application of the material, or cover too much information.

Improving Your Skills in 12-Lead ECG Interpretation is a text-workbook written by nurses for the clinical nurse and health practitioner. Using a step-by-step approach to this complicated and difficult subject makes it easier to understand. The emphasis is on developing speed and accuracy in 12-lead ECG analysis. The design of the book allows the learner to develop confidence in his/her interpretation and to use the information appropriately in the patient's plan of care. It stresses the comprehension of the information relative to the patient's plan of care and the nurse's role. The *systematic* approach in this book will make it a valuable reference.

ACKNOWLEDGMENTS

First, we would like to thank the nursing staff of the coronary care unit at the Lawrence and Memorial Hospital, New London, Connecticut, for collecting and sending us ECGs for the past 2 years. Without their assistance, this book would not have been possible.

We would like to thank Margaret Sexton Adams, RN, MSN, CNA, Bonnie S. Hoeper, BSPE, ASN, Richard Fazio, MD, and Timothy F. Brewer III, MD, for their help in reviewing this manuscript and Donna M. Cristadore for her graphic design assistance.

Finally, we would like to thank our husbands, Bob and Tim, who have both been extraordinarily patient and understanding and who supported us through the times we thought we would never complete this book.

CONTENTS

INTRODUCTION
Fundamental Principles

As a nurse or health care professional caring for cardiac patients, the knowledge and skill in quickly identifying normal from abnormal electrocardiograms (ECGs), and new from old ECG changes, are important to learn. This is considered advanced knowledge in cardiac care. Four things are essential in learning to interpret electrocardiograms:

1. Knowledge of the normal ECG features
2. Knowlege of common abnormal ECG features
3. Application of a systematic approach
4. Drill and practice

However, before your can add this knowledge, it is required that you have a thorough understanding and skill in assessing dysrhythmias.

The information contained in this book will assist you in accomplishing the above in a practical and logical way. Complex ECG examples and detailed explanations are purposely excluded. The book concentrates on the *how to* and provides self-assessment 12-lead ECG practice exercises at the end of each chapter, allowing the learner to immediately apply what is discussed.

12-LEAD ECG DEFINED

A 12-lead ECG is a common diagnostic test. It produces a graphic representation of the electrical forces of depolarization and repolarization of the heart. The electrical forces precede the contraction of the heart and are produced by its conduction system.

The ECG machine picks up the electrical activity of the heart and records it as positive (upright) and negative (inverted) deflections or waves on the ECG graph paper. The deflections caused when all of the cells of the heart are stimulated are called the P and QRS waves. The deflection caused by repolarization of the ventricles is the T wave. The distance between two waves is called a *segment*, and a wave and its accompanying segment is called an *interval*. The portion between the end of the T wave and the beginning of the next P wave is called the *baseline*. It is isoelectric meaning neither elevated nor depressed. The significance of each wave, segment, and interval is described below and labeled in Figure 1.

P Wave

The P wave represents atrial depolarization. It is produced by the firing of the sinoatrial (SA) node and the resultant spread of depolarization through the atria. The right atrium depolarizes first, then the left atrium. A P wave is generally positive, depending on the lead, and slightly rounded. It measures less than 0.11 sec in width and less than 2.5 mm in height.

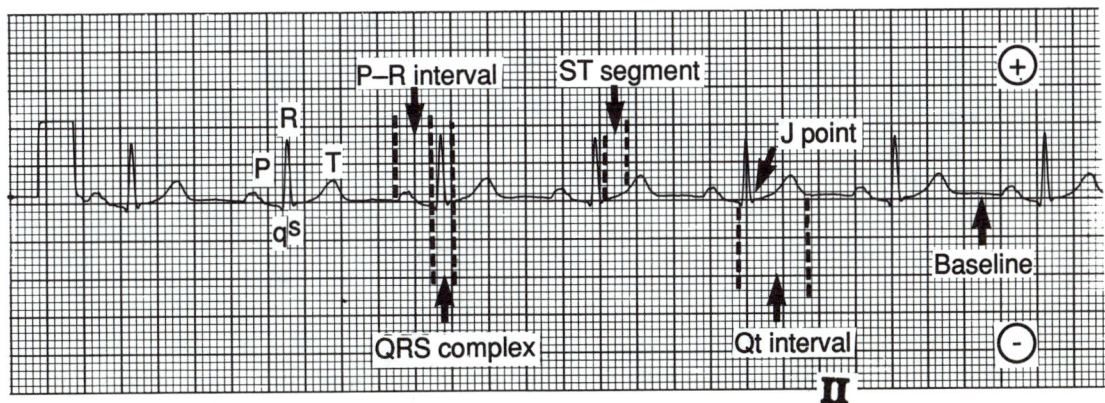

Figure 1. PQRST deflections, intervals, and segments. The U wave is not present in this diagram. The baseline is established by the line that runs between the end of the T wave to the beginning of the next P wave.

P-R Interval

The P-R interval indicates the time it takes the wave of depolarization to travel from the SA node through the atria to the start of ventricular depolarization. It includes a conduction delay of 0.04 sec at the atrioventricular (AV) node.

QRS Complex

The QRS complex represents ventricular depolarization. It can be composed of one, two, or three waves. The three waves are labeled Q, R, or S. The Q wave is the first negative deflection and is generally less than 0.04 sec in width. An R wave is the first positive deflection, and an S wave is a negative deflection after an R wave. When tall in amplitude, a wave is symbolized with capital letters. When small in amplitude, lower case letters are used.

ST Segment

The ST segment is the line that runs between the end of the QRS complex and the beginning of the T wave. It should be isoelectric and on the same level as the baseline. It is a sensitive indicator of myocardial ischemia and injury. The point where the ST segment departs from the QRS complex is known as the J point.

T Wave

A T wave represents ventricular repolarization. It is normally slightly rounded and asymmetrical in shape. T waves generally do not exceed 5 mm in height in the limb leads and 10 mm in the chest leads. A T wave is usually positive in leads that have a tall R wave. T wave abnormalities may indicate electrolyte and drug imbalances, or myocardial ischemia or infarction.

QT Interval

The QT interval represents the time it takes to complete ventricular depolarization and repolarization. It is measured from the beginning of the wave that composes the QRS complex to the end of the T wave.

U Wave

A U wave is a positive wave usually found after a T wave in the presence of bradycardia, hypokalemia, or ventricular hypertrophy.

Each of the 12 leads of an ECG records the electrical activity of the heart (depolarization and repolarization) from different view points. It must be understood that at any given instant the electrical activity of the heart is

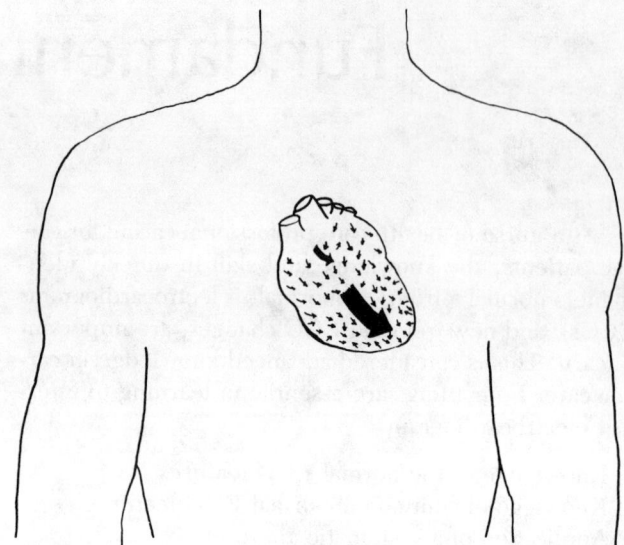

Figure 2. The mean cardiac vector or axis. Summation of multiple simultaneous forces equals the cardiac axis. Arrowhead = direction; arrowlength = amount. Used with permission from SJ Frye & P Lounsbury. *Cardiac rhythm disorders: An introduction using the nursing process.* Baltimore: Williams & Wilkins, 1988, p. 49.

being spread in many directions (up and down, right to left, front to back). Most of these forces are cancelled out by each other, and only the net force is recorded (Figure 2). The net force is called the *mean cardiac vector* or *cardiac axis*. It has magnitude and direction and is often represented by an arrow. The arrowhead points in the *direction* of the net wave of depolarization, and the arrow length denotes the *amount* of electrical activity. The amount of electrical activity is dependent on the number of heart cells depolarizing. A vector can be drawn for atrial depolarization (P wave), for ventricular depolarization (QRS waves) and for ventricular repolarization (T wave).

ECG GRAPH PAPER

The two things being recorded on the ECG graph paper are the *timing* of the electrical events in one cardiac cycle and the *amount* of current (voltage) being produced. *Timing* is measured on the horizontal axis of the graph paper. The graph paper should be moving at 25 mm per second. At this speed a 1 mm square on the horizontal axis equals 0.04 sec. *Voltage* is measured on the vertical axis. The calibration or standardization should be set at 1 mv, which equals a 10 mm deflection. At this standardization a 1-mm square on the vertical axis measures 0.1 mv. If the speed of the paper or the calibration is not as indicated, the measurements taken

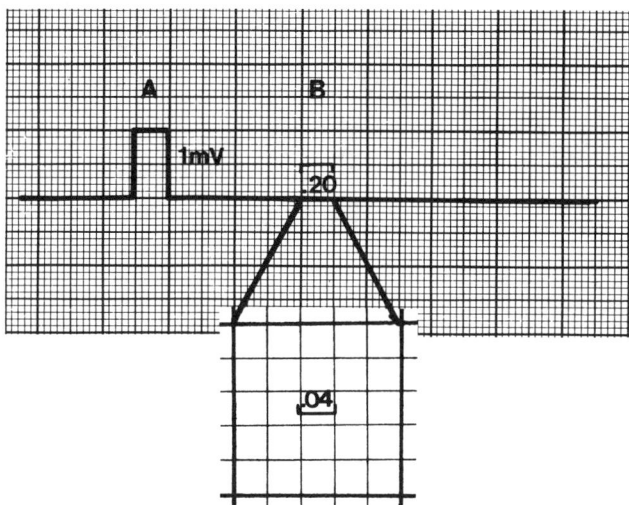

Figure 3. Time and voltage. *A,* vertical lines measure voltage. A 1 mv standardization mark writes a 10-mm deflection. *B,* horizontal lines represent time. One small square (1 mm) is equal to 0.04 sec. Five small squares are equal to 0.20 sec. Speed of recording paper is 25 mm per second. Used with permission from SJ Frye & P Lounsbury. *Cardiac rhythm disorders: An introduction using the nursing process.* Baltimore: Williams & Wilkins, 1988, p. 32.

will be incorrect. There are reasons it might be helpful to change the speed of the graph paper or the standardization calibration (Figure 3).

12 LEADS

A 12-lead ECG provides 12 different pictures of the electrical activity of the heart from either the frontal or horizontal plane. It does so by recording the difference in electrical activity between a positive (+) and a negative (−) electrode site that have been placed on the body. A combination of a positive and a negative electrode site is called a *lead.* The lead selected will determine which electrode is positive or negative by the ECG machine.

The electrodes placed on each extremity provide the electrode sites for the six limb leads. The electrode placed on the right leg (RL) serves as a reference electrode. Its function is to reduce interference from extraneous electrical activity. The *six limb leads* include the three bipolar standard limb leads *I, II, and III* and the three unipolar augmented limb leads *aVR, aVL, and aVF* (Figure 4). They record frontal plane activity. That is, they record the electrical activity traveling in two directions only from right to left and top to bottom. Each limb lead also examines certain surfaces of the heart differently.

Leads I, II, and III are bipolar leads because they look at the electrical activity between a positive and a negative electrode site. Lead I is looking at the electrical activity of the heart between the negative right arm (RA) and positive left arm (LA) electrode sites. Lead II is looking between the negative right arm (RA) and positive

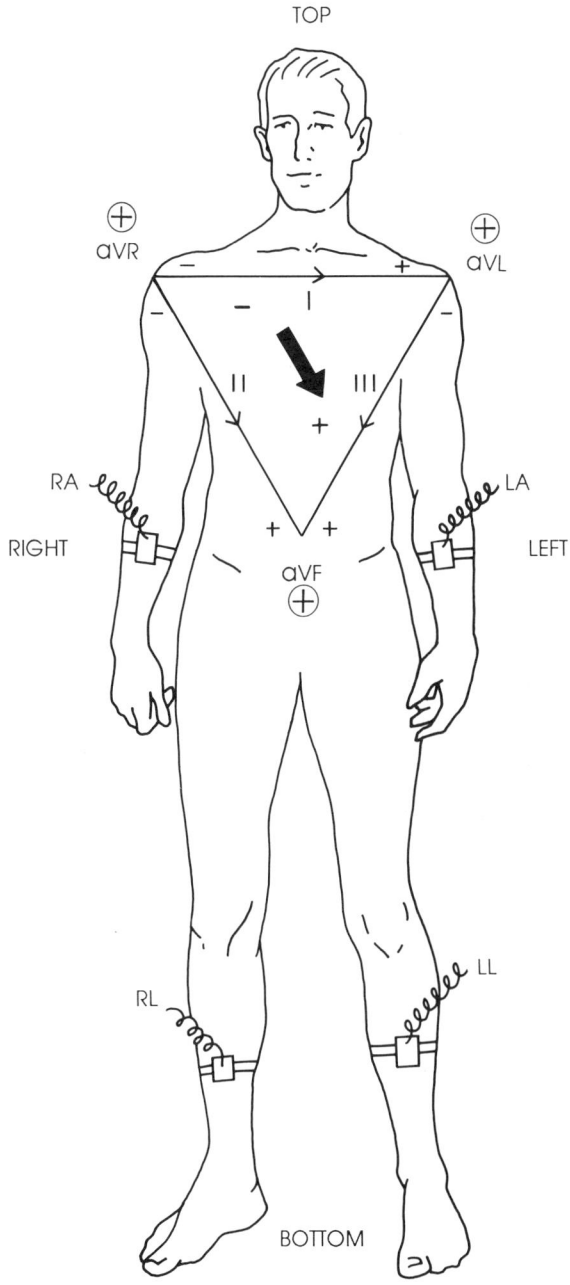

Figure 4. Limb lead placement records frontal plane activity (right to left, top to bottom): I = RA (−) to LA (+); II = RA (−) to LL (+); III = LA (−) to LL (+); aVR = RA (+); aVL = LA (+); aVF = LL (+). *Arrow,* mean cardiac axis. Adapted with permission from RM Berne & MN Levy. *Cardiovascular physiology.* St. Louis: CV Mosby Co., 1986, p. 39.

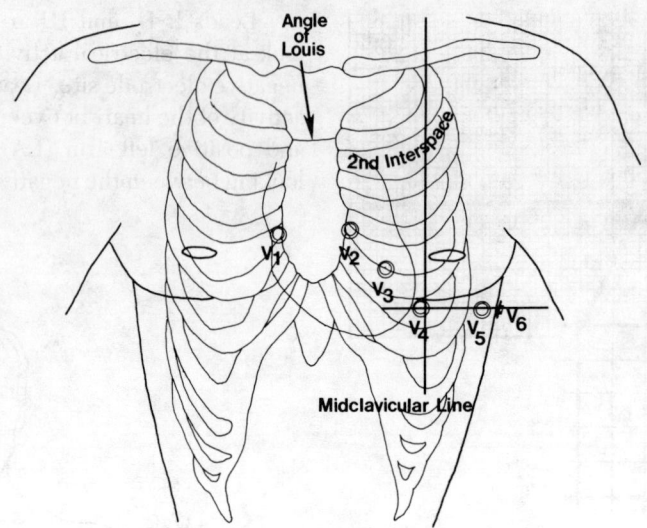

Figure 5. Chest lead placement records horizontal plane activity (right to left, back to front): V1 = 4th intercostal space (ICS) right side of sternum; V2 = 4th ICS left side of sternum; V3 = midway between V2 and V4; V4 = 5th ICS left midclavicular line (MCL); V5 = 5th ICS left anterior axillary line (AAL); V6 = 5th ICS left midaxillary line (MAL). Used with permission from SJ Frye & P Lounsbury. *Cardiac rhythm disorders: An introduction using the nursing process.* Baltimore: Williams & Wilkins, 1988, p. 58.

left leg (LL) electrode sites. Lead III is looking between the negative left arm (LA) and positive left leg (LL) electrode sites.

Leads aVR, aVL, and aVF are different from I, II, III in that they are unipolar and require the ECG machine to amplify the signal before recording it. Unipolar means it records the electrical activity from a single positive site. To complete the electrical circuit the ECG machine makes all of the other extremity electrode sites negative. Lead aVR is recorded from the positive RA electrode site. Lead aVL is recorded from the positive LA site. Lead aVF is recorded from the positive LL site.

The six electrodes placed on the chest provide the electrode sites for the six chest or precordial leads. The

chest leads are positioned on the chest in specific places (Figure 5). The *six chest* unipolar leads are *V1, V2, V3, V4, V5, and V6.* To complete the lead circuit the ECG machine considers the center of the heart negative. The chest leads record the electrical activity traveling on a horizontal plane that is from a right to left and a front to back direction.

To summarize, the 12-lead ECG consists of three bipolar standard limb leads, three augmented limb leads, and six chest leads. They provide a look at the electrical activity of the heart from 12 different viewpoints. Learn the positive pole of each of the 12 leads. Study the text and figures to determine how the P, QRS, and T waves in each lead should look.

1

Systematic Approach to 12-Lead Interpretation

This chapter describes the normal configurations of each of the 12 leads that must be learned before interpreting an electrocardiogram (ECG) accurately. Its main function is to outline one systematic approach to use in reading ECGs.

NORMAL 12-LEAD CONFIGURATIONS

What are the normal configurations of the P wave, QRS complex, T wave, and ST segment of the 12 leads?

The following *principles of electrocardiography* are necessary to comprehend why a specific lead has a positive or negative wave configuration, or is small or large in amplitude.

1. If the wave of depolarization of the heart is traveling toward the positive electrode site of the recording lead, a positive or upright deflection is produced on the ECG (Figure 1.1).
2. If the wave of depolarization of the heart is traveling away from the positive electrode site of the recording lead, a negative or inverted deflection is produced on the ECG (Figure 1.2).
3. If the wave of depolarization of the heart is traveling toward the positive electrode and then away from it, a diphasic or partially positive and negative deflection is produced on the ECG (Figure 1.3).
4. If the wave of depolarization being produced is small, the deflection on the ECG will be small in amplitude.
5. If the wave of depolarization being produced is large, the deflection on the ECG will be large in amplitude.

Next is a discussion of the normal deflections (P wave, QRS complex, T wave, and ST segment) in each lead. Remember to apply the principles of electrocardiography to your understanding of why a wave is positive or negative in certain leads. Also, it is important to know and relate the direction of the mean cardiac axis

of the heart to the positive recording site of the lead. The mean cardiac axis of the heart is oriented downward and to the left, and it is in the direction of the apex.

Generally, the P wave in the limb leads should be less than 0.11 seconds in width and less than 2.5 mm in height. The QRS complex should be less than 26 mm in amplitude. The ST segment should be isoelectric, not varying more than 1 mm above or 0.5 mm below the baseline in all leads. The T wave should be positive in leads with a positive R wave and a normal QRS duration.

Limb Leads (Figure 1.4)

Lead I is looking from the right arm (RA) (−) to the left arm (LA) (+). The wave of depolarization of the heart is moving downward and to the left, toward the positive pole of lead I, so the P wave, QRS complex, and T wave will be mainly positive. The QRS complex is generally composed of a small q (negative) wave, a large R (positive) wave, and an S (negative) wave that is smaller than the R wave.

Lead II is looking from the RA (−) to the left leg (LL) (+). The wave of depolarization is moving directly toward the positive LL electrode, so the P wave, QRS complex, and T wave will be positive. The P wave generally is taller and more positive in Lead II than the other limb leads. The QRS complex is composed of a small q wave, a large R wave, and an S wave that is always smaller than the R wave.

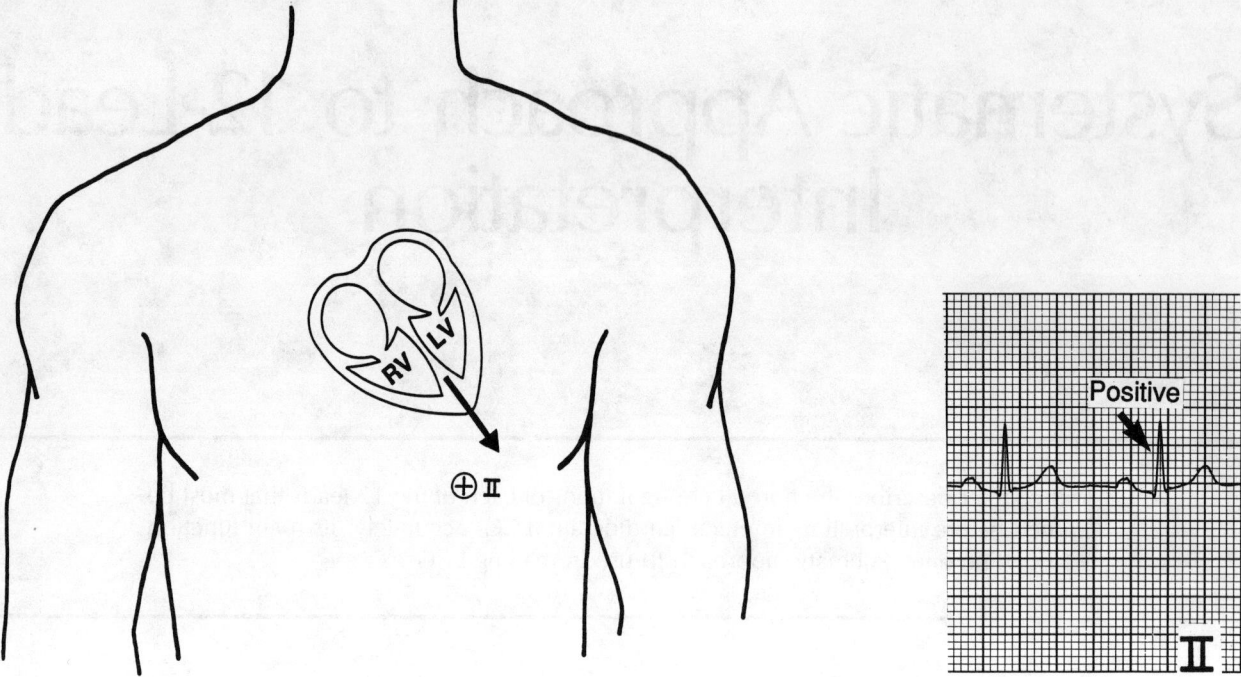

Figure 1.1. Wave traveling toward positive pole = Positive Deflections.

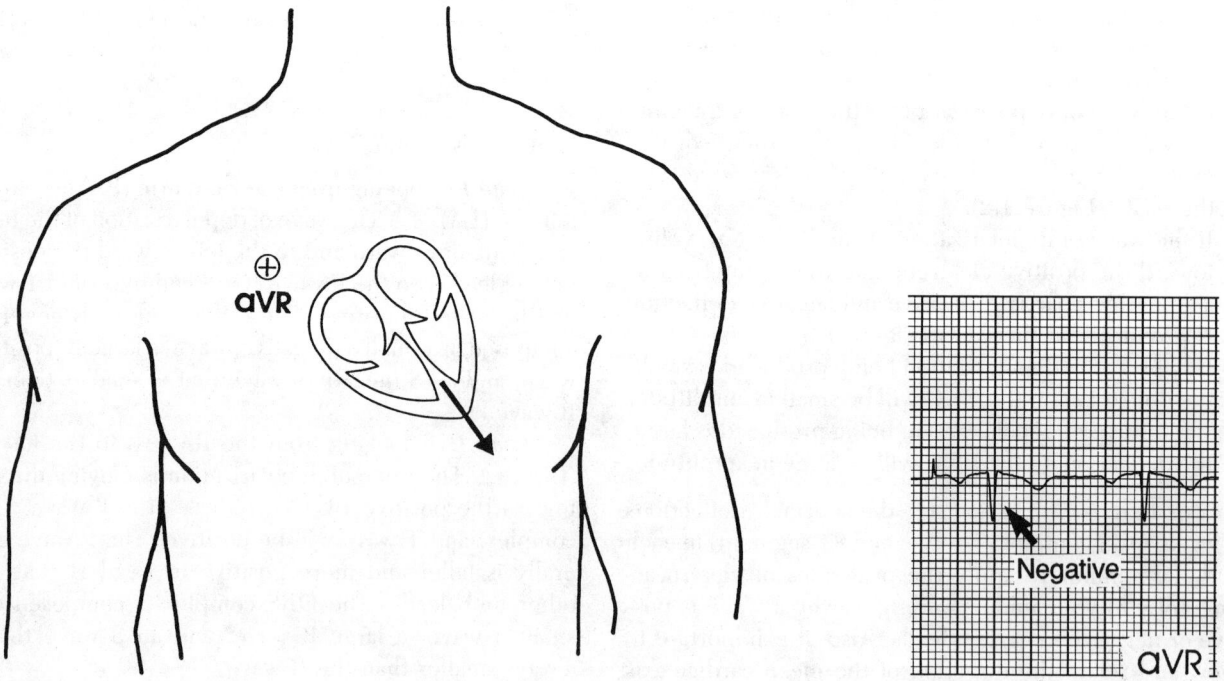

Figure 1.2. Wave traveling away from positive pole = Negative Deflections.

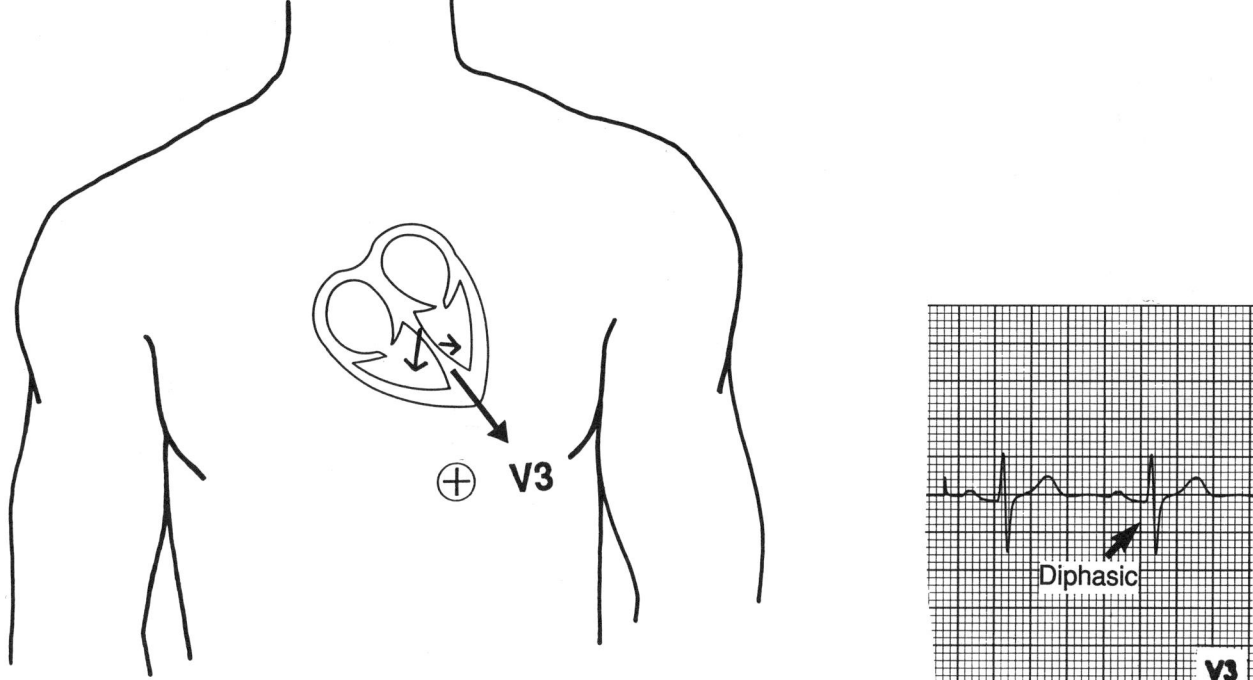

Figure 1.3.   Wave traveling toward positive pole then away from it = Diphasic Deflections.

Lead III is looking from the LA (−) to the LL (+). The sum of electrical activity travels toward the positive LL electrode and then away from it. The P and T waves will be variable in shape and direction. Because it is variable it could be either positive, flat, diphasic, or negative, depending on the cardiac axis. The P wave is generally smaller than in lead II. The QRS complex will be mainly positive. The QRS complex consists of a small or absent q wave, a large R wave, and a small s wave. Depending on the electrical axis of the heart, the S wave may be larger than the R wave and still be normal.

Lead *aVR* is looking at the electrical activity from the RA (+). Because the wave of depolarization is moving away from the positive electrode, the P wave and QRS complex will always be negative. The QRS complex could be composed of either a small, absent, or large Q wave, a very small or absent R wave, and generally a large S wave. It is often referred to as a large QS complex. The T wave will also be negative.

Lead *aVL* looks at the electrical activity from the LA (+). The electrical activity approaches the positive LA electrode and then recedes away from it producing a diphasic deflection, first positive then negative. P waves are small and vary in shape and direction. The QRS complex may have either a small, absent, or large Q wave and R wave. The S wave may be absent or large, and the T wave will be variable in shape and direction.

Lead *aVF* looks at the electrical activity from the LL (+). The wave is directed toward the positive LL electrode, so the P wave and the QRS complex will be positive. The QRS complex may have either a small or absent q wave, a small, absent, or large R wave, and an absent to large S wave. The T wave will vary in shape and direction.

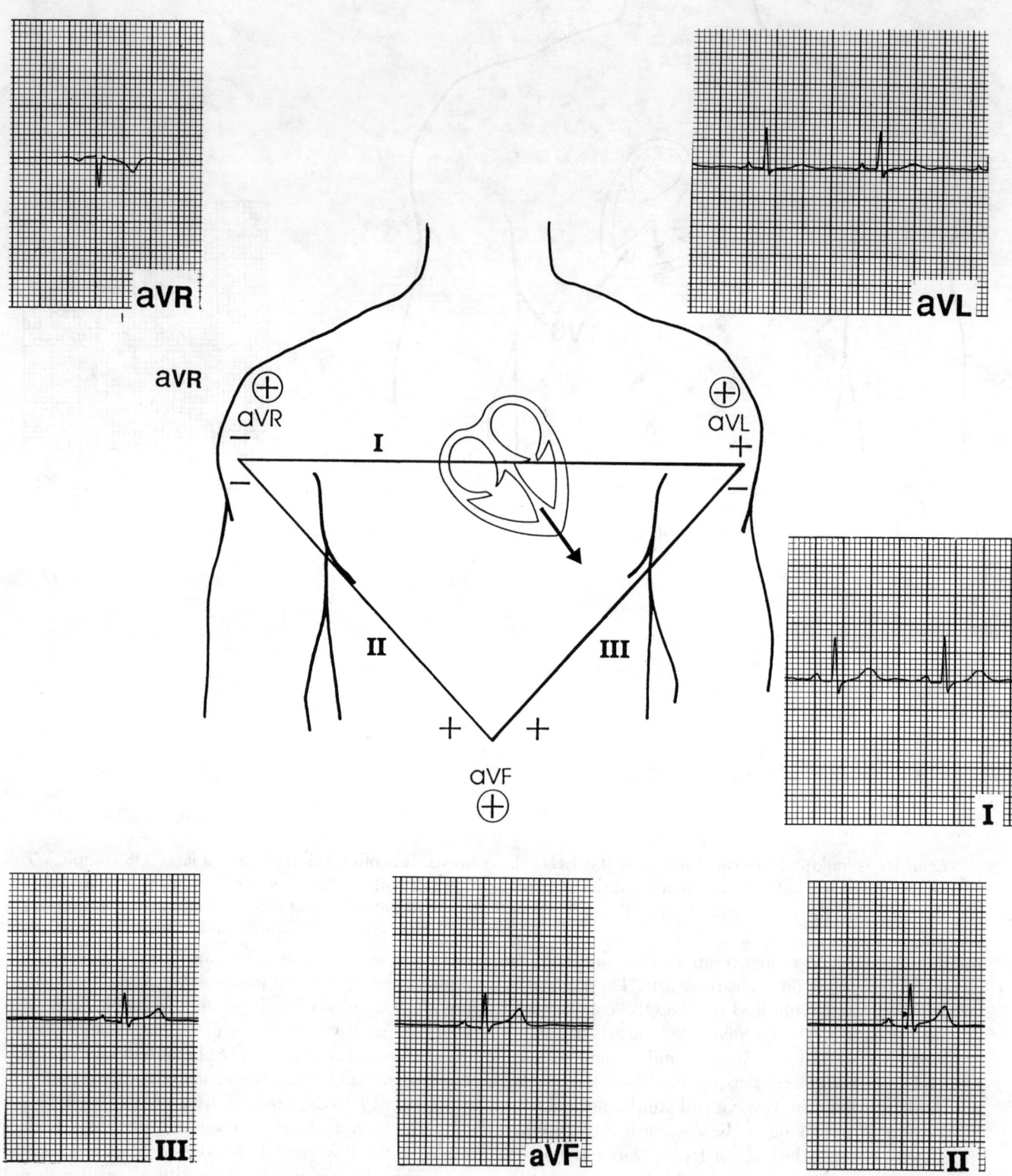

Figure 1.4.   Limb leads and their respective recordings.

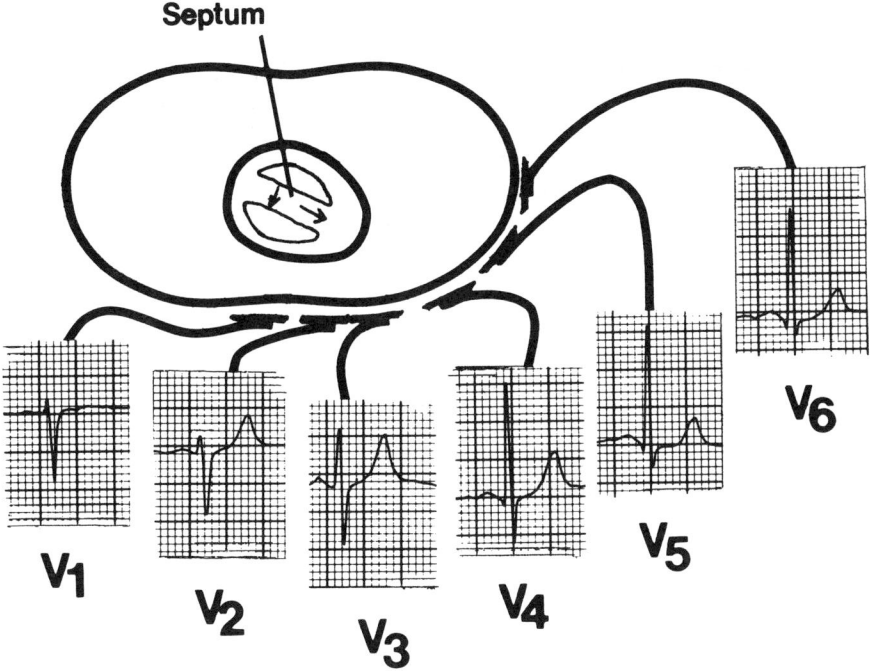

Septum

Figure 1.5. Chest leads and their respective recordings. Used wih permission from SJ Frye & P Lounsbury. *Cardiac rhythm disorders: An introduction using the nursing process.* Baltimore: Williams & Wilkins, 1988, p. 59.

Chest Leads (Figure 1.5)

The deflections in the precordial leads change as the electrode site moves from right to left around the chest wall. The V leads are single positive electrode sites. The deflections in the V leads vary because the wave of depolarization stimulates the ventricles in a very specific pattern. The first part of the ventricular myocardium to be activated is the interventricular septum. The impulse then spreads down the septum and stimulates both right and left ventricles. The R wave in V1 is small and becomes progressively larger in leads V2–V6. This is called normal R wave progression through the chest leads.

V1 and V2 will have similar appearances because they are close together. They are primarily negative and are referred to as *right* chest leads. They see the initial wave through the septum, from left to right, coming toward them, and produce a small r wave. Then the wave proceeds through the left ventricle, away from them, producing a deep S wave. The R wave in V2 will be slightly taller than in V1. The QRS complex may have either an absent q wave, absent or small r wave, or a large S wave. The P wave and T wave will be variable. They can be positive, flat, negative, or diphasic.

V3 and V4 also may be similar in configuration. They are diphasic and are referred to as *transitional* leads. Because of their location, they do not see the initial septal wave from left to right, but they do see the wave as it comes down the septum straight toward them, which produces a large R wave. Then the wave moves up through the left ventricular wall, away from V3 and V4, producing a deep S wave. The R wave is taller in these leads than in V1 and V2. The QRS complex may have either a small or absent q wave and an R wave that is less than, greater than, or equal to the S wave in size. The R in V4 is greater than in V3. The P wave in V3 is variable, whereas it is generally positive in V4. The T wave is positive in both leads.

V5 and V6 are primarily positive and are referred to as *left* chest leads. They are located laterally and view the initial wave through the interventricular septum moving from left to right away from them producing a small q wave. Then the wave comes down the septum and begins to move toward V5 and V6, producing a large R wave. The QRS in these leads will normally have exactly the opposite configuration to V1 and V2. Both the P and T waves will be positive.

Table 1.1 summarizes the normal configurations for the 12 leads.

Table 1.1.
Normal 12-Lead Configurations[a]
Listed below are the normal and some normal variations of adult 12-lead ECG configurations. The waves described below will vary depending on the axis of the heart. The configurations may also represent abnormal findings depending on the clinical situation.

Lead	P Wave	QRS Complex Waves	T Wave[b]	ST Segment[c]
I	Positive	Small q. R > S	Positive	Isoelectric
II	Positive	Small q. R > S	Positive	Isoelectric
III	Variable	Small or absent q. R > S	Variable	Isoelectric
aVR	Negative	Small, absent, or large Q Small or absent r Large S (may be QS)	Negative	Isoelectric
aVL	Variable	Small, absent, or large Q Small, absent, or large R Absent to large S	Variable	Isoelectric
aVF	Positive	Small or absent q Small, absent, or large R Absent to large S	Variable	Isoelectric
V1	Variable	Absent Q Absent or small r R < S Large S (QS)	Variable	Isoelectric
V2	Variable	Same as V1 R > R in V1	Variable	Isoelectric
V3	Variable	Small or absent q R <, >, or = S R > R in V2	Positive	Isoelectric
V4	Positive	Small or absent q R > S R > R in V3	Positive	Isoelectric
V5	Positive	Small q Large R (<26 mm) R > R in V4 S < S in V4	Positive	Isoelectric
V6	Positive	Small q Large R (<26 mm) S < S in V5	Positive	Isoelectric

[a]Adapted with permission from MJ Goodman, *Principles of Clinical Electrocardiography.* Los Altos, California: Lange Medical, 1982.
[b]Positive = upright; negative = inverted; variable = either positive, flat, diphasic, or negative.
[c]The ST Segment is isoelectric but may vary from +1 to −0.5 mm.

CLINICAL SIGNIFICANCE

Interpreting a 12-lead ECG requires a considerable amount of knowledge and skill. Accurate interpretation requires knowledge of the patient's clinical and drug history, and comparison of baseline and serial ECG tracings for trends. An ECG must be interpreted in conjunction with the clinical situation. A normal ECG does not equal absence of heart disease, and an abnormal ECG does not equal heart disease.

Each lead is looking at the heart from different angles and surfaces. Thus each lead has a specific function that can provide valuable information in caring for your car-

diac patients. The specific functions of each lead are as follows:

Lead I—Axis determination
   Cardiac monitoring
   Lateral wall changes
   Hemiblocks
Lead II—Axis determination
   Cardiac monitoring
   Inferior wall changes
   Atrial abnormalities
Lead III—Same as Lead II
   Hemiblocks

Lead aVR—Axis determination
Lead aVL—Axis determination
  Lateral wall changes
Lead aVF—Axis determination
  Inferior wall changes
Lead V1—Bundle branch block (BBB) determination
  Anteroseptal/posterior wall changes
  Ventricular ectopy versus aberrancy
  Atrial abnormalities
  Ventricular hypertrophy
Lead V2—Anteroseptal/posterior wall changes
  Ventricular hypertrophy
Lead V3—Anteroseptal wall changes
Lead V4—Anteroseptal wall changes
Lead V5—Anterior/lateral wall changes
  Ventricular hypertrophy
Lead V6—Bundle branch block determination
  Lateral wall changes
  Ventricular ectopy versus aberrancy
  Ventricular hypertrophy

Knowledge of the specific function of each of the 12 leads above is important because the location of an infarction can predict what type of complication the patient might develop. This will be made clear in ensuing chapters. For example, if your patient was admitted with an anterior wall myocardial infarction (MI), you would most likely monitor on V1. This is because an anterior wall MI is often associated with the development of a bundle branch block.

SYSTEMATIC APPROACH

Where to begin? The steps in analyzing a 12-lead ECG are listed below.

Step 1. Rhythm Determination

In this step you must be able to calculate the atrial and ventricular heart rates, measure the P-R interval and the duration of the QRS complex, and describe the shape of the individual waves. The result of this step is the determination of the rhythm diagnosis.

Step 2. Axis Determination

In this step you will determine the cardiac axis. Is the axis normal, deviated to the right or left, or indeterminate? The normal axis is generally considered between 0 and 90 degrees.

Step 3. Chamber Enlargement Determination

In this step, you will determine whether there is right or left atrial abnormality or right or left ventricular hypertrophy.

Step 4. Intraventricular Conduction Blocks Determination

In this step you will determine the presence of right bundle branch block (RBBB), left bundle branch block (LBBB), incomplete bundle branch blocks, intraventricular conduction delays, left anterior hemiblock (LAH), or left posterior hemiblock (LPH).

Step 5. Ischemia, Injury, and Infarction Determination

In this step you will determine the presence of myocardial ischemia, injury, or infarction. You will also determine the location of the problem identified.

Step 6. Miscellaneous ECG Changes

In this step, you will examine the ECG for the presence of common electrolyte imbalances, drug effects, and cardiac conditions that affect the 12-lead ECG.

Step 7. Final Interpretation

In this final step, you will establish a 12-lead ECG interpretation and combine it with the rhythm diagnosis determined in Step 1.

Each of the steps above in the systematic process will be described in detail in the ensuing chapters. Table 1.2, a self-assessment analysis form, outlines the steps of the process and is used throughout the book (Brown & Jacobson, 1988; Smith-Marker, 1982). A tear-out sample is also provided at the back of this book for future use in your clinical practice.

SELF-ASSESSMENT EXERCISES

Each chapter will provide self-assessment exercises for you to analyze using the systematic process. All of the ECGs were recorded on a triple channel machine except where noted. A triple channel ECG machine records three leads simultaneously. Leads appear to run together without obvious demarcation between them and display only 2.5 sec of information. The ECGs should be read down each row and from left to right. Figure 1.6 is an example of a normal triple channel ECG recording.

It is standard practice to run a 10 sec rhythm strip of either leads II, V1, or V6 when performing a 12-lead ECG to assist in rhythm determination. Rhythm strips will not be reproduced with the ECG examples except in Chapter 2 and where necessary.

It is important to verify that a ECG is technically correct before analyzing the tracing. To quickly verify, scan leads I, II, and III. The R wave voltage in lead II should equal the sum of the R wave voltage in leads I and III (lead II = lead 1 + lead III). If not, the ECG

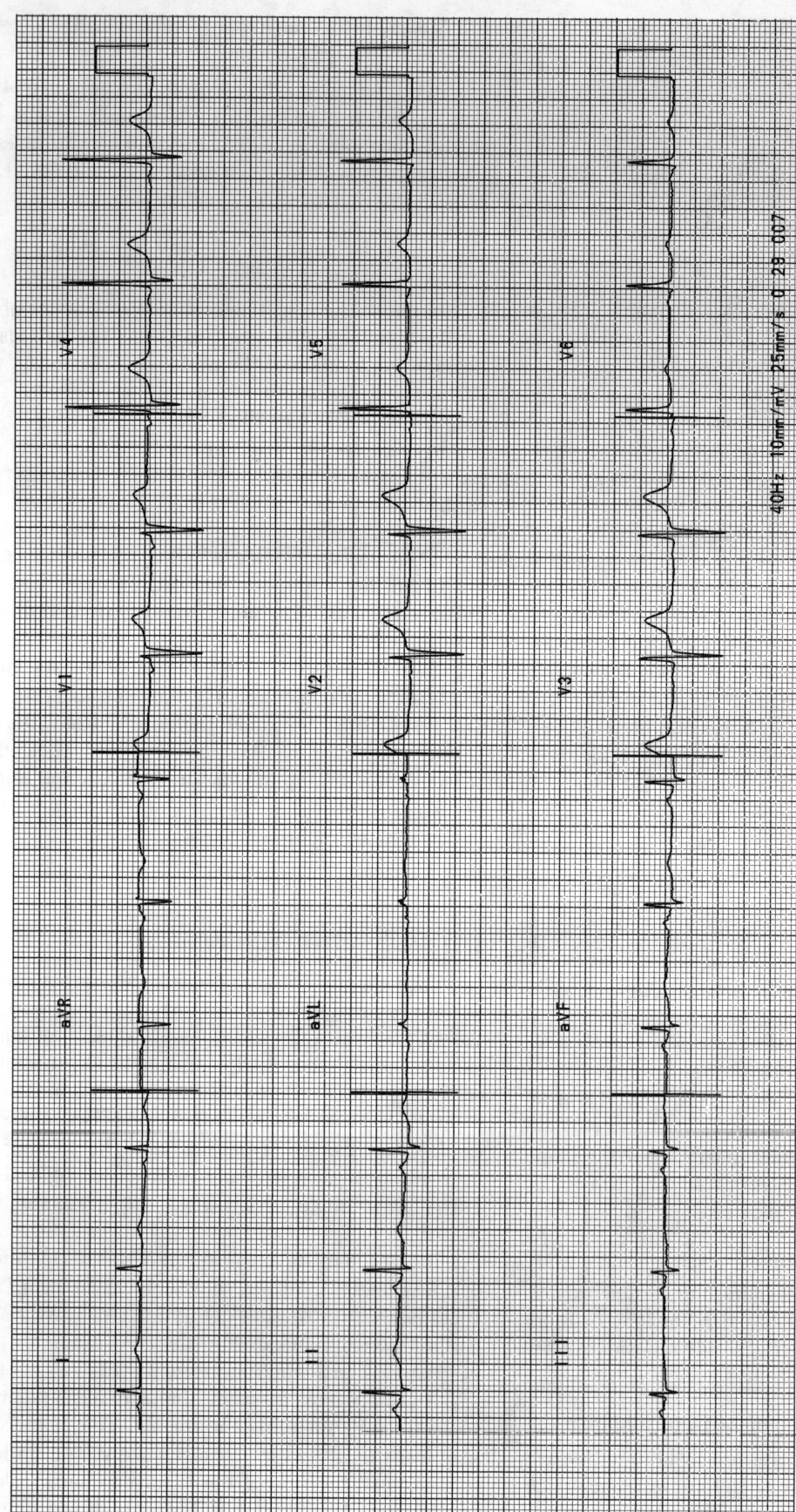

Figure 1.6. Normal ECG example run on a triple channel ECG machine. Read down each row and from left to right.

Table 1.2.
Self-Assessment Analysis Form

STEP 1. *Rhythm Determination*
- Ventricular rate _____
- QRS shape _____
- R-R rhythm _____
- QRS interval _____
- QT interval _____
- Dominant pacemaker site _____
- Interpretation _____
- Atrial rate _____
- P wave shape _____
- P-P rhythm _____
- P-R interval _____
- P:R conduction ratio _____

STEP 2. *Axis Determination*
Normal ___   Right ___   Left ___   Indeterminate ___

STEP 3. *Chamber Enlargement Determination*
Atrial Abnormality: Right ___   Left ___
Ventricular Hypertrophy: Right ___   Left ___

STEP 4. *Intraventricular Conduction Blocks Determination*
RBBB ___   LBBB ___
Incomplete RBBB ___   Incomplete LBBB ___   IVCD ___
LAH ___   LPH ___

STEP 5. *Ischemia, Injury, and Infarction Determination*
Inferior leads (II, III, aVF): _____
Anterior leads (V1–V6): _____
Lateral leads (I, aVL, V5–V6): _____
Anteroseptal leads (V1–V4): _____
Posterior leads (V1–V2 Reciprocal): _____
Diffuse _____

STEP 6: *Miscellaneous ECG Changes*
Electrolytes: _____
Drugs: _____
Pericarditis: _____
Other: _____

STEP 7. *Final Interpretation*
_____
_____

possibly was recorded incorrectly. Lead aVR will always be negative.

SELF-ASSESSMENT EXERCISES 1–6

The following 12-lead ECGs all are normal. Analyze each ECG by comparing the P waves, QRS complexes, ST segments, and T wave configurations in each of the 12 leads with that identified in this chapter as normal for that lead. You must be able to recognize normal before you can learn the abnormal changes and their significance.

When you have completed all of the exercises in this book, come back to this exercise and apply the systematic process. Check your answers with the suggested interpretation found at the end of this chapter. Answers for remaining steps will be found in Appendix A.

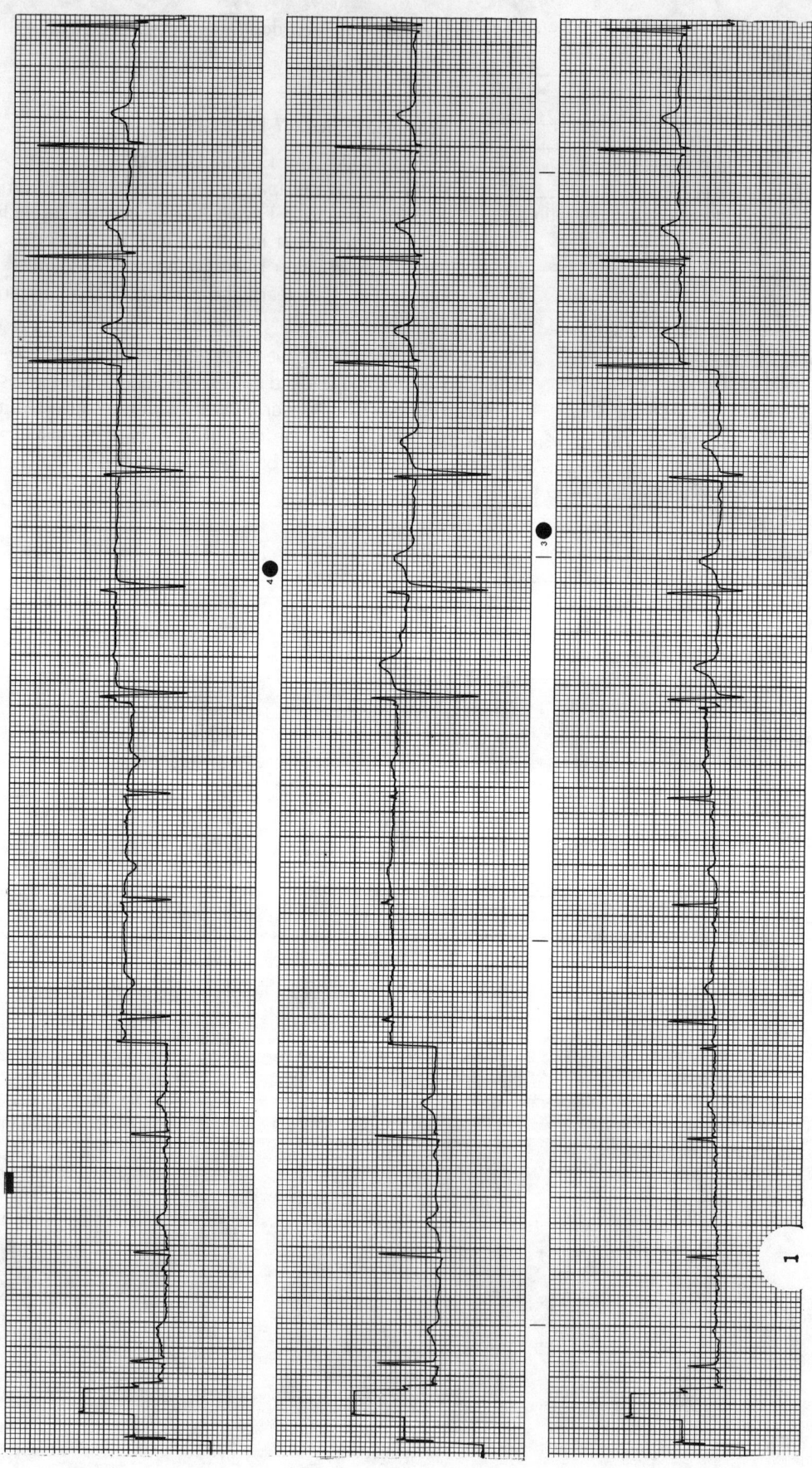

Exercise 1. A 24-year-old female college student with no history of cardiac disease or smoking.

Exercise 2. A 34-year-old woman with no history of cardiac problems. Positive cigarette smoking history.

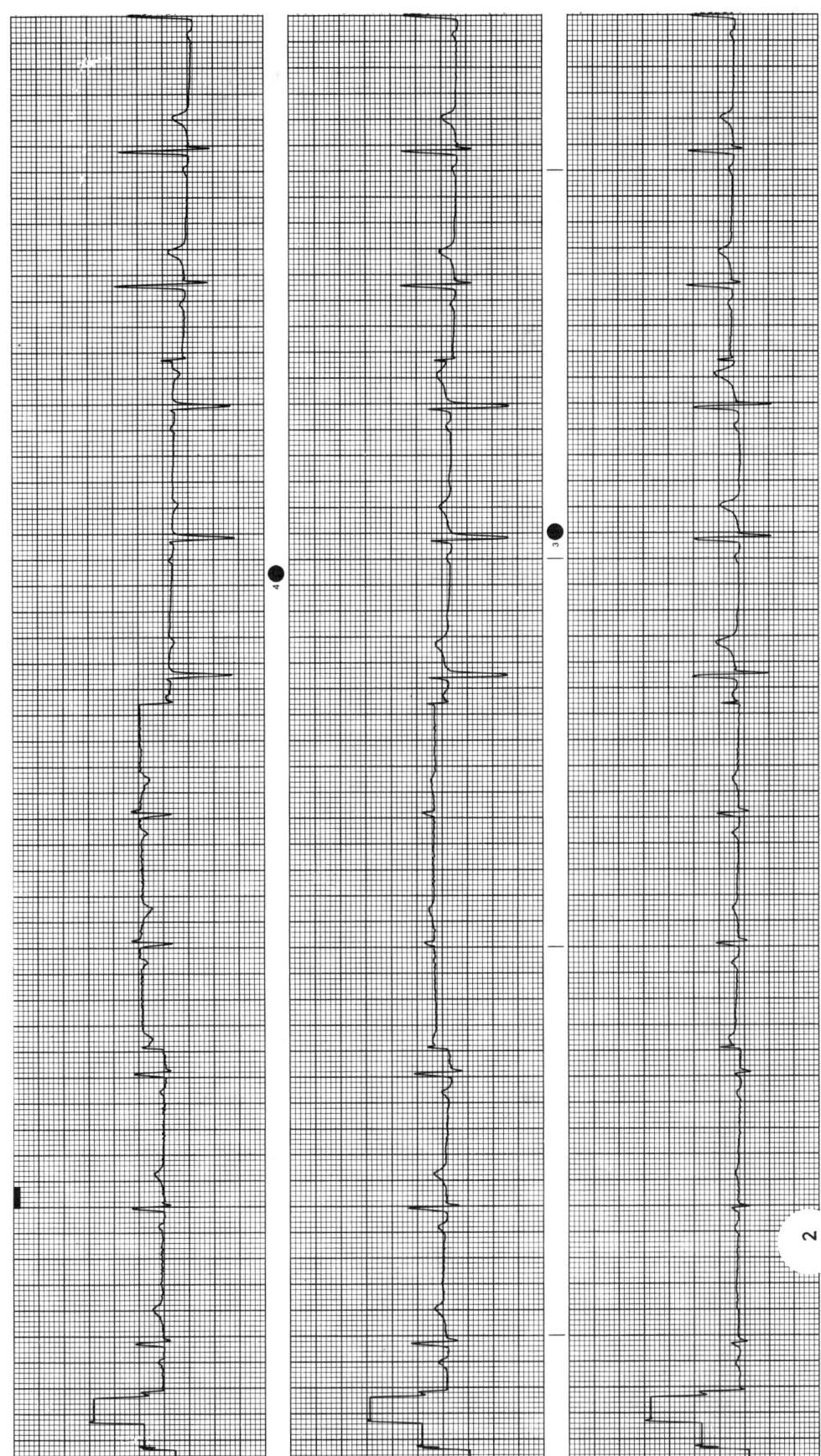

Exercise 3. A 60-year-old man admitted to the coronary care unit (CCU) with a 4-hour history of substernal chest pain. He described the pain as stabbing in nature. Does not smoke. Cardiac enzymes normal.

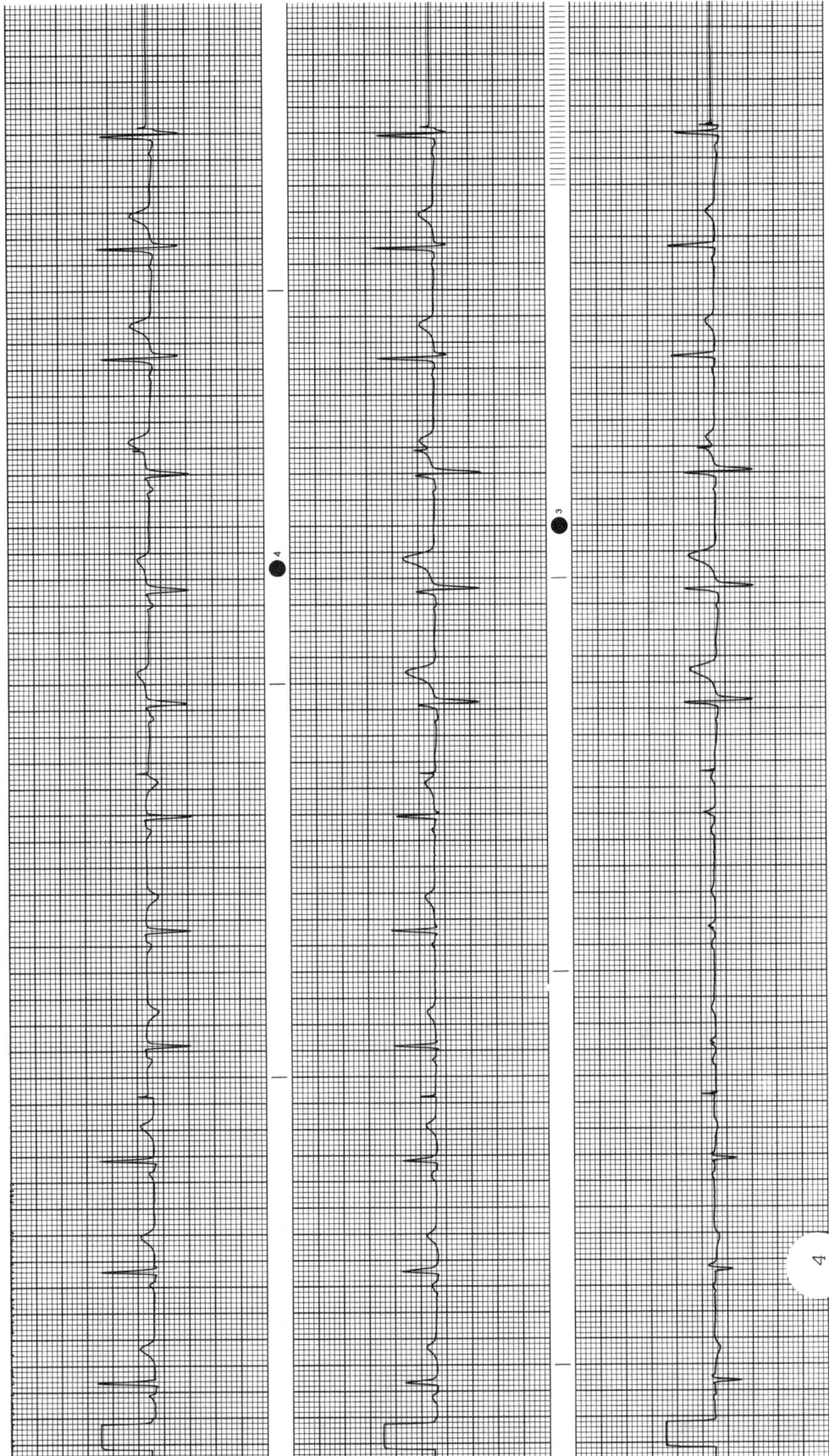

Exercise 4. A 43-year-old man admitted to the CCU with a 2-hour history of retrosternal chest heaviness. Positive smoking history and positive family history for cardiac disease. Cardiac enzymes normal.

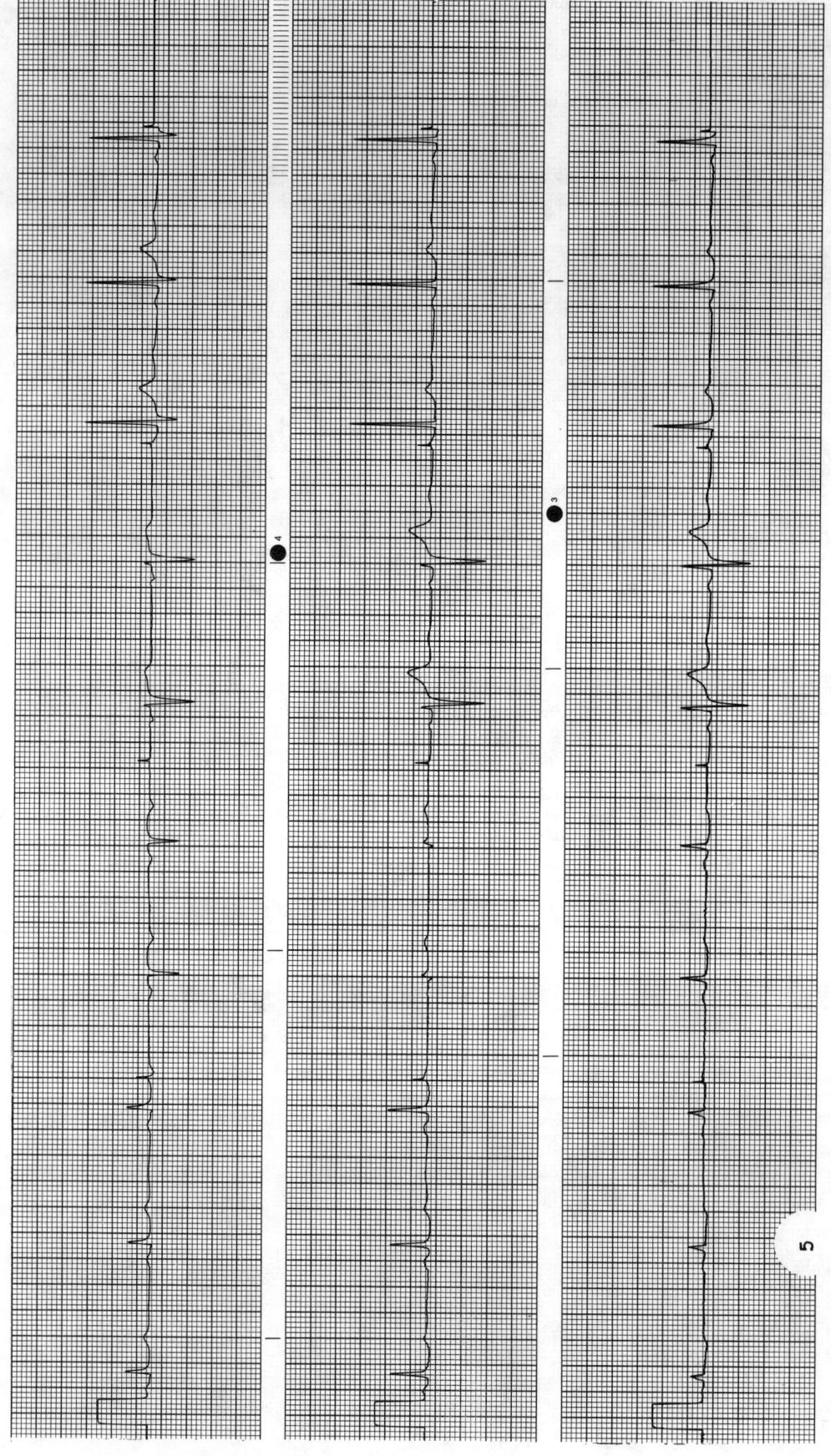

Exercise 5. A 78-year-old man admitted complaining of prolonged chest pain. Positive smoking history. Status post-non-Q wave anterior infarction 1 year ago. Cardiac enzymes negative. On the following daily medications: Digoxin, Tenormin, Nitro paste, Procardia, ASA.

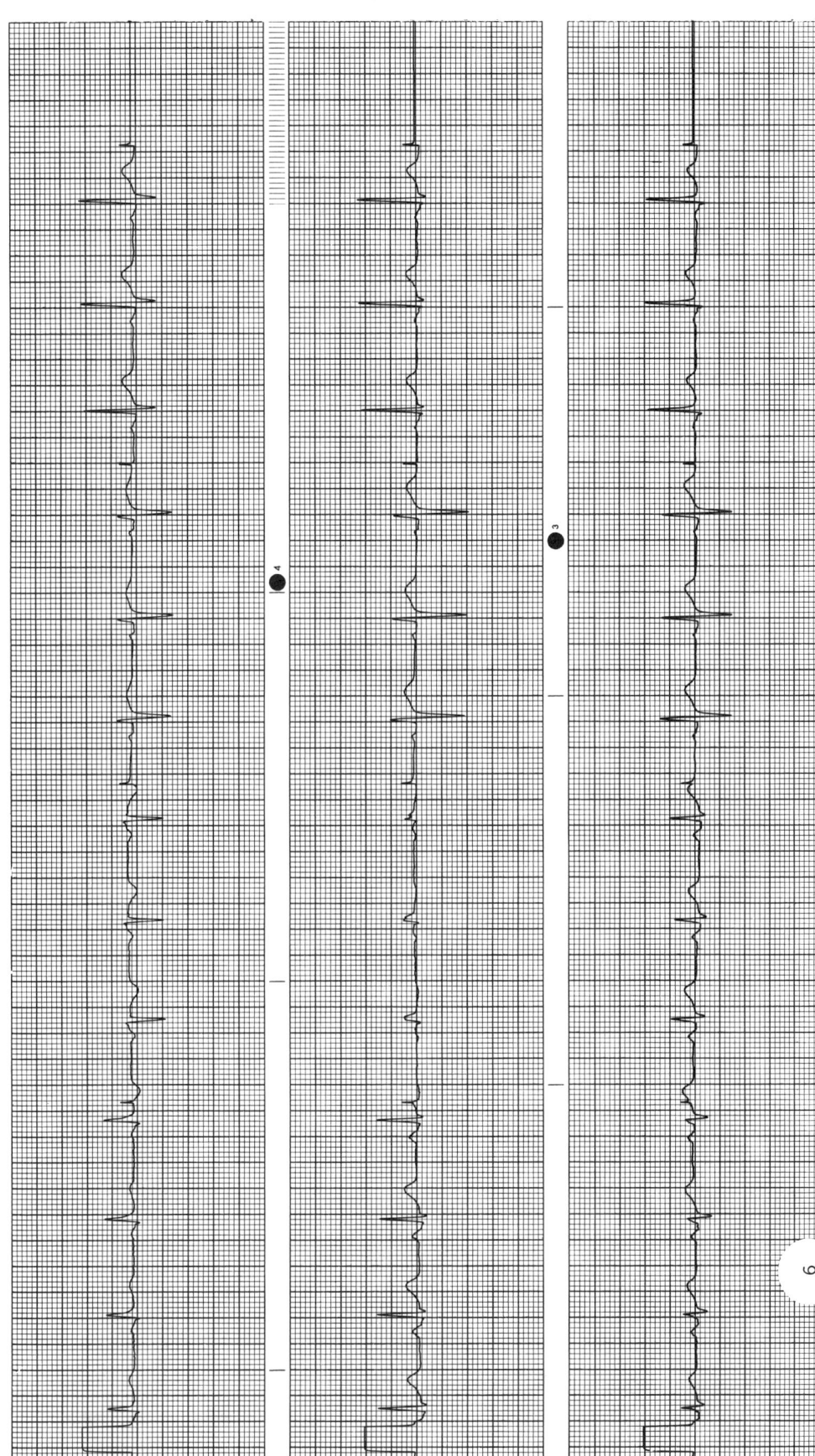

Exercise 6. A 63-year-old man arrived in emergency department complaining of severe substernal chest pain. Cardiac enzymes negative.

SELF-ASSESSMENT ANSWERS TO EXERCISES 1–6

Exercise 1. P waves are positive in all leads except aVR.
- QRS normal configurations. Normal R wave progression through chest leads.
- ST segment is isoelectric in all leads.
- T wave is positive in all leads except negative in aVR.

Exercise 2. P waves are positive in all leads except negative in aVR and flat in aVL.
- QRS normal configurations. Normal R wave progression through chest leads.
- ST segment is isoelectric in all leads.
- T wave is positive in all leads except negative in aVR and V1.

Exercise 3. P waves are positive in all leads except negative in aVR and flat in aVL.
- QRS normal configurations. Normal R wave progression through chest leads.
- ST segment is isoelectric in all leads.
- T wave is positive in all leads except negative in aVR and flat in aVL.

Exercise 4. P waves are positive in all leads except negative in aVR and diphasic in V1.
- QRS normal configurations. Normal R wave progression through chest leads.
- ST segment is isoelectric in all leads.
- T wave is positive in all leads except negative in aVR and III.

Exercise 5. P waves are positive in all leads except negative in aVR, diphasic in V1, and flattened in aVL.
- QRS normal configurations. Normal R wave progression through chest leads.
- ST segment is isoelectric in all leads but sagging in leads with tall R wave.
- T wave is positive in all leads except negative in aVR.

Exercise 6. P waves are positive in all leads except negative in aVR and aVL.
- QRS normal configurations. Normal R wave progression through chest leads.
- ST segment is isoelectric in all leads.
- T wave is positive in all leads except negative in aVR and negative and flattened in aVL.

2
Rhythm Determination

$$\boxed{\text{STEP 1}}$$

Rhythm Determination is the *first step* in the systematic process. Before you can proceed in analyzing 12-lead electrocardiograms (ECGs), it is necessary to have a thorough understanding and skill in interpreting dysrhythmias (arrhythmias). The main purpose of this chapter is to review the steps in rhythm diagnosis, briefly outline the ECG features for selected dysrhythmias, and discuss the clinical significance for this step.

RHYTHM DETERMINATION

In this step, you will analyze selected features listed in Table 2.1 (Brown & Jacobson, 1988; Frye & Lounsbury, 1988). To interpret a rhythm, compare the ECG information collected in this step with the features of normal sinus rhythm (NSR) and dysrhythmias. For a description of the ECG features of NSR see Table 2.2 and for those of dysrhythmias see the description later in this chapter.

It is routine practice to use leads II, V1, or V6 in this process. Lead II is selected because it provides large, positive P waves and QRS complexes. Leads V1 and V6 are chosen because they provide detailed information

Table 2.2.
ECG Features of Normal Sinus Rhythm (NSR)

- Ventricular rate: Normal (60–100 BPM)
- QRS shape: Normal for lead
  Positive in Lead II
- R-R rhythm: Regular
- QRS interval: 0.06–0.09 seconds
- QT interval: <0.44 seconds
- Atrial rate: Normal
  Same as ventricular
- P wave shape: Normal for lead
  Positive in Lead II
- P-P rhythm: Regular
- P-R interval: 0.12–0.20 seconds
- P:R conduction ratio: 1:1
- Dominant pacemaker site: Sinus
- Interpretation: Normal sinus rhythm

Table 2.1.
Step One of Systematic Process: Rhythm Determination[a]

- Ventricular rate _____
- QRS shape _____
- R-R rhythm _____
- QRS interval _____
- QT interval _____
- Dominant pacemaker site _____
- Interpretation _____
- Atrial rate _____
- P wave shape _____
- P-P rhythm _____
- P-R interval _____
- P:R conduction ratio _____

[a]Adapted with permission of K Brown and S Jacobson. *Mastering dysrhythmias: A problem solving guide.* **Philadelphia: F. A. Davis Co., 1988.**

about ventricular conduction abnormalities. They assist in distinguishing supraventricular dysrhythmias from ventricular, and in identifying bundle branch blocks. The normal shape of the P-QRS complex in these leads is summarized in Table 2.3.

Each feature required for the completion of step one is described below in more detail. Application of each component is performed using Figure 2.1 as an example. Remember each small (1 mm) horizontal square on the ECG graph paper represents 0.04 sec and each large one (5 mm) equals 0.20 seconds. Usually on the ECG graph paper, there are vertical lines that are 3 inches apart, and represent 3 seconds of time.

Table 2.3.
Comparison of Leads II, V1, and V6[a]

Lead	P Wave	QRS Complex	T Wave
II	Positive	Positive	Positive
V1	Variable	Negative	Variable
V6	Positive	Positive	Positive

[a]Positive = upright; negative = inverted; variable = either positive, negative, flat, or diphasic.

Ventricular Rate: Calculate the ventricular rate.
- Is the rate normal (60–100 BPM)?
- Is the rate bradycardic (less than 60 BPM)?
- Is the rate tachycardic (greater than 100 BPM)?

Methods for calculating the ventricular rate are (Brown & Jacobson, 1988):

1. Count the number of R waves or QRS complexes in a 6 second rhythm strip and then multiply by 10.
2. Count the number of large boxes between two consecutive QRS complexes and divide the number into 300.
3. Memorize this scale based on the number of large boxes between QRS complexes.
   - 1 = 300
   - 2 = 150
   - 3 = 100
   - 4 = 75
   - 5 = 60
   - 6 = 50
4. Use an ECG ruler designed for this purpose.

In Figure 2.1, the ventricular rate is 70 BPM.

QRS Shape: Describe the morphology of the QRS complex in each lead.
- Is the QRS shape normal, notched, positive, negative, diphasic, wide, slurred, or absent?

- Is the QRS shape consistent with each beat?
- How does the QRS shape compare with what is normal for that lead?
- Are any of the QRS complexes abnormal in shape?

Remember the morphology of a QRS is specific to the lead you are studying. The shape will help in determining whether the origin of the dysrhythmia is ventricular, or if a ventricular conduction problem exists.

In Figure 2.1 the QRS morphology consists of a tall R wave, which is normal for that lead.

R-R Rhythm: Assess the regularity of the R-R interval.
- Is the ventricular rhythm regular or irregular?
- Is there a pattern to the irregular rhythm?

Use calipers or an edge of a piece of paper to determine the R-R rhythm. To be irregular, R-R intervals must differ by three (0.12 seconds) or more small squares (Meltzer, Pinneo, & Kitchell, 1987). If irregular, look for one of the following reasons in descending order:

1. Premature or ectopic beats
2. Atrial Fibrillation
3. AV heart blocks
4. Irregular sinus rhythms

QRS Interval: Measure the QRS interval.
- Is it normal (0.06–0.09 seconds), slightly widened (0.10–0.11 seconds), or wide (0.12 seconds or greater)?
- Are all QRS intervals the same?

The QRS interval is measured from the beginning of the initial QRS wave to the J point or where the ST segment begins. A QRS interval ≥0.12 seconds may signify a ventricular dysrhythmia or a bundle branch block. A QRS interval between 0.10 to 0.11 seconds may represent an intraventricular conduction delay (IVCD).

In Figure 2.1 the QRS interval is normal (0.06 seconds).

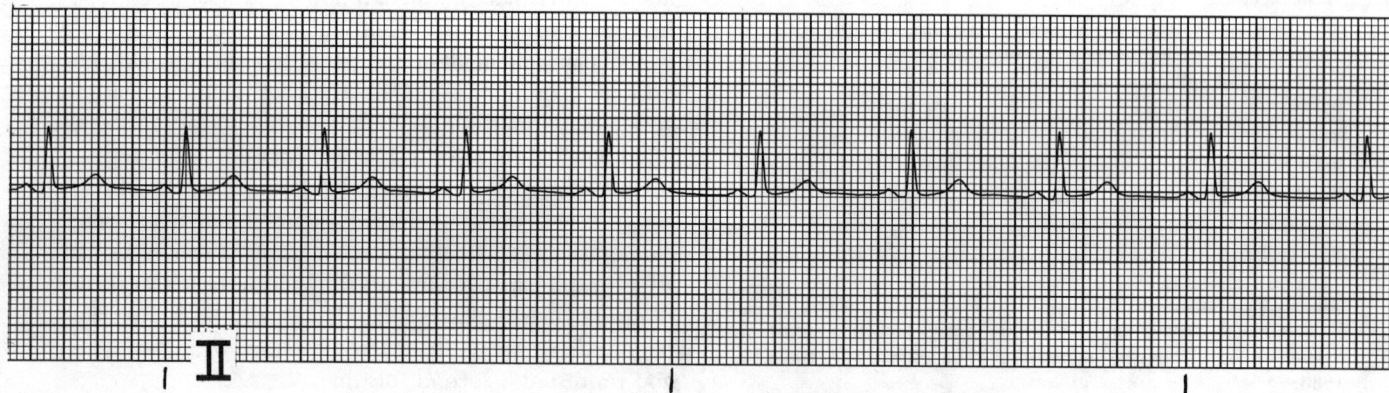

Figure 2.1.   Rhythm strip lead II sample for use as directed in text.

QT Interval: Measure the QT interval.
- What is the measured QT interval?
- Has the QT interval been corrected based on the patient's heart rate?
- How does the measured QT interval compare with the corrected QT interval (QTc)?

The QT interval is measured from the beginning of the QRS complex to the end of the T wave. It varies with the heart rate and must be corrected for the heart rate. One simple procedure to determine a corrected QT interval is (Frye & Lounsbury, 1988):

1. Count the number of small boxes between two QRS complexes, then
2. Add 18 to the number, then
3. Place a decimal in front of the number.

A QT interval greater than 0.44 seconds is generally considered abnormal.

In Figure 2.1 the QT interval is 0.40 seconds. The corrected QT interval is 21 boxes + 18 = 39 or 0.39 seconds, and is similar to the measured QT interval, and is therefore normal.

Atrial Rate: Calculate the atrial rate.
- Is the atrial rate the same or different from the ventricular rate?

Use the same methods described for calculating the ventricular rates, only substitute P for R waves.

In Figure 2.1 the atrial rate is 70 BPM.

P Wave Shape: Describe the morphology of the P wave in each lead.
- Is the P wave shape normal, widened, tall and pointed, notched, a wavy line, or absent?
- Do all P waves look the same?
- Are there different P waves in the same lead or in just one beat? Look for ectopic beats.

Remember, P waves look different in certain leads and are still considered normal. Different P waves in the same lead indicate shifting pacemaker sites. A supraventricular origin is probable if a P wave is present and coupled to a QRS complex.

In Figure 2.1 the P waves are positive.

P-P Rhythm: Assess the regularity of the P-P interval.
- Is the atrial rhythm regular or irregular?
- Where are the P waves in relation to the QRS?

In Figure 2.1, the P-P rhythm is regular and the P waves are related to the QRS.

P-R Interval: Measure the P-R interval.
- Is the P-R interval normal (0.12–0.20 seconds) or prolonged (greater than 0.22 seconds)?
- Is the P-R interval consistent throughout the rhythm strip?
- Does the P-R interval vary from beat to beat, or does it get progressively longer?

It is measured from the beginning of the P wave to the beginning of the QRS complex. A P-R interval greater than 0.20 seconds suggests a delay in conduction at the AV node.

In Figure 2.1 the P-R interval is 0.16 seconds.

P:R Conduction Ratio: Determine the relationship between the P waves and the QRS complexes.
- Are there more P waves than QRS complexes?

In Figure 2.1, the P:R conduction ratio is 1 to 1.

Dominant Pacemaker Site: Determine the dominant pacemaker site.
- Is it sinus, atrial, junctional, or ventricular?
- Is there a secondary pacemaker site? ·

A P wave indicates the rhythm is either sinus, atrial, or junctional depending on its shape. If there are no related P waves and a widened QRS complex, the rhythm is probably ventricular in origin.

In Figure 2.1 the dominant pacemaker site is sinus.

Interpretation: Analyze the data and determine a rhythm interpretation or diagnosis.

Consider the consequences of that rhythm diagnosis for the patient.
- What is its effect on the patient's cardiac output?
- What are the patient's blood pressure and pulse?
- Is the patient complaining of chest pain (angina) or dyspnea?
- On lung auscultation, do you hear crackles at the bases?

In Figure 2.1 the rhythm interpretation is normal sinus rhythm.

DYSRHYTHMIA ECG FEATURES

The key features of selected dysrhythmias and their effect on the patient's heart rate determine the correct rhythm diagnosis and are recorded in Table 2.4 (Hurst, 1986; Brown & Jacobson, 1988; Frye & Lounsbury, 1988). In the table, all sinus, supraventricular, ventricular, and AV conduction dysrhythmias are grouped together. The effect on the patient's heart rate determines how serious it is and how quickly it should be treated. The effects are classified as either normal (60–100 BPM), bradycardia (less than 60 BPM), tachycardia (greater than 100 BPM), or death producing.

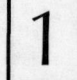

Table 2.4.
Dysrhythmias Catalogued as to Type, Key Features, and Heart Rate[a]

Type of Dysrhythmia		Key Features	Heart Rate
S I N U S	Sinus bradycardia	■ VR = <60 BPM ■ P wave shape = Normal	Bradycardia
	Sinus tachycardia	■ VR = 100–150 BPM ■ P wave shape = Normal	Tachycardia
	Sinus arrest/block	■ R-R Rhythm = Irregular due to missing PQRST for one or more beats ■ P wave shape = Normal in other beats	Normal to bradycardia
	Sinus arrhythmia	■ R-R Rhythm = Irregular due to slowing and speeding up of heart rate caused by respiratory effect	Normal
S U P R A V E N T R I C U L A R	Atrial premature beat (APB or PAC)	■ R-R Rhythm = Irregular due to early beat. ■ P wave shape = Of early beat different from sinus P wave ■ If no QRS follows early P wave called *Blocked APB* ■ If comes after a pause called *Escape atrial beat*	Normal
	Junctional premature beat (JPB or PJC)	■ R-R Rhythm = Irregular due to early beat ■ P wave shape of early beat = absent, inverted before or after the QRS complex in Lead II ■ PRI = none or <0.12 seconds ■ If come after a pause called an *Escape junctional beat*	Normal
	Junctional rhythm (JR)	■ VR = 40–60 BPM ■ P wave shape = absent, inverted before or after the QRS complex in Lead II ■ PRI = none or <0.12 seconds	Bradycardia
		■ If VR = 60–100 called *Accelerated junctional rhythm (AJR)*	Normal
		■ If VR = >100 called *Junctional tachycardia*	Tachycardia
	Supraventricular tachycardia (SVT) or Atrial tachycardia (AT)	■ VR = 150–250 BPM ■ R-R rhythm = Regular ■ P waves present but buried in T wave ■ PRI = unmeasurable ■ If occurs suddenly called Paroxysmal ■ Junk term used when unable to tell if sinus, atrial or junctional in origin (Hurst, 1986)	Tachycardia
	Atrial flutter	■ VR = Varies 80–150 BPM, less than atrial ■ R-R Rhythm = Regular or irregular ■ AR = 250–350 BPM ■ P wave shape = Saw-toothed pattern ■ P-P Rhythm = Regular	Normal to tachycardia

Table 2.4. Continued.
Dysrhyhmias Catalogued as to Type, Key Features, and Heart Rate[a]

Type of Dysrhythmia	Key Features	Heart Rate
Atrial fibrillation	■ VR = Varies; < or > 100 BPM ■ R-R Rhythm = Grossly irregular ■ AR = >360 BPM ■ P wave shape = None to wavy line	Normal to tachycardia
Multifocal atrial tachycardia (MAT)	■ VR = 100–200 BPM ■ R-R Rhythm = Irregular ■ P wave shape = Varies, three different shapes but dominant sinus P wave ■ PRI = Varies ■ P:R ratio = 1:1	Tachycardia
Wandering atrial pacemaker (WAP)	■ VR = < or > 60 BPM ■ R-R Rhythm = Regular ■ P wave shape = Varies three different shapes but dominant sinus P wave ■ P:R ratio = 1:1	Normal to bradycardia
VENTRICULAR Ventricular premature beat (VPB or PVC)	■ QRS shape = Widened/Distorted. T wave in opposite direction from QRS complex ■ R-R Rhythm = Irregular due to premature beat ■ QRS interval = >0.12 seconds ■ P wave = None relate to beat	Normal
Ventricular rhythm	■ VR = <40 BPM ■ QRS shape = Widened/Distorted ■ R-R Rhythm = Regular ■ QRS interval = >0.12 seconds ■ P wave = None related ■ If VR = 40–100 called *Accelerated ventricular rhythm*	Bradycardia Normal
Ventricular tachycardia (VT)	■ VR = 100–250 BPM ■ See features under VPBs ■ If VR = 250–350 BPM with zig zag appearance called *Ventricular flutter* ■ If QRS changes direction and size frequently and has prolonged QT interval called *Torsades de Pointes*	Tachycardia to death producing
Ventricular fibrillation (VF)	■ Shape = grossly distorted ■ No clearly defined P-QRS	Death producing
Ventricular asystole	■ VR = None ■ QRS shape = None ■ AR = Some or none ■ P wave = Some or none ■ P-P Rhythm = Normal or none ■ PRI = None ■ If no P wave = Straight line ■ Can have P waves, but no QRS	Death producing

1

Table 2.4. Continued.
Dysrhythmias Catalogued as to Type, Key Features, and Heart Rate[a]

Type of Dysrhythmia	Key Features	Heart Rate
A First degree AV **V** block	■ P wave = Normal ■ PRI = >0.20 seconds ■ P:R ratio = 1:1	Normal

B
L Second degree
O   AV block
C   (Mobitz I)
K   (Wenckebach)
S
	■ VR < AR
	■ R-R Rhythm = Irregular due to dropped
	   beat
	■ P wave = Normal but not all conducted
	■ PRI = Progressively longer until a QRS is
	   dropped
		Normal to
		bradycardia

Second degree AV block (Mobitz II)	■ VR < AR ■ QRS shape = Can be widened ■ R-R rhythm = Regular. (Can be irregular if dropped QRS presented) ■ P-P Rhythm = Regular ■ PRI = Normal or prolonged but constant ■ P:R ratio = More Ps than QRSs	Normal to bradycardia
Third degree AV block	■ VR = <40 BPM ■ QRS shape = Widened. If normal then junctional escape pacer site ■ R-R Rhythm = Regular ■ AR = Normal ■ P-P Rhythm = Regular ■ PRI = Varies, Not consistent	Bradycardia

[a]VR = ventricular heart rate; AR = atrial heart rate; PRI = PR interval; BPM = beats per minute.

Aberrancy

Aberrancy is defined as a temporary intraventricular conduction delay found in a supraventricular beat or rhythm. It produces a wide distorted QRS complex resembling a bundle branch block. The wide QRS complex makes it difficult to distinguish an aberrantly conducted supraventricular beat or rhythm from one of ventricular origin. The ability to distinguish is clinically important as ventricular beats and rhythms usually require treatment. Some key ECG features that favor a rhythm diagnosis of supraventricular beat with aberrancy are (ACLS, 1987; Karnes, 1987; Frye & Lounsbury, 1988):

1. Premature P wave buried on preceding T wave
2. QRS complex <0.14 seconds
3. Triphasic QRS complex or RBBB Pattern (RSR) in V1
4. Triphasic QRS complex (qRS) in V6
5. In the presence of atrial fibrillation, a wide QRS complex with a RBBB pattern after a short or normal R-R interval that is preceded by a long R-R interval (Ashman phenomena) in V1 (ACLS, 1987)

Some key ECG features that favor a rhythm diagnosis of ventricular tachycardia are (ACLS, 1987; Karnes, 1987; Frye & Lounsbury, 1988):

1. AV dissociation
2. QRS complex >0.14 seconds
3. Monophasic R wave or biphasic "RBBB-like" QRS complex (qR, RS) in V1
4. rs, QS, QR in V6
5. Left rabbit ear of QRS taller than right in V1
6. Left axis deviation

CLINICAL SIGNIFICANCE

The advantages of performing rhythm determination first is three-fold. *First* some dysrhythmias adversely affect the cardiac output (CO) and require treatment. Dysrhythmias require treatment because they are either bradycardic, tachycardic, ventricular, or death producing. Potential consequences on the heart rate of selected dysrhythmias are listed in Table 2.4. If the dysrhythmia is causing symptoms of hypotension, angina, palpitation, unconsciousness, or pulselessness, it must be treated immediately. Symptomatic bradycardic rhythms are treated with atropine, a noninvasive external pacemaker, a temporary transvenous pacemaker, or with Isuprel. Sinus tachycardia is treated based on its etiology. Supraventricular tachycardias are treated with vagal maneuvers,

1

digoxin, verapamil, inderal, brevibloc, and/or cardioversion. Ventricular rhythms especially in the setting of an acute myocardial infarction (MI) are treated with lidocaine, pronestyl, or bretylium. Death producing rhythms are treated with cardiopulmonary resuscitation (CPR), medication, or defibrillation as indicated. If the rhythm does not affect the patient's hemodynamic status, plan to continue with the interpretation of the 12-lead ECG.

In addition dysrhythmias may mask or make it difficult to interpret the rest of the ECG. For example, a 100% paced rhythm makes it impossible to document the presence of an MI via the ECG. The occurrence of aberrancy may interfere with the interpretation of a bundle branch block (BBB).

Second, the dysrhythmias identified may lead you to inspect the ECG closer for signs of myocardial ischemia, myocardial infarction, drug effects, electrolyte imbalances, and other etiologies. Table 2.5 catalogues selected dysrhythmias as to their possible cardiac, electrolyte imbalance, drug effect, and miscellaneous etiologies (Meltzer et al., 1987; Frye & Lounsbury, 1988).

Third, some of the information obtained in this step may offer you a clue to other abnormalities in the ECG, such as atrial abnormalities, ventricular conduction blocks, electrolyte imbalances, or adverse drug effects. What to analyze and its significance is condensed below.

- *Abnormal QRS shape and QRS intervals* greater than 0.12 seconds may signify an intraventricular

Table 2.5.
Cardiac and Other Etiological Causes for Selected Dysrhythmias[a]

Dysrhythmias	Cardiac	Drug	Electrolyte	Other
Premature beats (atrial or junctional)	Healthy heart CHF Ischemia Valvular disease Pericarditis	Digoxin	Hypokalemia Hypomagnesemia	Pulmonary embolism Metabolic alkalosis
Sinus bradycardia	Inferior wall MI Myocardial ischemia	Digoxin Beta-blockers	Hyperkalemia	Hypothyroidism Increased ICP Pain
Sinus tachycardia	MI CHF Pericarditis	Caffeine Aminophylline		Hypovolemia Infection Pain Hyperthyroidism Stress
SVT (Atrial tachycardia/Flutter/Fibrillation)	Healthy heart MI Valvular disease Pericarditis	Caffeine		Stress Pulmonary emboli Hyperthyroidism
MAT			Hypokalemia	COPD
Ventricular	Myocardial ischemia MI	Digoxin toxicity	Hypokalemia Hyperkalemia Hypomagnesemia Hypocalcemia Hypercalcemia	Stress Hypothermia Hypoxia Acidosis
AV blocks (Wenckebach) (Type II)	Increased vagal tone Inferior MI Anterior MI	Digoxin Beta-blockers Ca-channel blockers		

[a]MI = myocardial infarction; CHF = congestive heart failure; COPD = chronic obstructive pulmonary disease; ICP = intracranial pressure.

conduction block. This may be due to the presence of a bundle branch block.

- *Abnormal P wave shape* may indicate some defect in atrial conduction. A notched or widened P wave may reflect an atrial abnormality.
- *Absence of P waves* may suggest hyperkalemia.
- *Prolonged QT intervals* may represent a drug imbalance from such drugs as quinidine or pronestyl. It may also denote hypokalemia ($\downarrow$ K), hypocalcemia ($\downarrow$ Ca), or hypomagnesemia ($\downarrow$ Mg).
- *Shortened QT intervals* are often present in patients who are taking digoxin or who have hypercalcemia ($\uparrow$ Ca).

Key questions to ask yourself once you have identified the rhythm are:

How does the monitor rhythm strip or 12-lead ECG compare with a previous rhythm or ECG?
- Report significant rhythm changes or P-QRS changes to the physician. An increased number of atrial premature beats (APBs) may warn of impending atrial dysrhythmias.
- A change in the QRS interval ≥ 0.12 seconds may warn of the development of BBB.

What is the effect on the heart rate or cardiac output?
- Monitor for signs and symptoms of dizziness, syncope, palpitations, loss of consciousness, pulse deficit, etc.

What is the clinical situation in which the dysrhythmia is appearing?
- Assess for history of chronic obstructive pulmonary disease (COPD), hypertension, anxiety, myocardial infarction or ischemia, overindulgence in caffeine or an infection.

Are there signs and symptoms of heart failure?
- Monitor heart and lung sounds, daily weights, intake and output, and vital signs.
- Assess for crackles at bases of lungs, third heart sound (S3), peripheral edema, and shortness of breath.

Does the patient show signs and symptoms of myocardial ischemia?
- Assess for angina and cardiac enzyme changes.
- Look for ST segment and T wave changes on monitor rhythm strip or in the 12-lead ECG.

Does the dysrhythmia suggest the possibility of further problems such as drug or electrolyte imbalances?
- Assess the patient's drug therapy.
- Monitor serum drug and electrolyte levels, especially digoxin and potassium (K).

- Assess ECG or rhythm strip for changes in QT interval.

What monitor or rhythm lead should be used in caring for this patient?
- Use multiple leads as needed.
- V1 + V6 if looking for difference between supraventricular beats and ventricular beats or the development of BBBs.
- Leads II + V1 if looking for P waves and rhythm diagnosis.
- Limb leads if looking for axis changes and hemiblocks.

What treatment should I prepare for?
- Provide O_2.
- Establish an intravenous or heparin lock for drug administration.
- Initiate treatment protocols as established by standing orders.
- Initiate treatments as ordered by physician.
- Be prepared for drug or electrical treatments (Lidocaine, defibrillation, pacing).

SELF-ASSESSMENT EXERCISES 7–12

In the following six ECG samples, perform step one of the systematic process:

Step One. Determination of Rhythm

- Ventricular rate _____
- QRS Shape _____
- R-R rhythm _____
- QRS interval _____
- QT interval _____
- Atrial rate _____
- P wave shape _____
- P-P rhythm _____
- P-R interval _____
- P:R conduction ratio _____

- Dominant pacemaker site _____
- Interpretation _____

Remember to use a rhythm strip that usually accompanies a standard 12-lead ECG tracing and the self-assessment analysis form referenced in Chapter 1. This is the only chapter that will provide rhythm strips with the ECG tracings.

You must be able to perform this step successfully before proceeding. When you have completed all of the exercises in this book, come back to this exercise and complete the remaining steps of the *systematic approach*.

Check your answers with the suggested interpretations found at the end of this chapter. Answers for remaining steps will be found in Appendix A.

1

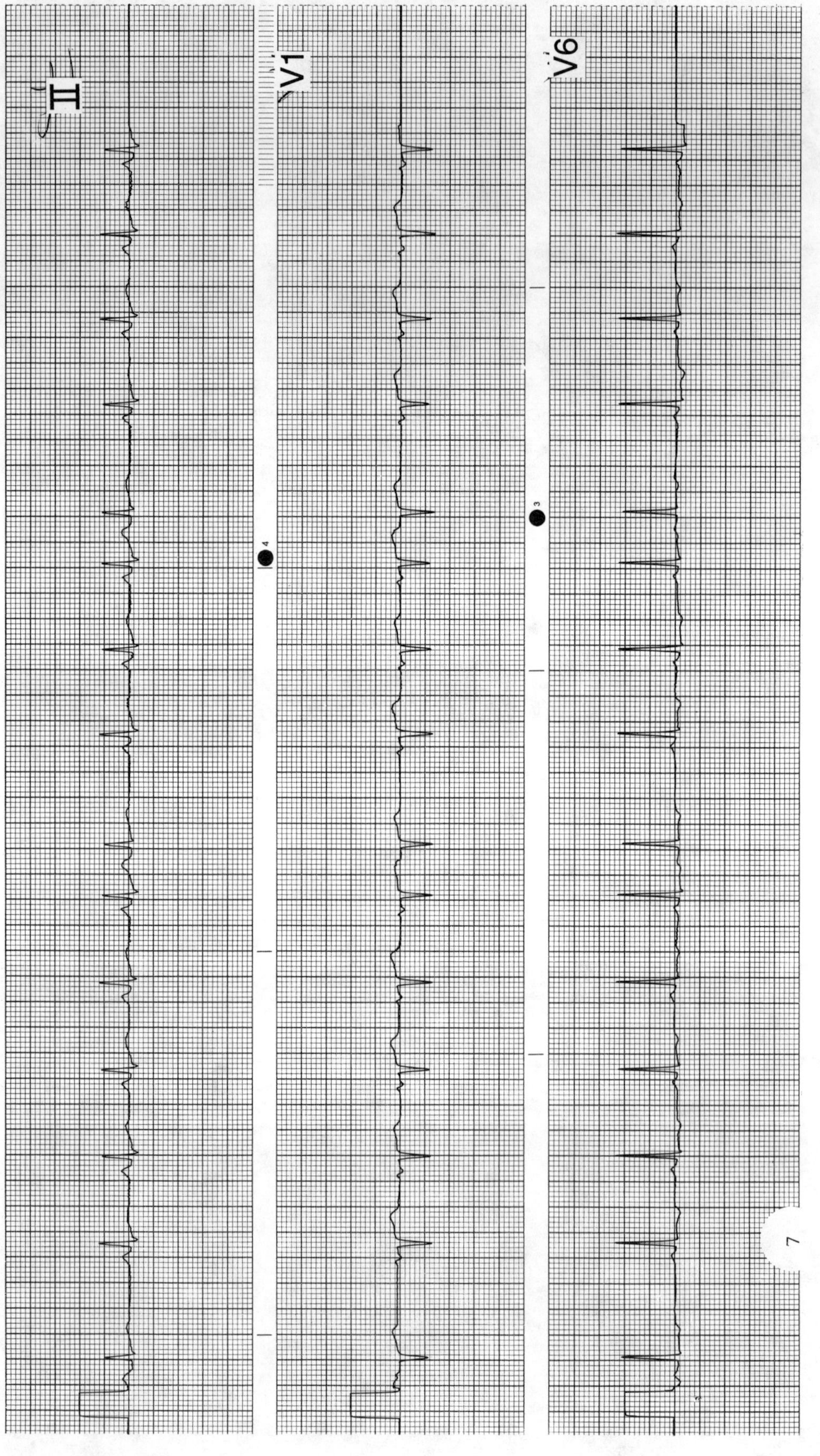

Exercise 7. Rhythm strips of leads II, V1, and V6.

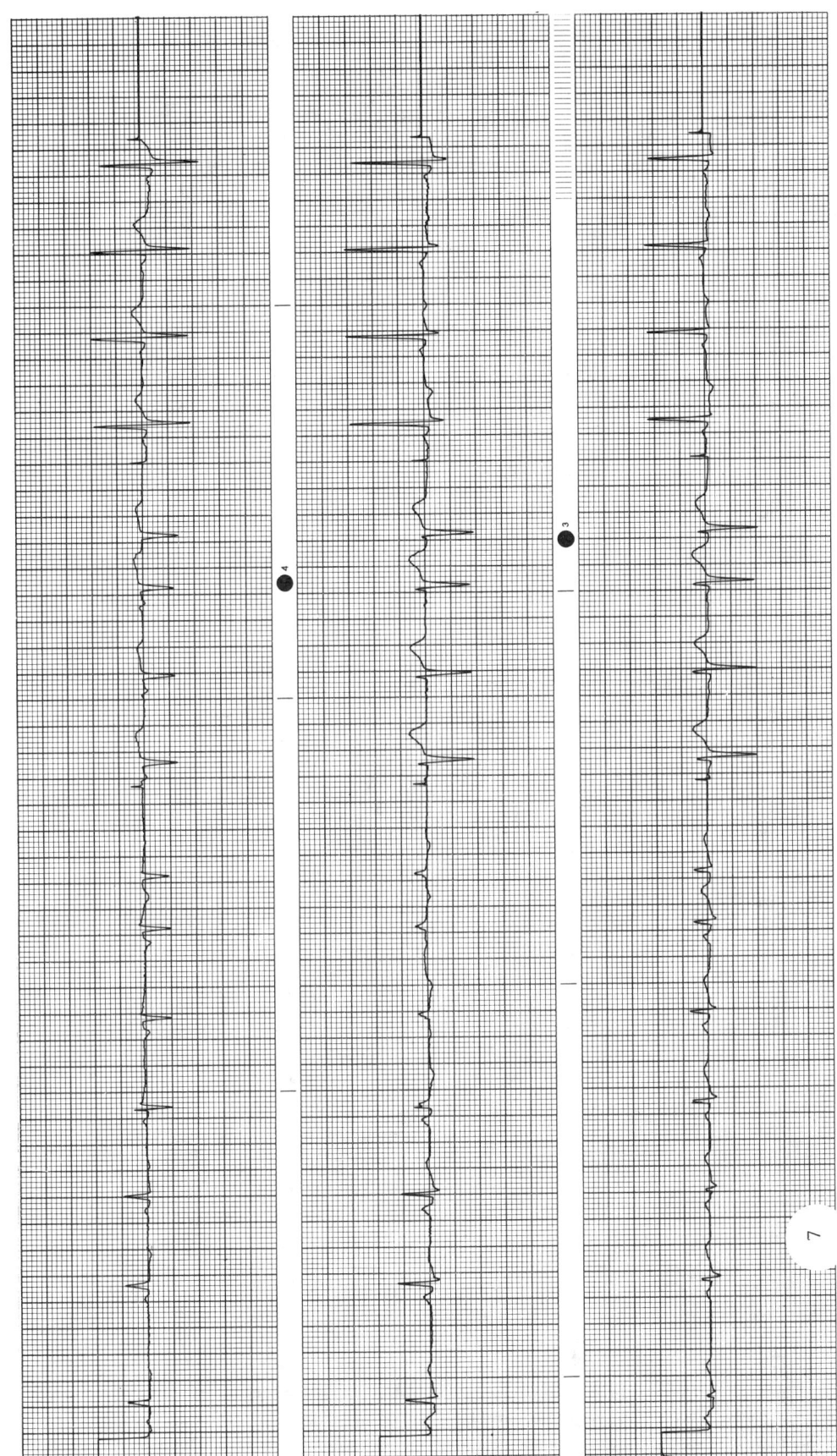

Exercise 7. A 71-year-old woman with a history of hypertension admitted with constellation of chest pain, hypoxemia, high fever, and right leg pain. Admitting diagnosis was cellulitis of the right leg.

II

V1

V6

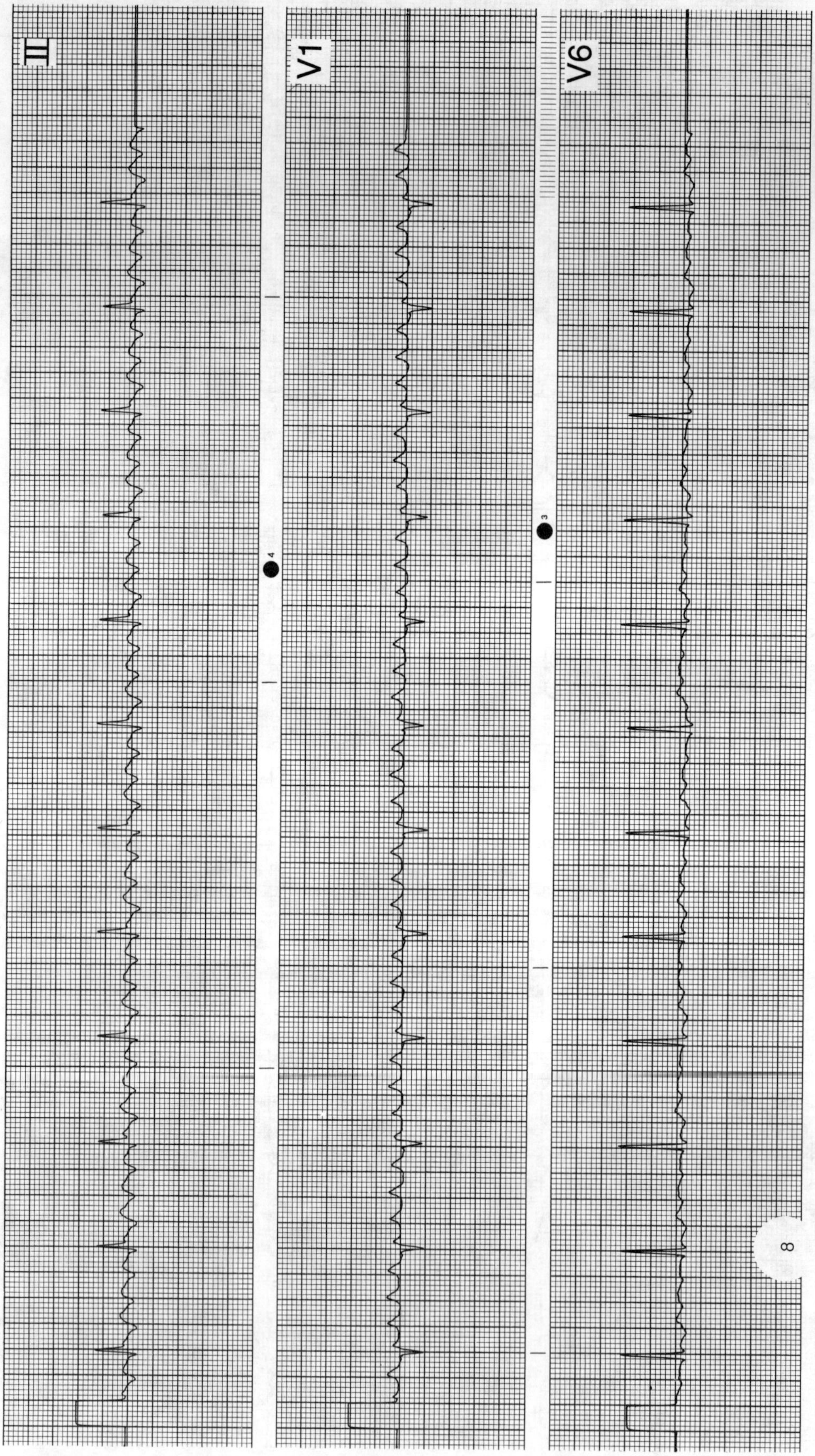

Exercise 8.   Rhythm strips of leads II, V1 and V6.

1

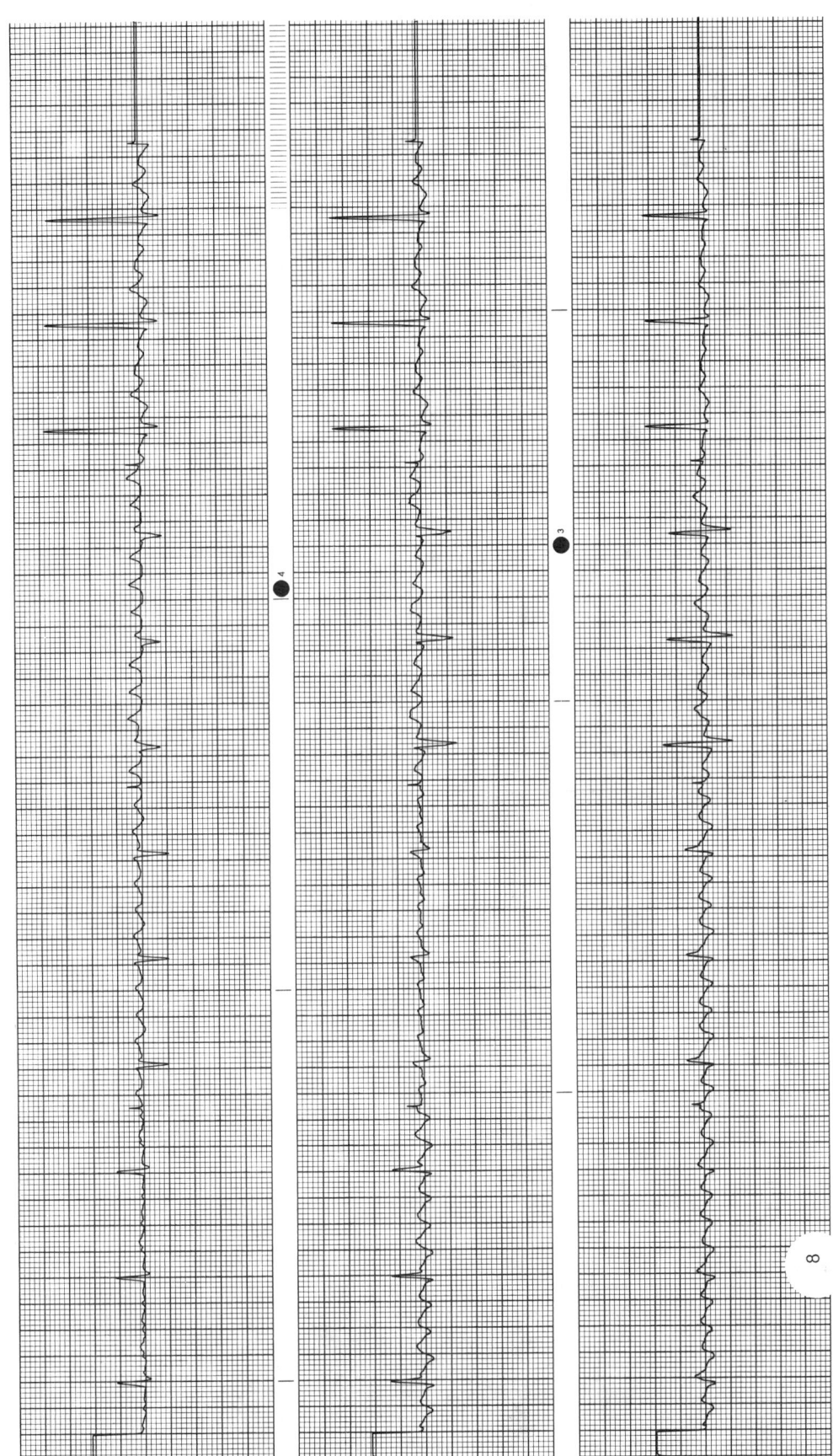

Exercise 8. A 54-year-old man admitted complaining of chest pain. History of sick sinus syndrome and permanent pacemaker insertion. Cardiac enzymes negative.

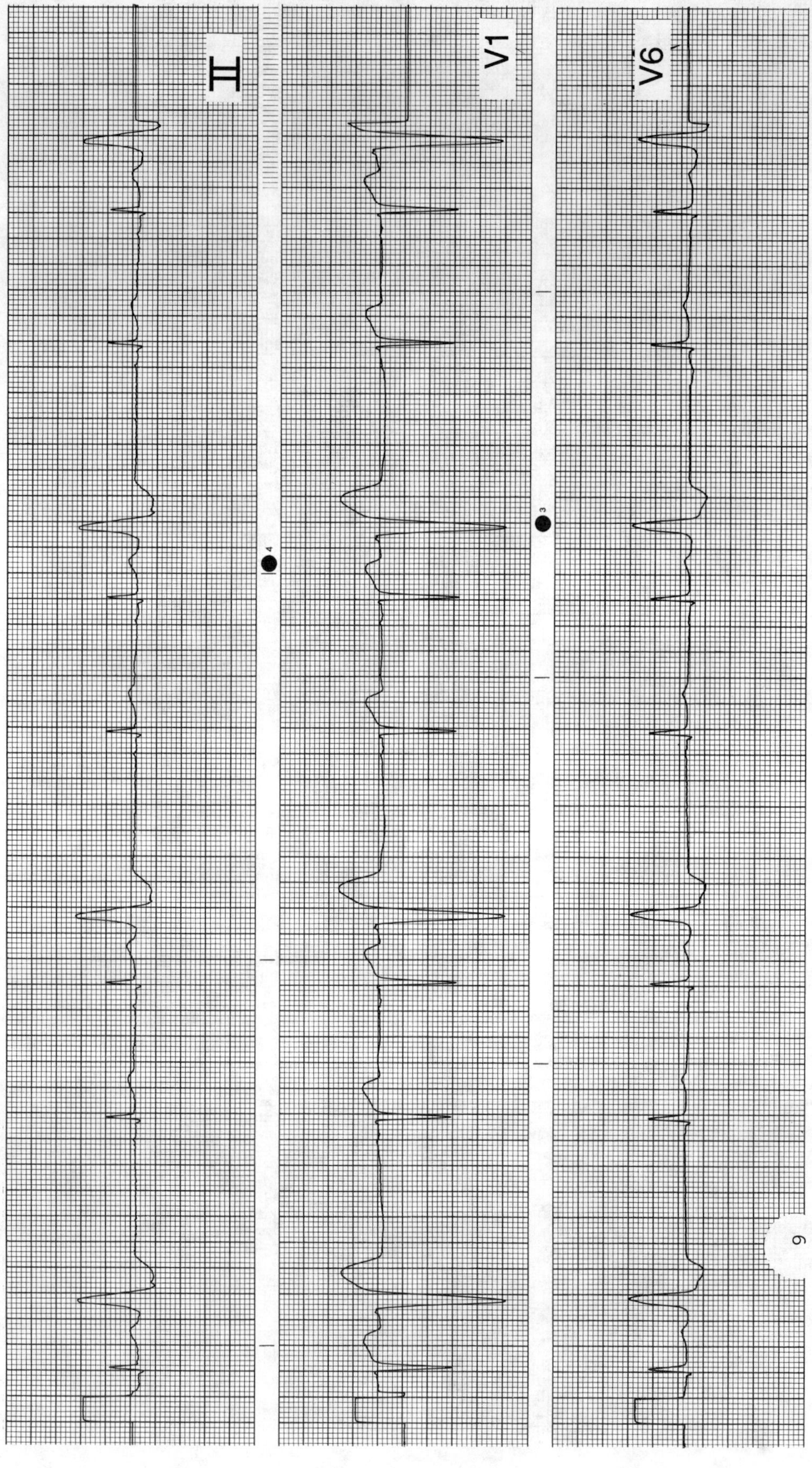

II

V1

V6

Exercise 9.   Rhythm strips of leads II, V1, and V6.

1

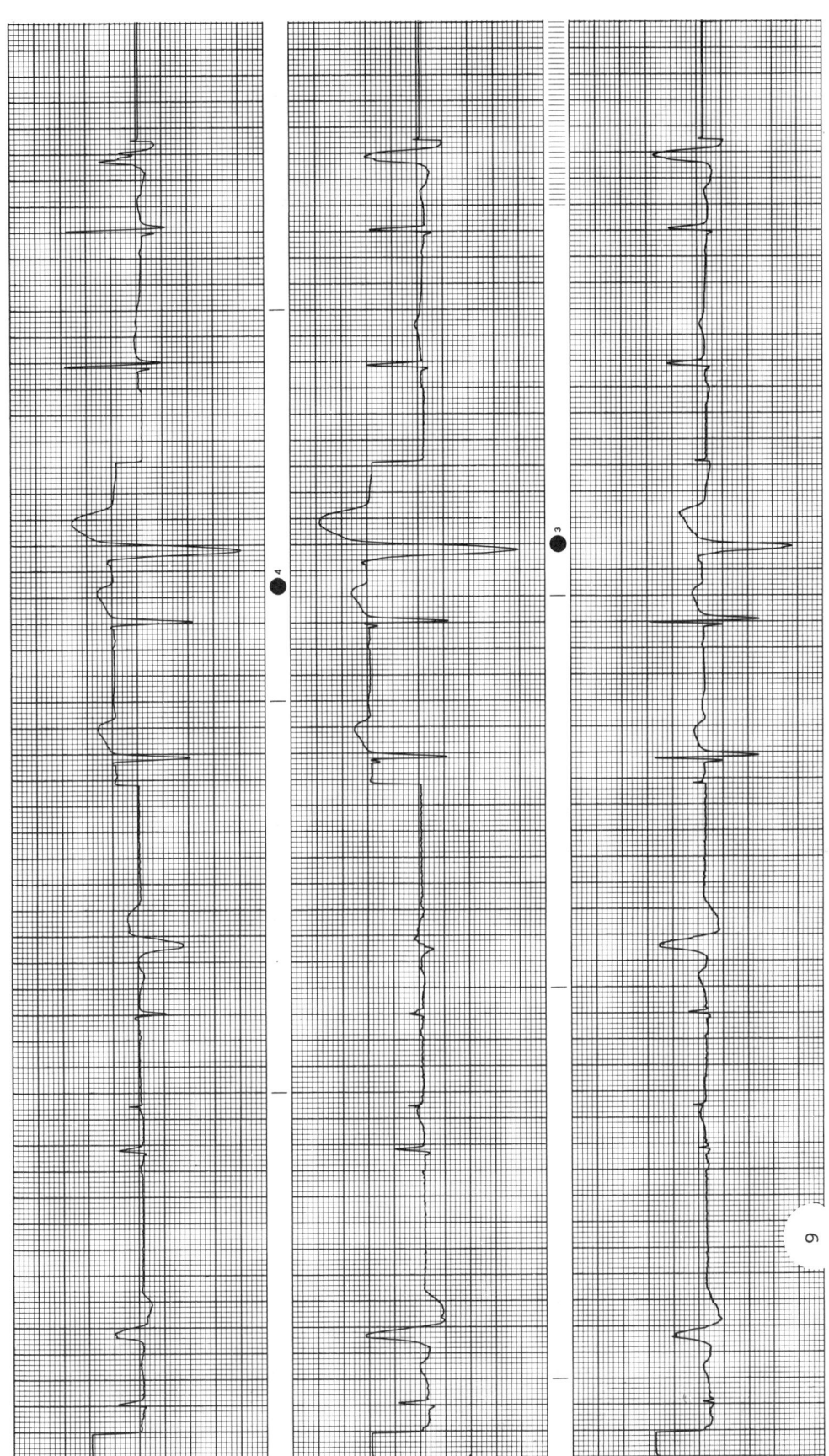

Exercise 9. A 64-year-old man admitted to CCU with sudden onset substernal chest pain with diaphoresis and shortness of breath on exertion. Status post-MI 2 years ago. Cardiac enzymes negative.

II

V1

V6

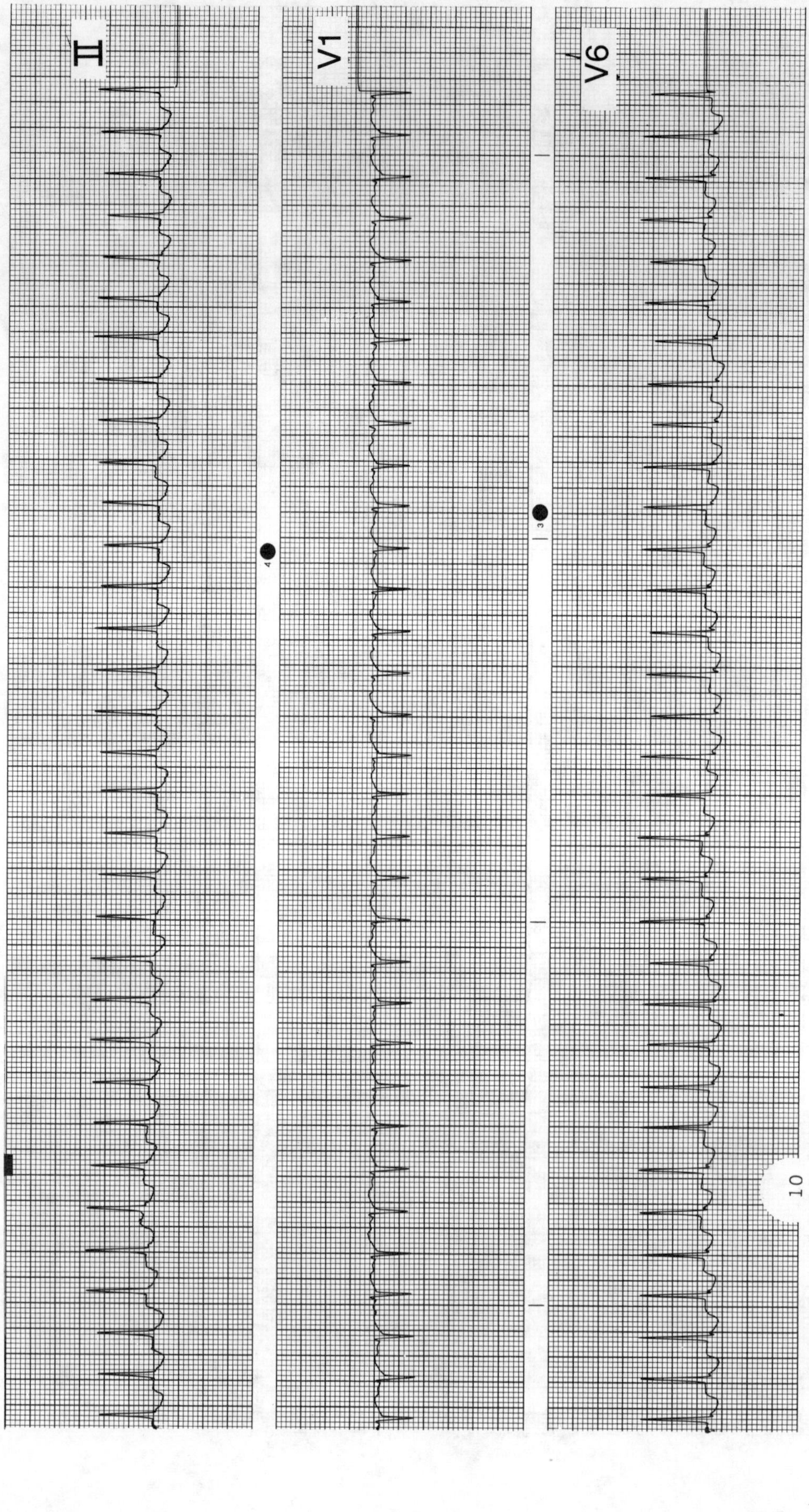

Exercise 10.   Rhythm strips of leads II, V1, and V6.

10

Exercise 10. An 81-year-old woman admitted to CCU complaining of palpitations and to rule out (R/O) an MI.

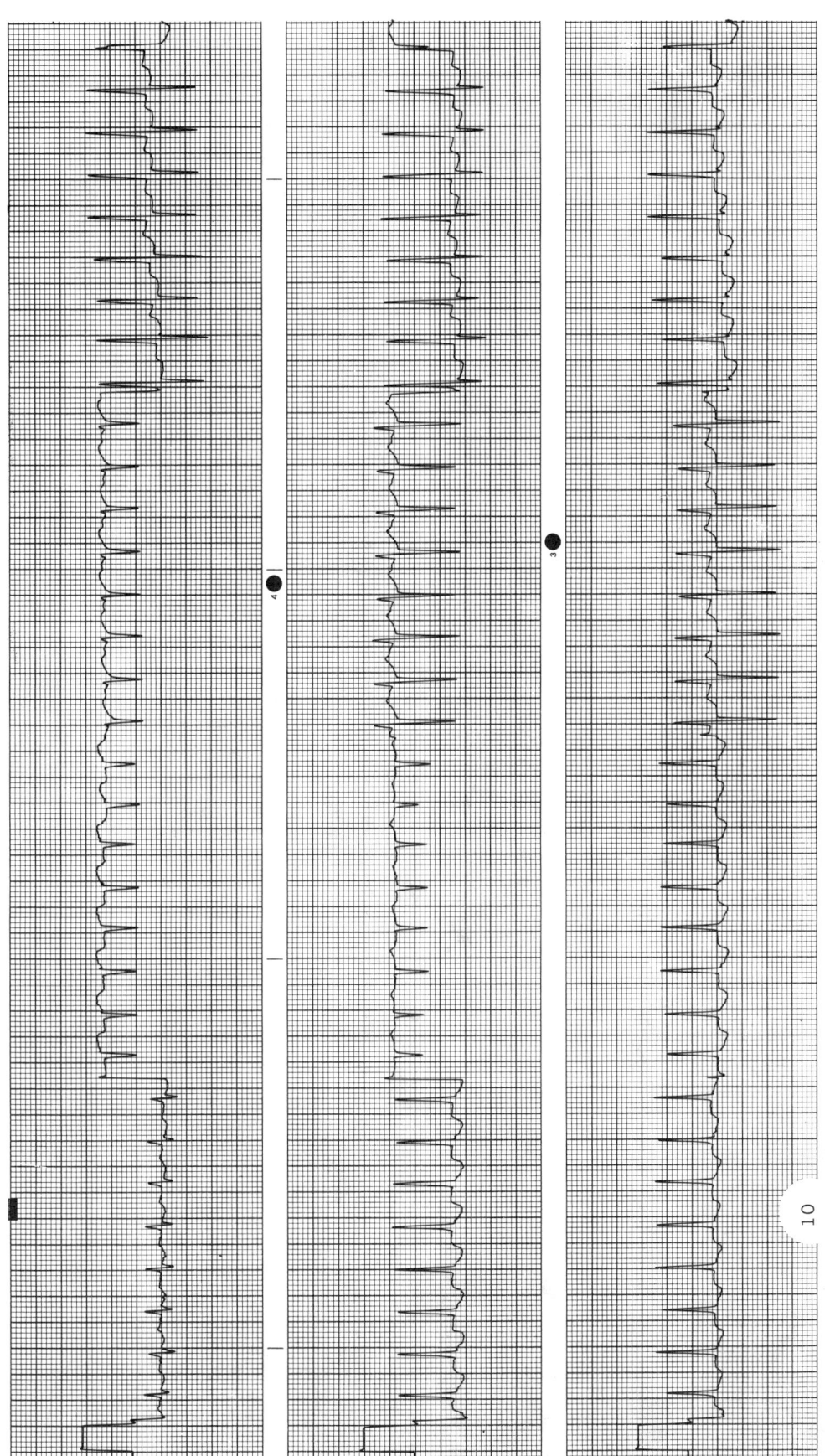

II

V1

V6

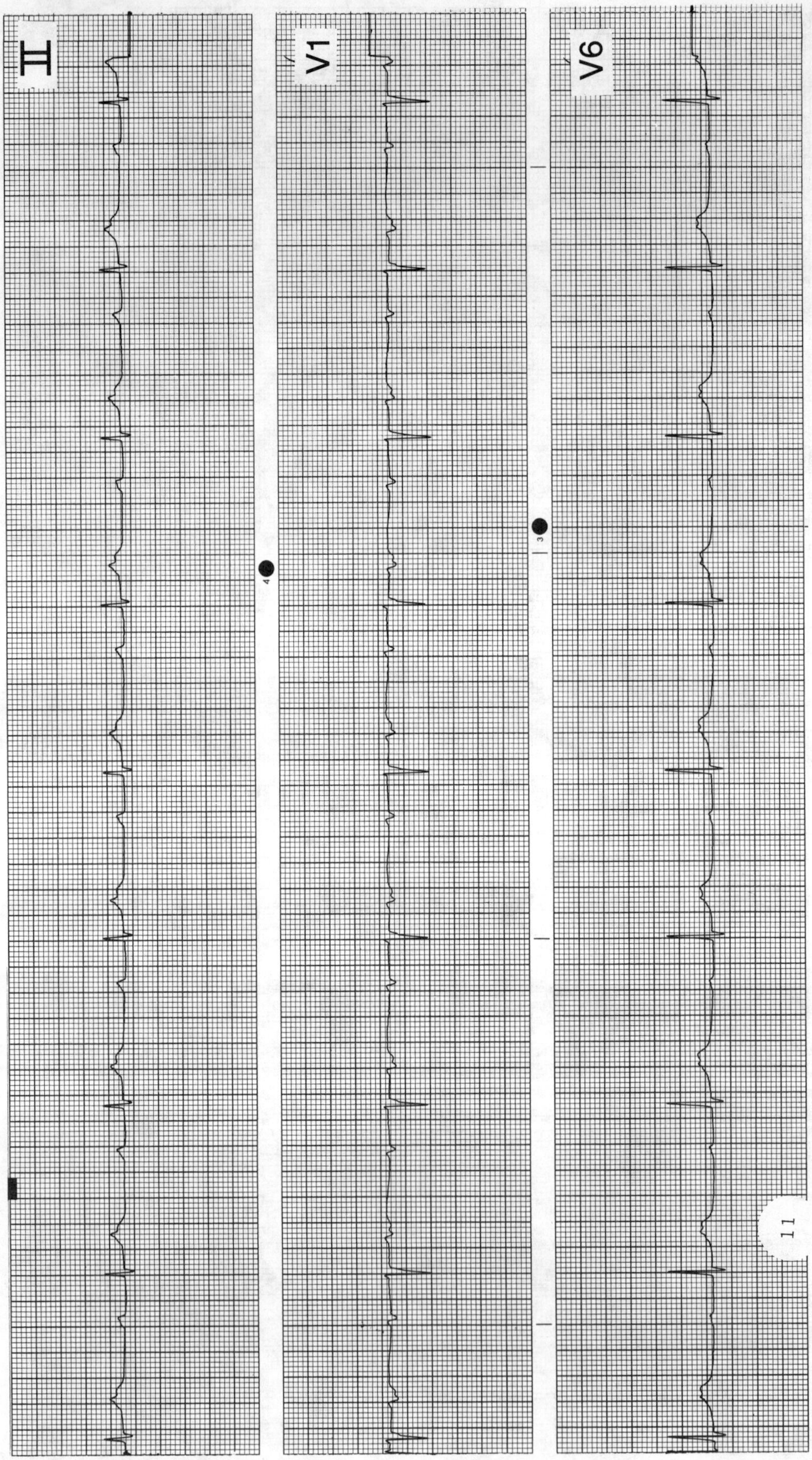

Exercise 11. Rhythm strips of leads II, V1, and V6.

1

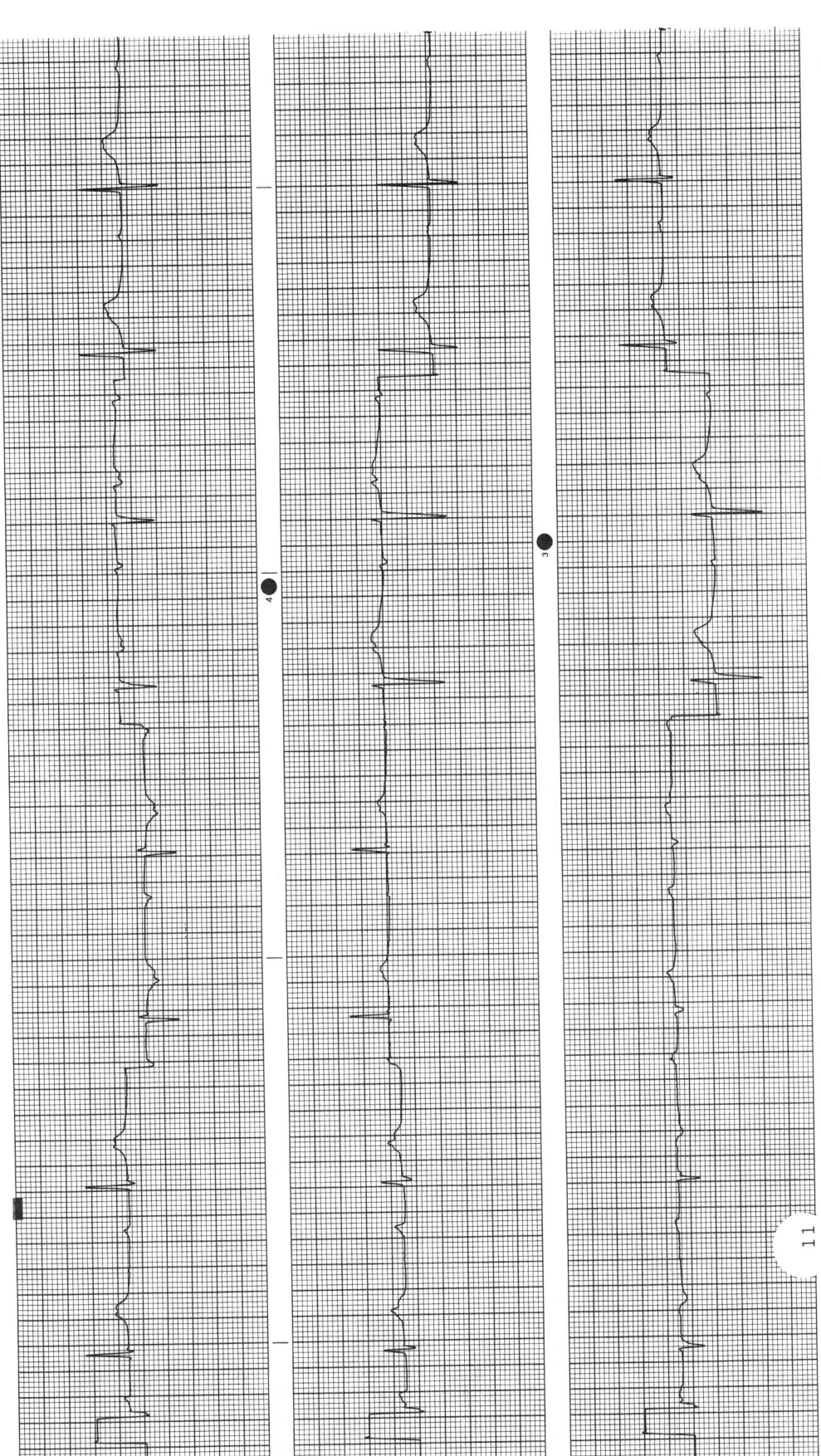

Exercise 11. A 64-year-old man complaining of dizziness and chest pain.

II

V1

V6

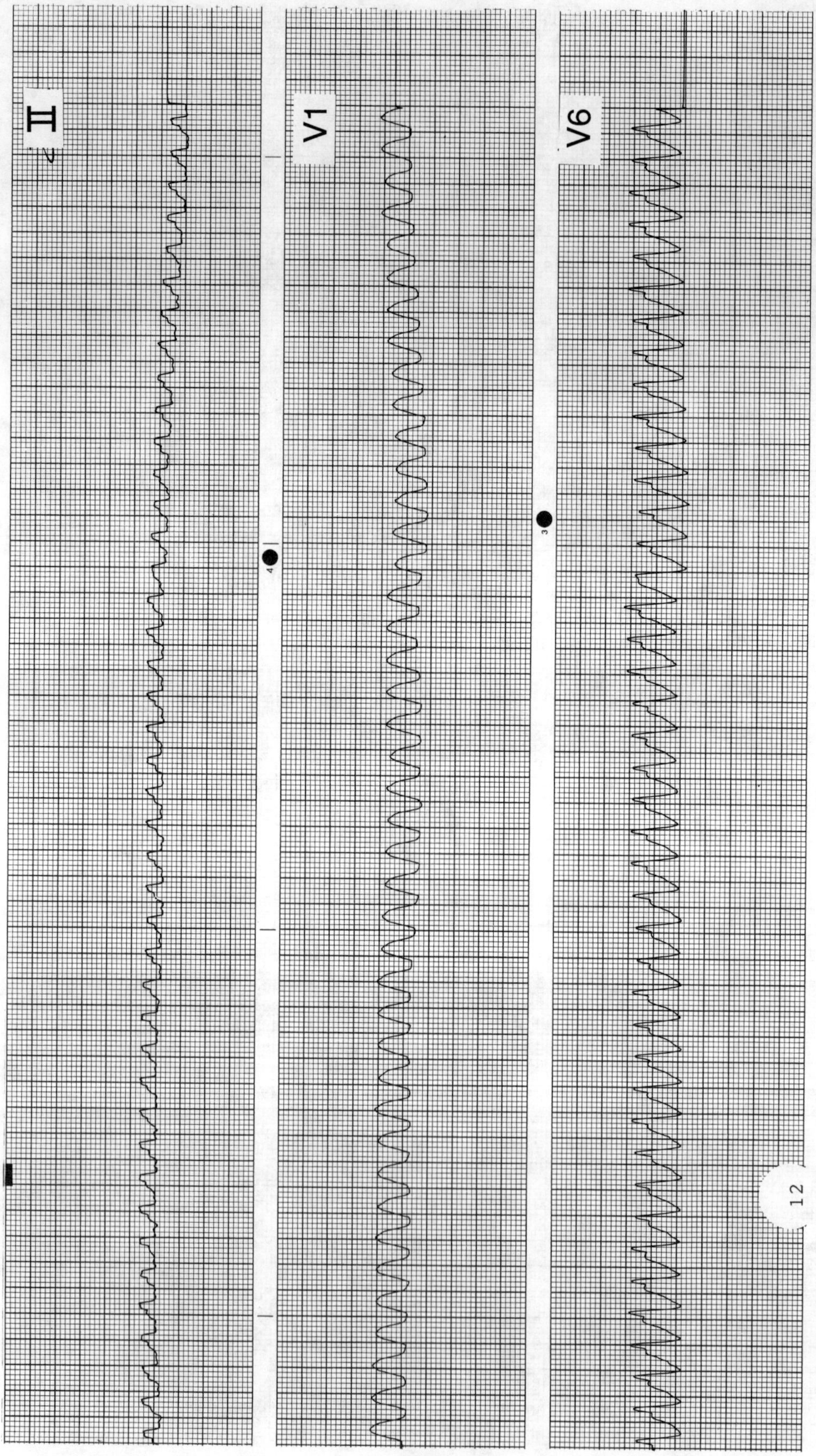

Exercise 12.   Rhythm strips of leads II, V1, and V6.

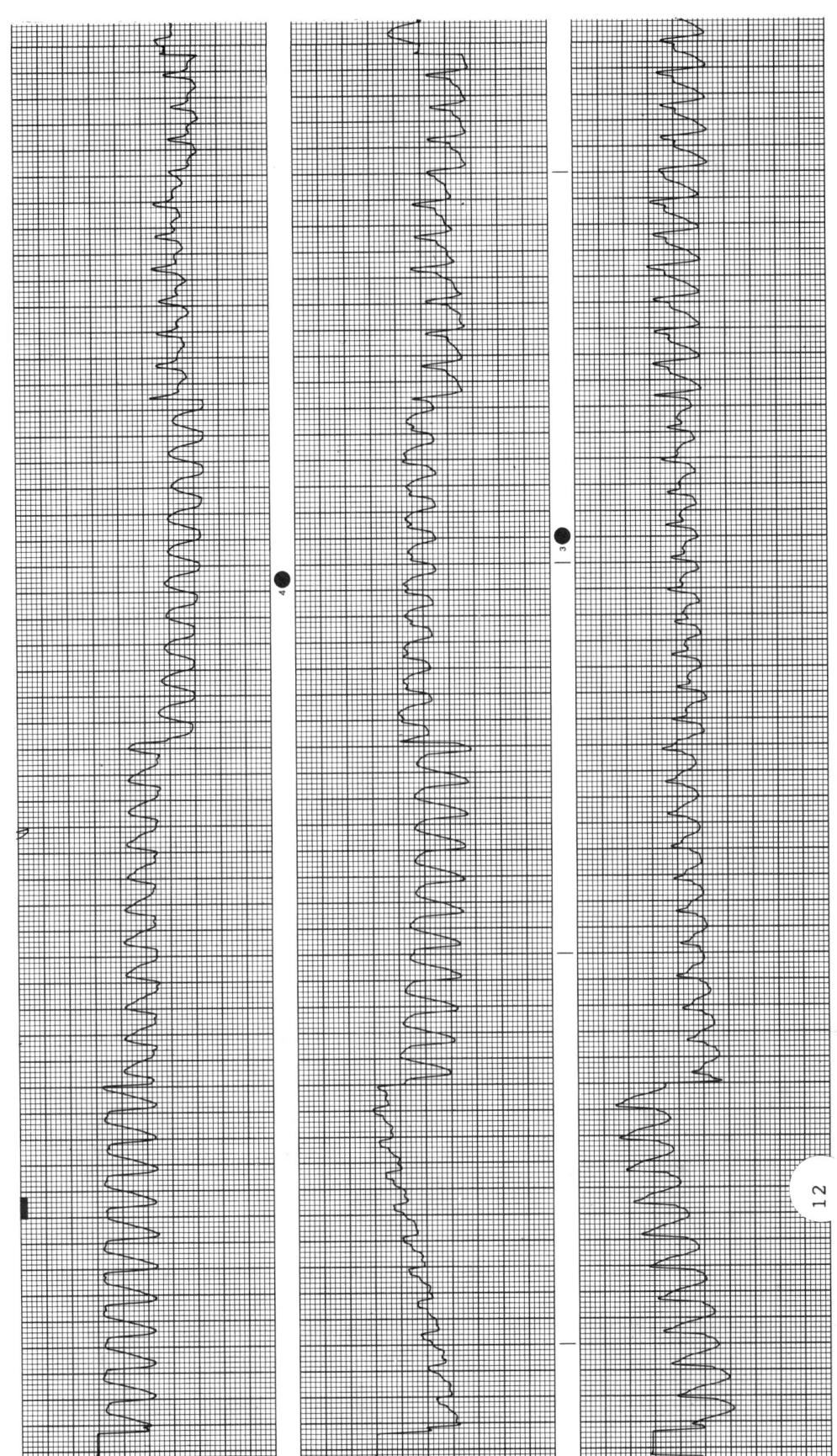

Exercise 12. A 55-year-old man presented in the emergency department complaining of lightheadedness and blurred vision. BP 60 systolic. No history of cardiac problems.

12

1

SELF-ASSESSMENT ANSWERS TO EXERCISES 7–12

EXERCISE 7

STEP 1. Rhythm Determination

- Ventricular rate 90
- QRS shape *Normal*

- Atrial rate 90
- P wave shape *Positive except negative in aVR and aVL, and diphasic in V1, V2*

- R-R rhythm *Mostly regular*
- QRS interval 0.08
- QT interval 0.32

- P-P rhythm *Mostly regular*
- P-R interval 0.14
- P:R conduction ratio *1:1*

- Dominant pacemaker site *Sinus*
- Interpretation *NSR with occasional APBs*

EXERCISE 8

STEP 1. Rhythm Determination

- Ventricular rate 78
- QRS shape *Normal*

- Atrial rate 320
- P wave shape *Saw toothed*

- R-R interval *Regular*
- QRS interval *.10 sec*
- QT interval *Cannot measure*
- Dominant pacemaker site *Atrial*

- P-P rhythm *Regular*
- P-R interval *Absent*
- P:R conduction ratio *4:1*

- Interpretation *Atrial flutter with a controlled ventricular response*

EXERCISE 9

STEP 1. Rhythm Determination

- Ventricular rate 58
- QRS shape *Normal with occasional wide beats*
- R-R rhythm *Irregular due to premature beats*
- QRS interval 0.08
- QT interval 0.42

- Atrial rate 58
- P wave shape *Positive except aVR negative*
- P-P rhythm *Regular except occasional absent P wave*
- P-R interval 0.16
- P:R conduction ratio *1:1*

- Dominant pacemaker site *Sinus*
- Interpretation *Sinus bradycardia with ventricular trigeminy*

EXERCISE 10

STEP 1. Rhythm Determination

- Ventricular rate 190

- QRS shape *Normal*
- R-R rhythm *Regular*
- QRS interval 0.06
- QT interval 0.22

- Atrial rate *Unable to measure*
- P wave shape *Buried*
- P-P rhythm _____
- P-R interval _____
- P:R conduction ratio _____

- Dominant pacemaker site *Atrial*
- Interpretation *Supraventricular tachycardia (SVT)*

EXERCISE 11

STEP 1. Rhythm Determination

- Ventricular rate 46
- QRS shape *Normal*

- Atrial rate 92
- P wave shape *Positive except negative in aVR and diphasic in V1 and V2*

- R-R rhythm *Regular*
- QRS interval 0.08
- QT interval 0.48

- P-P rhythm *Regular*
- P-R interval 0.36
- P:R conduction ratio *2:1*

- Dominant pacemaker site *Sinus*
- Interpretation *Second degree AV block with 2:1 conduction*

EXERCISE 12

STEP 1. Rhythm Determination

- Ventricular rate 240

- QRS shape *Wide and bizarre*
- R-R rhythm *Regular*
- QRS interval 0.22
- QT interval _____

- Atrial rate *Cannot measure*
- P wave shape _____
- P-P rhythm _____
- P-R interval _____
- P:R conduction ratio _____

- Dominant pacemaker site *Ventricular*
- Interpretation *Ventricular tachycardia*

3
Axis Determination

STEP 2

Axis determination is the *second step* in the systematic process. This step determines the *QRS*, or ventricular depolarization *axis* of the heart. The P wave, or atrial depolarization and the T wave, or ventricular repolarization axis will not be considered here. Because precise calculation methods are generally too complicated for daily use, only two approximate methods for axis determination are discussed. Axis deviations can occur in persons with normal electrocardiograms (ECGs), or could occur in persons with ventricular hypertrophy, acute myocardial infarctions, and hemiblocks.

AXIS

Axis indicates the average direction of the electrical activity of the heart during ventricular (QRS) depolarization. Ventricular depolarization normally occurs in three successive stages (Hurst, 1986; Alspach, 1979) (Figure 3.1). *In stage one*, depolarization of the ventricles begins at the bundle of His and travels through the interventricular septum toward the right ventricle in a left then right direction. This is often referred to as the septal depolarization stage. *In stage two*, the wave of depolarization travels toward the apical regions of the ventricles and stimulates both ventricles almost simultaneously. Because the left ventricle has the largest muscle mass, it dominates. *In stage three*, the wave of electrical activity progresses posteriorly and superiorly to depolarize the upper posterior portions of the ventricles. As a result, the electrical activity of the ventricles are being spread in many different directions. Most of these waves of electrical activity are being canceled out by each other, and only the net direction is recorded. The net direction is called the *mean QRS cardiac axis*. The *normal axis* is oriented downward (inferiorly) and to the left because the left ventricle has the most muscle mass.

The cardiac axis is determined by looking at the six frontal plane leads (I, II, III, aVR, aVL, and aVF). Each of the leads can be drawn to intersect in the center of the heart. The point in the center of the heart where the leads intersect is the AV node. This is known as the

hexaxial reference system. When a circle is drawn around these intersecting lines, degrees can be assigned to each lead (Duke, 1982; Alspach, 1979; Davis, 1985). The positive pole of lead I is assigned 0°. Moving clockwise in

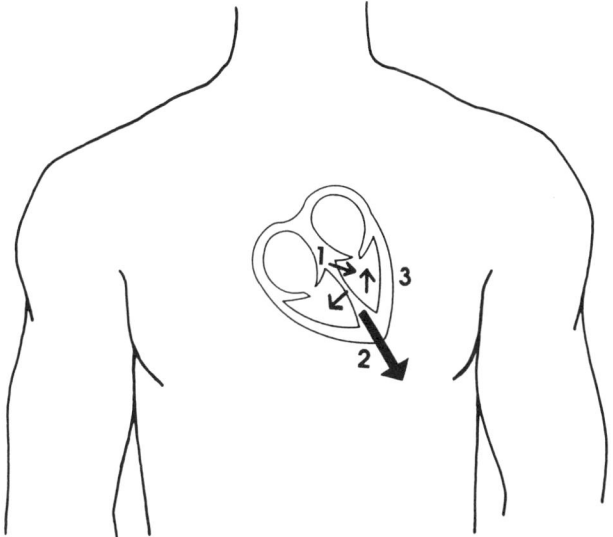

Figure 3.1. Stages and direction of mean QRS axis in relation to the left ventricle. *Arrows*, direction and magnitude: *1* = septal depolarization (left then right direction); *2* = Apical depolarization; points in a downward and leftward direction and equals mean QRS axis; *3* = posterior depolarization (terminal stage).

2

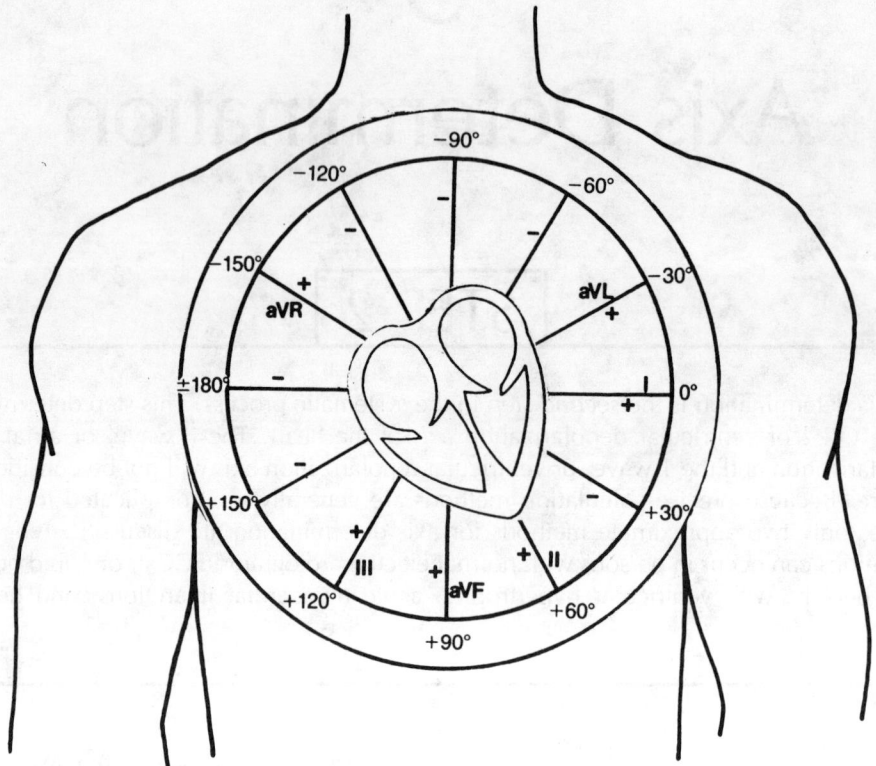

Figure 3.2. Hexaxial reference system. Degrees assigned to the leads of the frontal plane that intersect in the center of the heart. Leads are labeled on their positive poles. Adapted with permission from SJ Fry & P Lounsbury. *Cardiac rhythm disorders: An introduction using the nursing process.* Baltimore: Williams & Wilkins, 1988, p. 51.

30° increments, degrees are calculated as positive. Progressing counterclockwise in 30° increments, degrees are calculated as negative (Figure 3.2).

Axis is recorded as either normal axis (NA), right axis deviation (RAD), left axis deviation (LAD), or indeterminate axis (IA). Indeterminate axis is frequently labeled extreme right axis deviation. Ranges for normal axis and axis deviations are determined from the hexaxial reference system and summarized in Table 3.1. These ranges may vary with age, sex, body shape, and cardiologist. Many cardiologists extend the ranges. They consider the normal axis to range from +90 to −30°.

AXIS DETERMINATION METHODS

Two methods for determining the cardiac axis will be identified. Method one is an easy method utilizing leads I and aVF. It is often called the *easy quadrant method*. Method two is called the *null plane method*. It determines the axis in degrees, which is more accurate than the first method. There are numerous other methods that will not be covered. Knowledge of the hexaxial reference system is important in determining axis.

Easy Quadrant Method

Leads I and aVF are perpendicular to each other on the hexaxial reference system and divide the system into four quadrants (Duke, 1982). In this method, you determine the cardiac axis by examining leads I and aVF. It will localize the QRS axis into one of the four quadrants and lead to one of four combinations for axis determination (Figure 3.3).

Normal axis equals a POSITIVE QRS complex in lead I and a POSITIVE QRS complex in lead aVF. *Left axis deviation* equals a POSITIVE QRS complex in lead I and a NEGATIVE QRS complex in lead aVF. *Right axis deviation* equals a NEGATIVE QRS complex in lead

Table 3.1.
Degree Ranges for Normal Axis and Axis Deviations

Axis	Degrees
Normal	0 to +90
RAD	+90 to +/− 180
LAD	0 to −90
Indeterminate	−90 to +/− 180

2

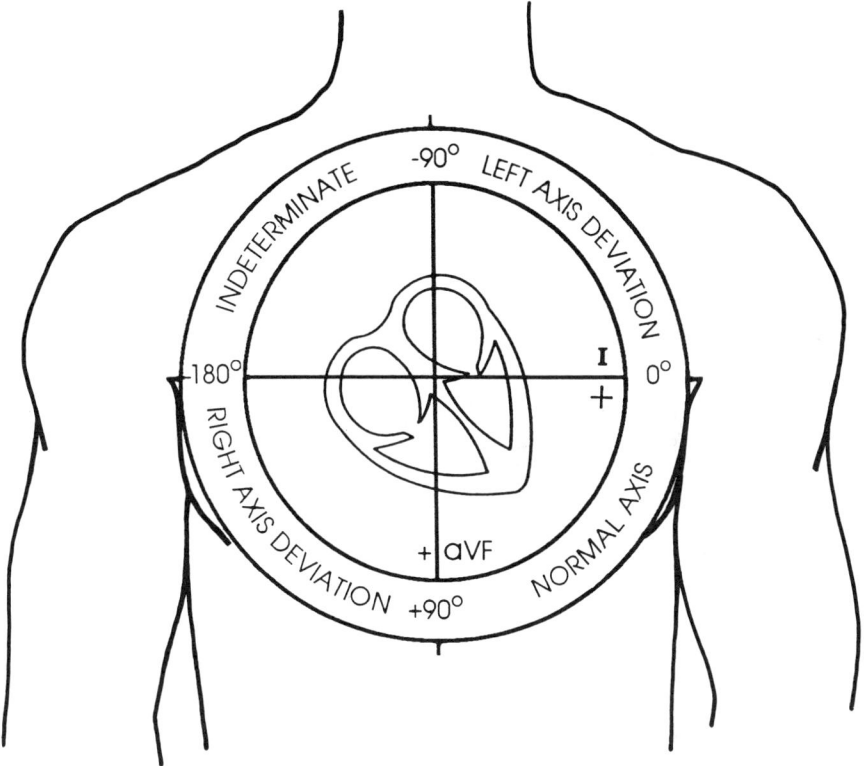

Figure 3.3. Easy quadrant method for determining axis using leads I and aVF of the hexaxial reference system.

I and a POSITIVE QRS complex in lead aVF. *Indeterminate axis* equals a NEGATIVE QRS complex in both leads I and aVF (Table 3.2). If complexes in leads I and aVF are equiphasic, try the null plane method to determine axis.

The three steps to the easy quadrant method are explained and demonstrated in Figure 3.4A–C using Figure 3.4D.

Step One: Determine whether the majority of the QRS complex in lead I is positive or negative. Then draw an arrow pointing toward the positive pole if lead I is positive, or toward the negative pole of lead I if it is negative. In the example, the QRS in lead I is mainly positive. Thus an arrow pointing toward the positive pole of lead I is depicted (Figure 3.4A).

Step Two: Determine whether the majority of the QRS complex in aVF is positive or negative. Then as in step one, draw an arrow pointing toward the pole of aVF as indicated by the direction of the QRS. In the example, the QRS in aVF is mainly positive. Thus an arrow is drawn pointing toward its positive pole (Figure 3.4B).

Step Three: Determine the QRS axis. The quadrant between the two arrow heads is the QRS axis. In Figure 3.4, leads I and aVF have positive QRS complexes. The

Table 3.2.
Axis Determined by Leads I and aVF

Axis	I	aVF
Normal axis (NA)	Positive	Positive
RAD	Negative	Positive
LAD	Positive	Negative
Indeterminate (IA)	Negative	Negative

area between the arrow heads depicts an axis that is normal (Figure 3.4C).

Null Plane Method

A second method for determining the mean QRS axis requires knowledge of three essential components. The first component is knowledge of which leads are perpendicular ($\perp$) to each other. Perpendicular leads are:

Lead I is $\perp$ to Lead aVF.
Lead II is $\perp$ to Lead aVL.
Lead III is $\perp$ to Lead aVR.

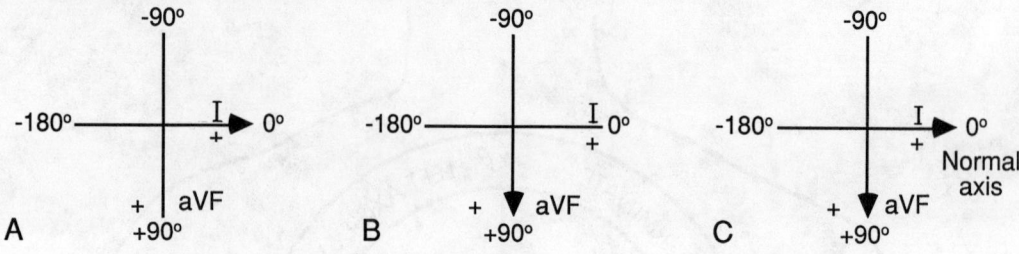

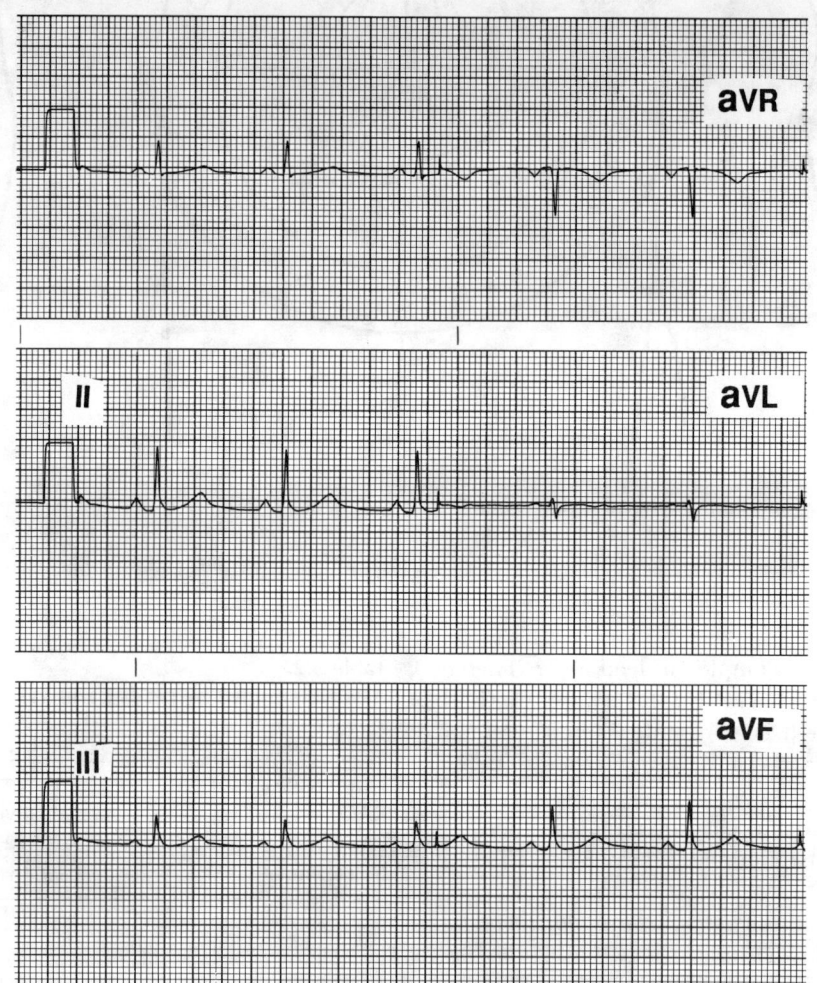

Figure 3.4.*A–C,* diagram for completing axis determination by the easy quadrant method using Figure 3.4*D.*

Figure 3.4.*D,* limb lead ECG example to be used for axis determination by the easy quadrant method.

One must memorize this information or use one of the following diagrams that relate perpendicular leads (Figure 3.5).

The second component is knowledge of the hexaxial reference system. The third component is knowledge of degrees and the degree range for each axis range. This

information can be found in Table 3.1. The null plane method calculates the approximate degree of the axis.

The three steps of the null plane method are described below and applied using Figure 3.6.

Step One: Look for the isoelectric lead. Examine the frontal plane leads and identify the QRS complex, which

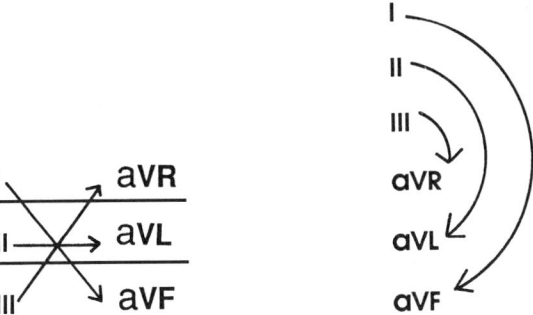

Figure 3.5. Perpendicular lead pairs. *Arrows* point to perpendicular lead pairs.

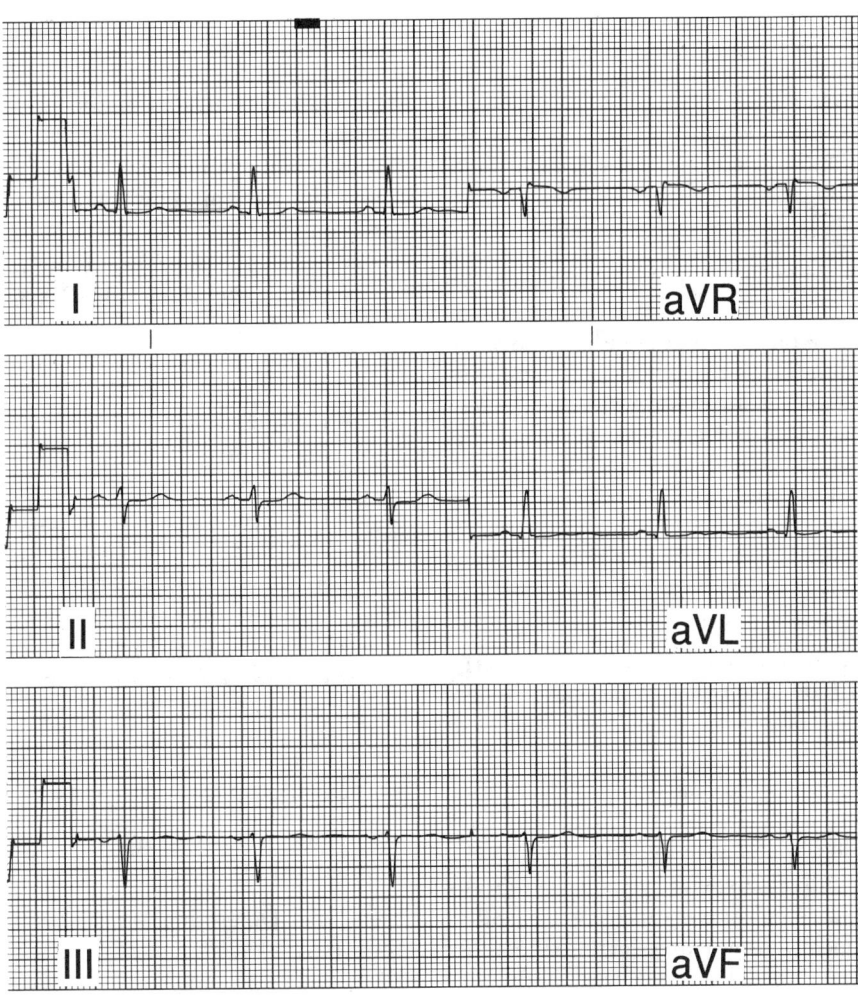

Figure 3.6. Limb lead examples for axis determination using the null plane method.

2

is either flat, diphasic, or isoelectric. The QRS complex of this lead is composed of equally negative and positive waveforms and is called the null plane lead. If all leads are equiphasic, the axis is indeterminate. In Figure 3.6, lead II is isoelectric and is thus the null plane lead.

Step Two: Find the lead that is perpendicular to the null plane lead. Locate the lead that is perpendicular or at right angles to the isoelectric lead determined in step one. In Figure 3.6, lead aVL is perpendicular to lead II.

Step Three: Look at the lead found in step two and determine its polarity. If the lead in step two is positive, read the axis directly. If the lead in step two is negative, the axis is 180° away. In Figure 3.6, aVL is positive so the axis is −30°. This is a left axis deviation.

CLINICAL SIGNIFICANCE

Axis determination is clinically useful in interpreting 12-lead ECGs because it warns you to look for other abnormalities. An abnormal axis is similar to the concept of ectopic beats. Ectopic beats put you on the alert to look for more serious dysrhythmias. Knowledge of the cardiac axis puts you on the alert to look for:

a. Ventricular hypertrophy
b. Acute myocardial infarction
c. Position changes of the heart due to mechanical shifts such as a pneumothorax
d. Hemiblocks

There will be more about these individual problems in later chapters.

An axis shift in general can occur in individuals without cardiac disease and thus is considered a normal variant. The three main causes for axis deviations are ventricular hypertrophy, a hemiblock, or a myocardial infarction. A key point regarding axis is that it generally will deviate toward hypertrophic areas and away from infarcted areas.

Right axis deviations can occur as the result of the development of a left posterior hemiblock (LPH) or a lateral myocardial infarction (MI). It also may develop in the presence of right ventricular hypertrophy (RVH), which can occur in individuals with pulmonary hypertension and chronic obstructive pulmonary disease (COPD).

Left axis deviations can be caused by left anterior hemiblocks (LAH) or an inferior MI. It also may develop in the presence of left ventricular hypertrophy (LVH), which can occur in individuals with systemic hypertension. Table 3.3 summarizes various causes of axis shifts.

Axis is also clinically useful in selecting the most appropriate monitoring lead based on the conduction problems presented. If a patient has a right bundle

Table 3.3.
Axis Causes

Right Axis Deviations	Left Axis Deviations
Normal variation	Normal variation
LPH	LAH
RVH	LVH
Lateral MI	Inferior MI

branch block (RBBB), monitor on any limb lead such as lead II to observe for a change in the QRS morphology. The QRS will likely change from a positive complex to a negative complex or vice versa. If the QRS morphology changes, determine the axis and look for the development of a hemiblock. If the patient has a left axis shift and LAH already, monitor on lead V1 to detect the development of a RBBB. Lastly, if the patient has a bifascicular block, monitor on any rhythm lead and assess for the development of complete heart block.

Key questions to ask yourself when performing this step of the systematic process are:

What is the clinical situation in which axis deviation is occurring?
- Monitor for hypertrophy, hemiblocks, or an MI.

Does the patient show signs of increasing conduction problems?
- Select the appropriate monitoring lead.
- If the patient has a RBBB, monitor on a limb lead and observe for changes in QRS configuration; if it changes, determine axis and look for the development of a hemiblock.
- If the patient has a LAH, monitor on lead V1 to observe for the development of a RBBB or completion of the LBBB.
- If the patient has a bifascicular block, monitor on a rhythm lead for complete heart block.

What treatment should you be prepared for in the presence of an axis change?
- Perform 12-lead ECG.
- Prepare for treatment of conduction problems (pacemaker).

SELF-ASSESSMENT EXERCISES 13–18

In the following six ECG examples complete the following steps:

Step One: Determination of rhythm
Step Two: Determination of axis

Normal _____ Right _____ Left _____
Indeterminate _____

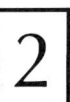

Remember generally we are interested only in whether the axis is left or right, not in the specific degrees. Thus, use the easy quadrant method. Also an abnormal axis leads you to suspect other problems that will be addressed in ensuing chapters.

You must be able to perform these steps successfully before proceeding. When you have completed all of the exercises in this book, come back to this exercise and complete the remaining steps.

Check your answers with the suggested interpretations found at the end of this chapter. Answers for remaining steps will be found in Appendix A.

2

Exercise 13.   A 64-year-old woman admitted to emergency department with complaints of dyspnea and chest pain. History of COPD and angina.

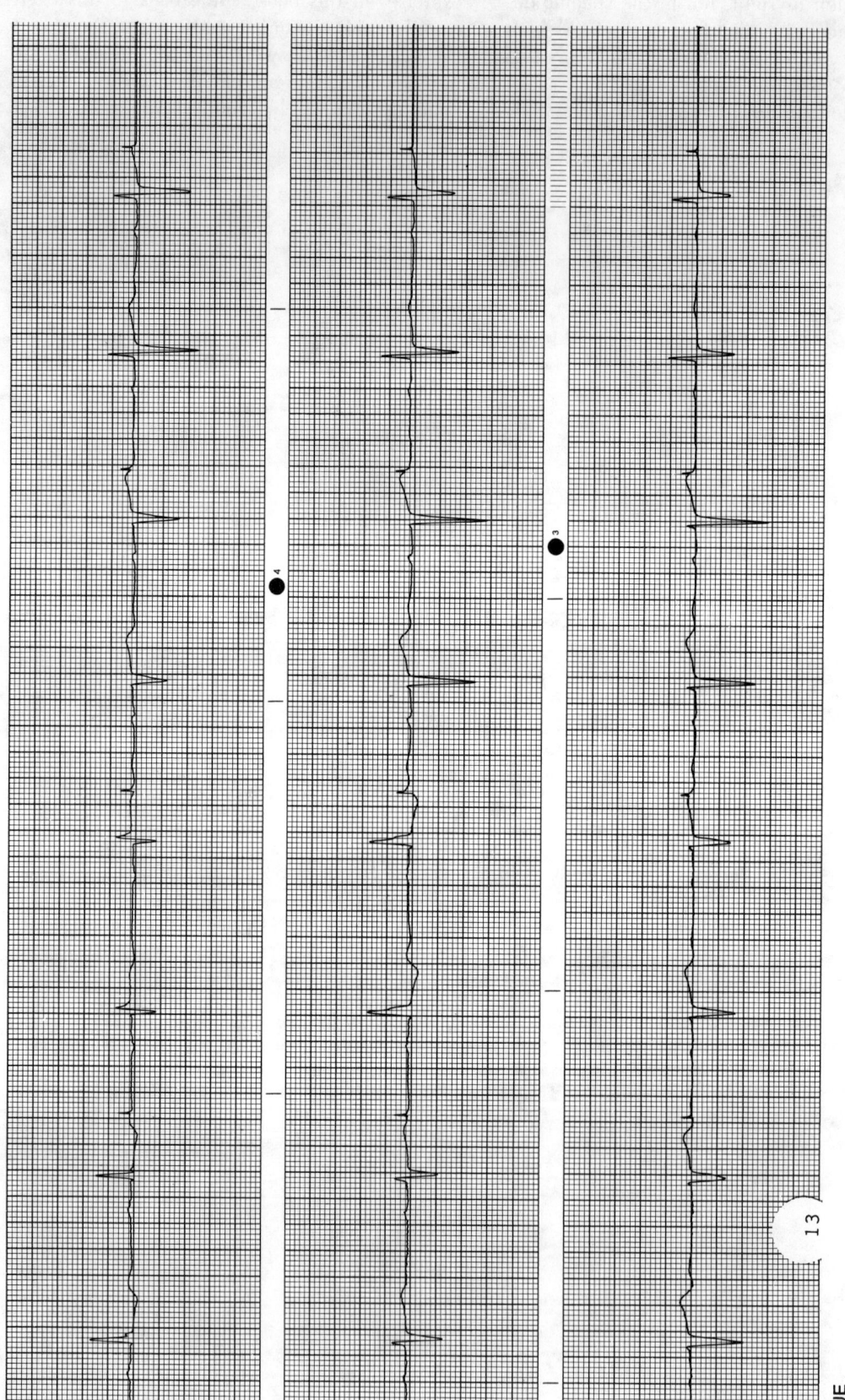

13

JE

Exercise 14. A 61-year-old man admitted to CCU complaining of sudden onset substernal chest pain at rest. History of COPD.

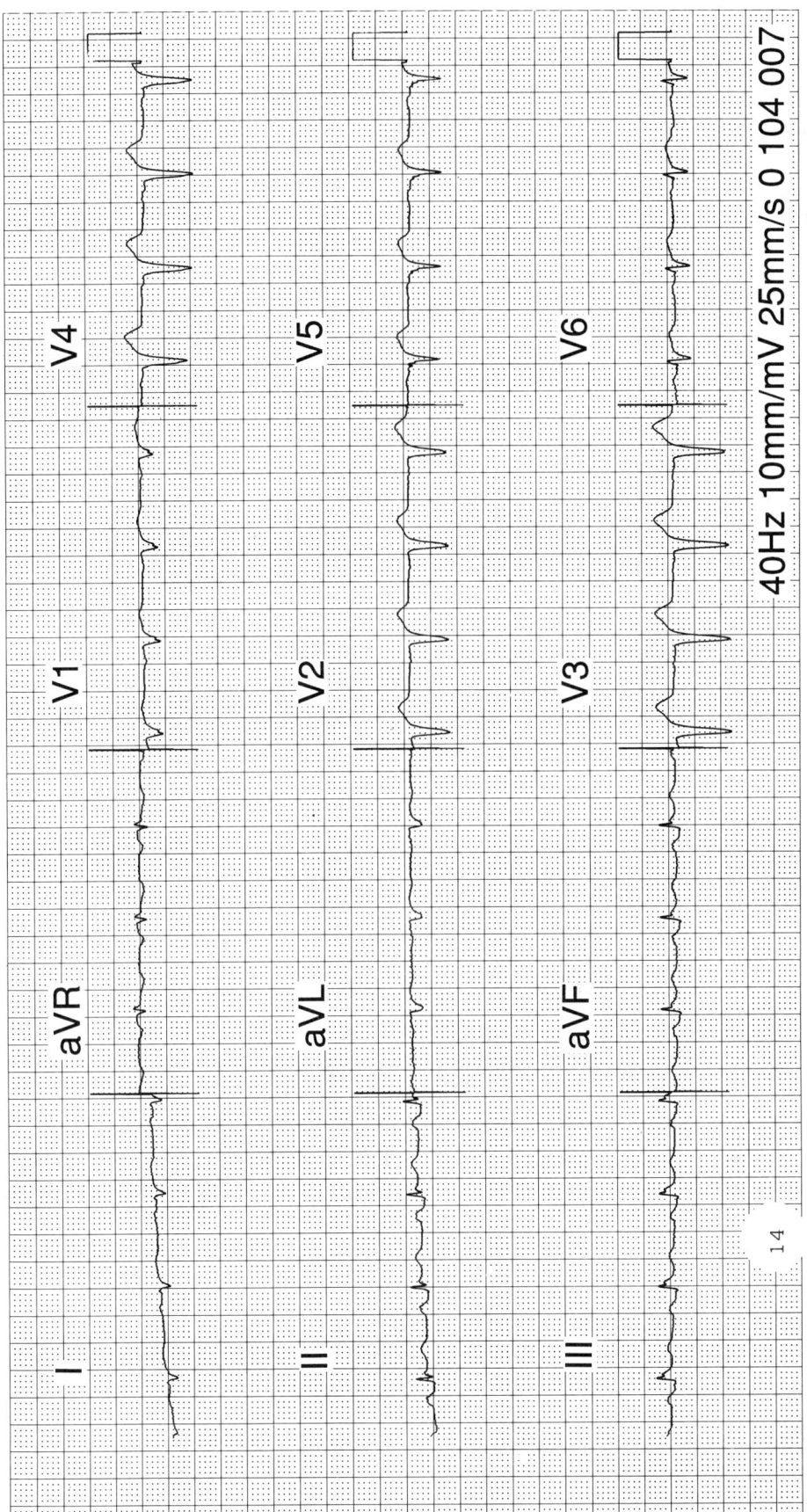

40Hz 10mm/mV 25mm/s 0 104 007

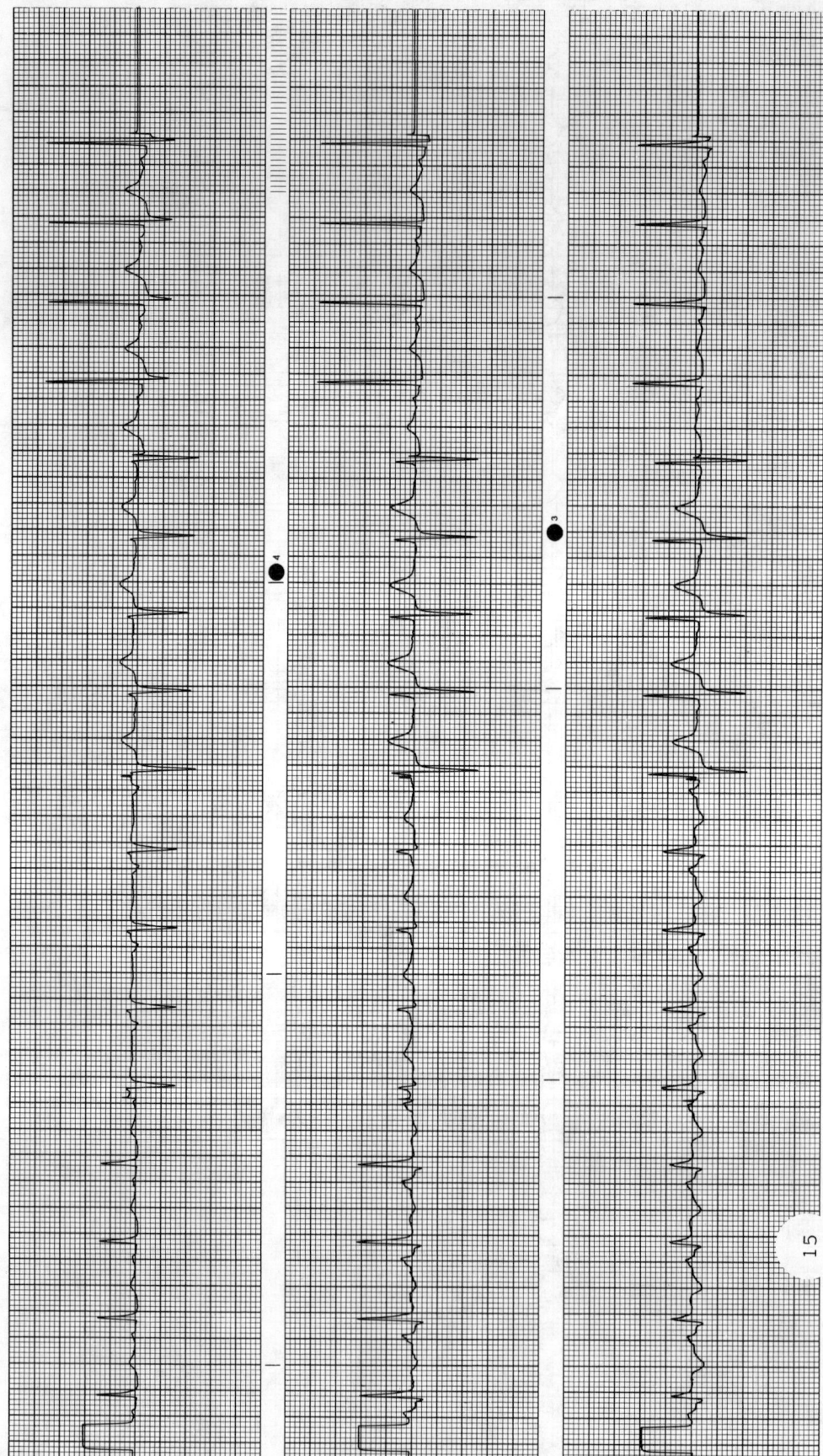

Exercise 15. A 62-year-old woman admitted because of recurrent midsternal chest pain. History of unstable angina. Positive cardiac enzymes.

15

2

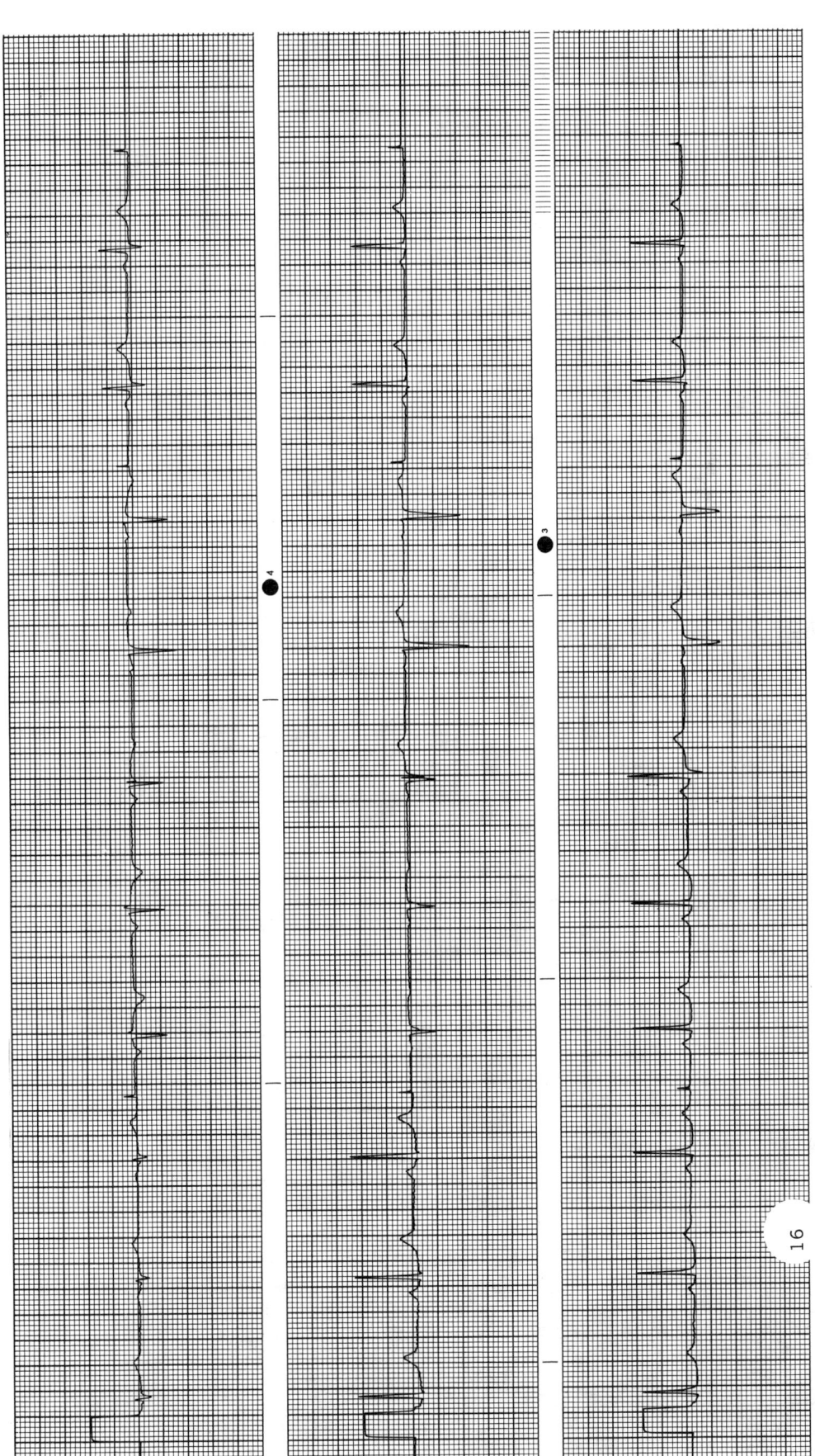

Exercise 16.   A 60-year-old woman admitted with chest pain.

16

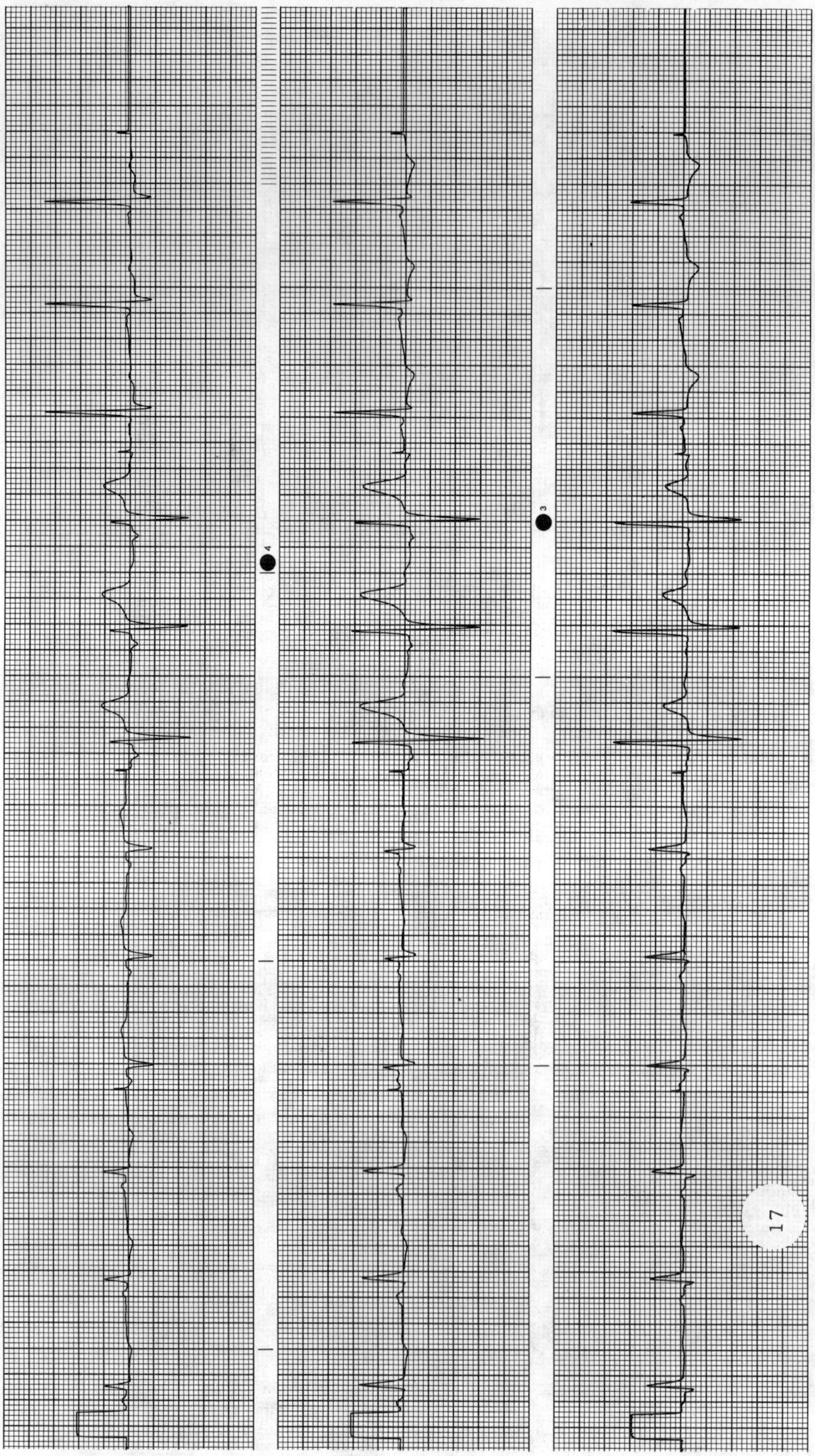

Exercise 17. A 66-year-old man admitted with chest pain. Cardiac enzymes negative.

2

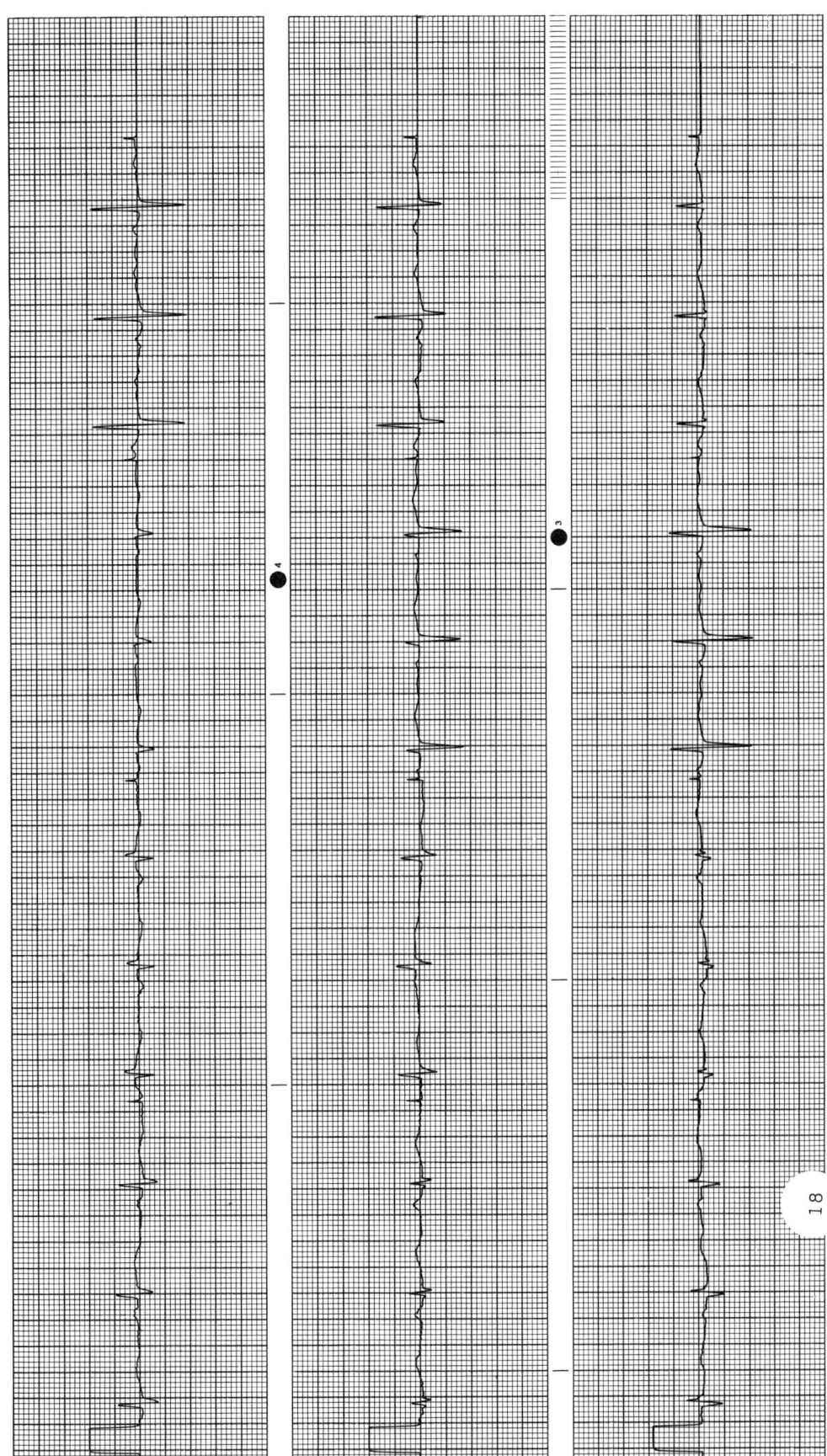

Exercise 18. A 66-year-old man with known coronary artery disease admitted with unstable angina. Cardiac enzymes negative.

2 SELF-ASSESSMENT ANSWERS TO EXERCISES 13–18

EXERCISE 13

STEP 1. Rhythm Determination

- Ventricular rate *47*
- QRS shape *Normal*

- Atrial rate *47*
- P wave shape *Positive except negative aVR and flat in III*

- R-R rhythm *Regular*
- QRS interval *0.11*
- QT interval *0.48*

- P-P rhythm *Regular*
- P-R interval *0.28*
- P:R conduction ratio *1:1*

- Dominant pacemaker site *Sinus*
- Interpretation *Sinus bradycardia with 1st degree AV block*

STEP 2. Axis Determination

Left axis

EXERCISE 14

STEP 1. Rhythm Determination

- Ventricular rate *90*
- QRS shape *Small and widened*

- Atrial rate *90*
- P wave shape *Positive except negative aVR, V1 and flattened in aVL*

- R-R rhythm *Regular*
- QRS interval *0.10*
- QT interval *0.32*

- P-P rhythm *Regular*
- P-R interval *0.16*
- P:R conduction ratio *1:1*

- Dominant pacemaker site *Sinus*
- Interpretation *NSR*

STEP 2. Axis Determination

Right axis deviation

EXERCISE 15

STEP 1. Rhythm Determination

- Ventricular rate *100*
- QRS shape *Normal*

- Atrial rate *100*
- P wave shape *Positive except negative in aVR and flat in aVL and V1– V3*

- R-R rhythm *Regular*
- QRS interval *0.09*
- QT interval *0.36*

- P-P rhythm *Regular*
- P-R interval *0.16*
- P:R conduction ratio *1:1*

- Dominant pacemaker site *Sinus*
- Interpretation *Sinus tachycardia*

STEP 2. Axis Determination

Normal

EXERCISE 16

STEP 1. Rhythm Determination

- Ventricular rate *64*
- QRS shape *Normal*

- Atrial rate *64*
- P wave shape *Positive except negative in aVR and aVL, and diphasic in V1*

- R-R rhythm, *Regular*
- QRS interval *0.08*
- QT interval *0.40*

- P-P rhythm *Regular*
- P-R interval *0.16*
- P:R conduction ratio *1:1*

- Dominant pacemaker site *Sinus*
- Interpretation *NSR*

STEP 2. Axis Determination

Normal. Because QRS complex equiphasic in lead I, cannot use easy quadrant method. Must use null plane method (axis 90°).

EXERCISE 17

STEP 1. Rhythm Determination

- Ventricular rate *72*
- QRS shape *Normal*

- R-R rhythm *Regular*
- QRS interval *0.10*
- QT interval *0.40*

- Dominant pacemaker site *Sinus*
- Interpretation *NSR*

- Atrial rate *72*
- P wave shape *Positive except negative in aVR and aVL, diphasic in V1 and V2*
- P-P rhythm *Regular*
- P-R interval *0.16*
- P:R conduction ratio *1:1*

STEP 2. Axis Determination

Normal

EXERCISE 18

STEP 1. Rhythm Determination

- Ventricular rate *72*
- QRS shape *Normal*

- R-R rhythm *Regular*
- QRS interval *0.08*
- QT interval *0.44*

- Dominant pacemaker site *Sinus*
- Interpretation *NSR*

- Atrial rate *72*
- P wave shape *Positive except negative aVR, V1*
- P-P rhythm *Regular*
- P-R interval *0.18*
- P:R conduction ratio *1:1*

STEP 2. Axis Determination

Indeterminate. Because all QRS complexes are diphasic neither the easy quadrant nor the null plane method can be used. It is impossible to determine the direction of the axis, therefore the axis is indeterminate.

4
Chamber Enlargement Determination

$$\boxed{\text{STEP 3}}$$

The *third step* in the systematic approach is to observe for chamber enlargement. This chapter will outline the electrocardiographic (ECG) changes that occur with right and left atrial abnormalities and ventricular hypertrophy.

Chamber enlargement occurs for two primary reasons, dilatation and hypertrophy. In dilatation, the chamber stretches to a size necessary to accommodate an increased volume of blood or pressure. When it must do so repeatedly as with chronic congestive heart failure, the chamber will adapt by increasing its inner radius. In hypertrophy, the chamber enlarges due to increased muscle mass. Muscle mass increases when the ventricle must eject its blood against higher pressures in such chronic conditions as hypertension and aortic stenosis. By increasing its muscle mass the chamber can generate a more forceful contraction, overcome the higher pressures, and eject its contents.

Although there are no ECG changes that are specific to chamber enlargement, changes that occur affect both the P wave and QRS complex. The changes relate to both the time it takes the electrical impulse to cross the chamber and the force of contraction.

ATRIAL ABNORMALITIES

Before discussing ECG changes found with a right atrial abnormality, it is important to review normal atrial events. To review, depolarization of the right and left atria are represented by the P wave. A P wave should be no taller than 2.5 mm and no wider than 0.11 seconds (Figure 4.1). Changes representing atrial repolarization usually cannot be visualized because they are buried in the QRS complex. Therefore, changes occurring due to atrial abnormalities will be seen in the P wave.

The atrial impulse originates in the right atrium and spreads from right to left. If the right atrium becomes enlarged, impulses will take longer to cross it. The P wave will not widen because the width of P waves is determined by the length of time the impulse needs to cross the left atrium. Therefore, the additional time the impulse needs to cross the right atrium will be buried in the left atrial portion of the P wave (Figure 4.2).

To identify atrial abnormalities, *examine leads II and V1 for height and width*. With a right atrial abnormality, the P wave in lead II will be pointed and taller than 2.5 mm. In left atrial abnormality, the P wave in lead II will be wider than 0.12 sec and look like the letter "m". In lead V1 with right atrial abnormality the P wave will be diphasic with the initial positive deflection taller than the second negative deflection. With left atrial abnormality, the P wave again will be diphasic in V1 but the terminal negative deflection will be deeper and wider than the initial positive deflection. Table 4.1 summarizes the features of right and left atrial abnormalities.

Now examine Figure 4.3. Are the P waves significant for right or left atrial abnormalities?

3

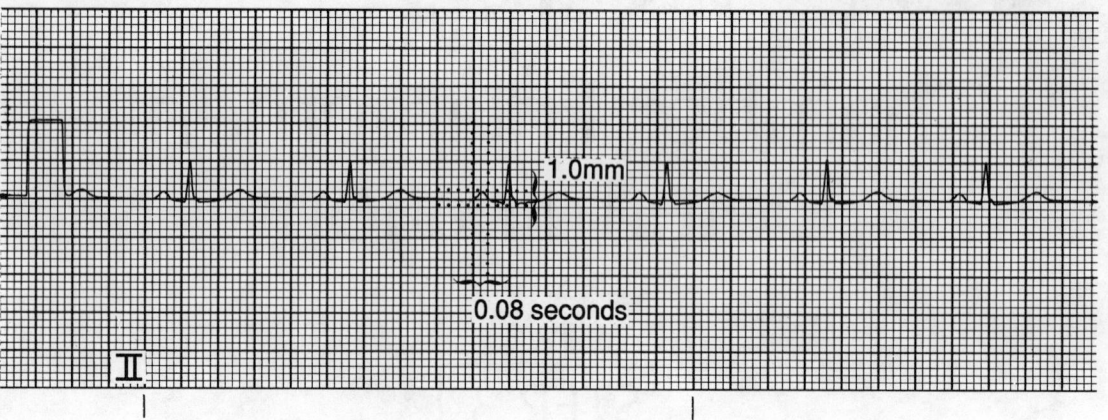

Figure 4.1. Height and width of normal P wave. Normal P wave = height ≤ 2.5 mm, width ≤ 0.11 seconds.

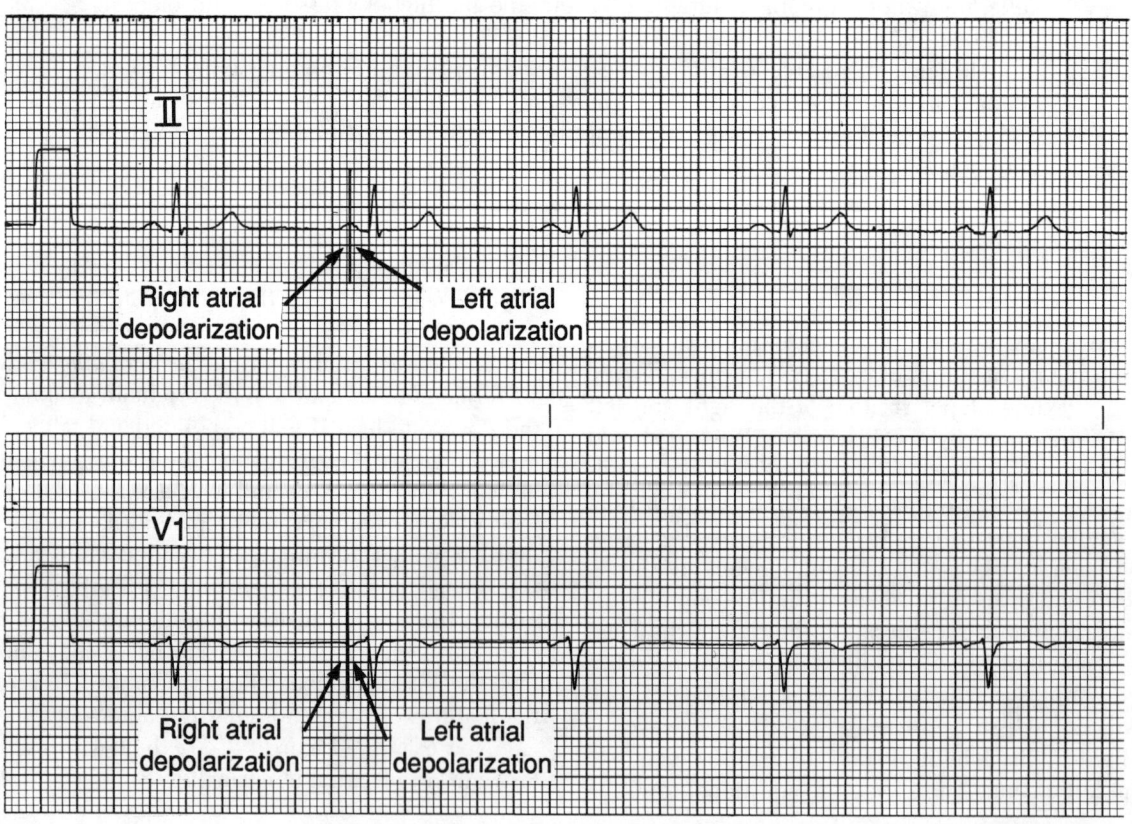

Figure 4.2. P wave depicting right and left Atrial depolarization utilizing leads II and V1. Adapted with permission from MS Thaler. *The only EKG book you'll ever need.* Philadelphia: JB Lippincott, 1988, p. 18.

3

Table 4.1.
Features of P Waves in Right and Left Atrial Abnormalities

	Right	Left
Lead II	Height >2.5 mm Pointed	Notched Looks like "m" Width >0.12 secs
Lead V1	Diphasic Initial positive deflection taller than terminal negative deflection	Diphasic Terminal negative deflection wider than initial positive deflection

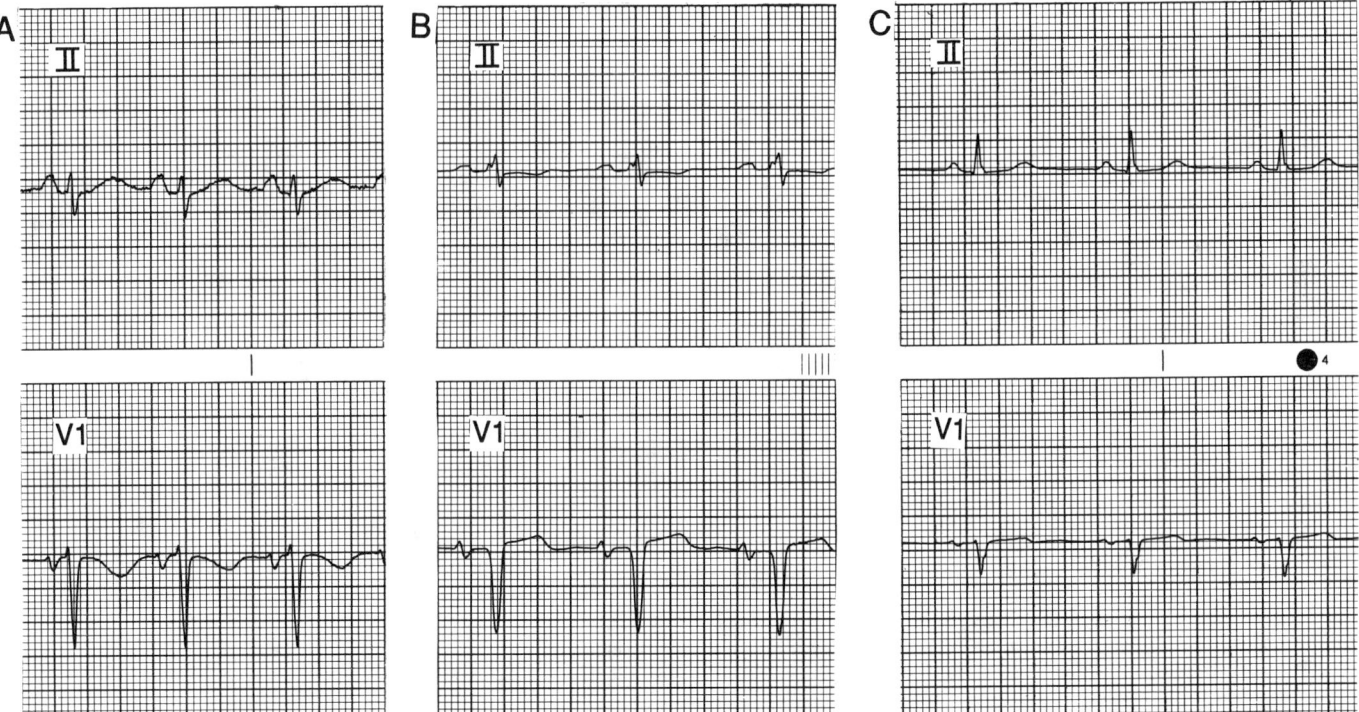

Figure 4.3.   Are the following P waves significant for right or
left atrial abnormalities?

3

VENTRICULAR HYPERTROPHIES

The ECG changes that occur with both right and left ventricular hypertrophies reflect the enlarged ventricular muscle mass. Unlike atrial abnormalities, both depolarization and repolarization changes occur with ventricular hypertrophies.

To identify hypertrophies, the best leads to *examine are the chest leads*, particularly leads V1 and V2 and leads V5 and V6. In *right ventricular hypertrophy (RVH)*, leads V1 and V2 may have a tall R wave. In fact the R wave will be larger than the S wave, which is normally larger in these leads. Leads reflecting the left side of the heart, V5 and V6, will have deep S waves (Figure 4.4). Probably the most important sign of right ventricular hypertrophy is right axis deviation. This occurs because the larger right ventricular muscle is able to generate greater force and thus shift the axis to the right.

In *left ventricular hypertrophy (LVH)*, the height of the R wave will be taller in leads reflecting the left side of the heart, leads V5 and V6. The depth of the S wave will be greater in those leads reflecting the right side of the heart, leads V1 and V2. A simple method to use to look for LVH is to add the depth of the S wave in either V1 or V2 to the height of the R wave in V5 or V6. If the sum is equal to or greater than 35 mm, LVH is present (Figure 4.5). Left ventricular hypertrophy cannot be identified when a left bundle branch block is present. A left bundle branch block distorts the amplitude of the waves in the QRS complex thus making this an invalid measure of hypertrophy.

Although it is unknown why, repolarization changes accompany hypertrophies. The repolarization change occurs as a strain pattern—downward sagging ST segments with inverted T waves that can be seen in any lead with tall R waves. In RVH, strain pattern occurs in any lead facing the right side of the heart—leads III, aVF, V1, and V2 (See Figure 4.4).

In LVH, strain pattern occurs in leads with a tall R wave reflecting the left side of the heart, leads I, aVL, V5, and V6 (See Figure 4.5). Table 4.2 summarizes the features of right and left ventricular hypertrophies.

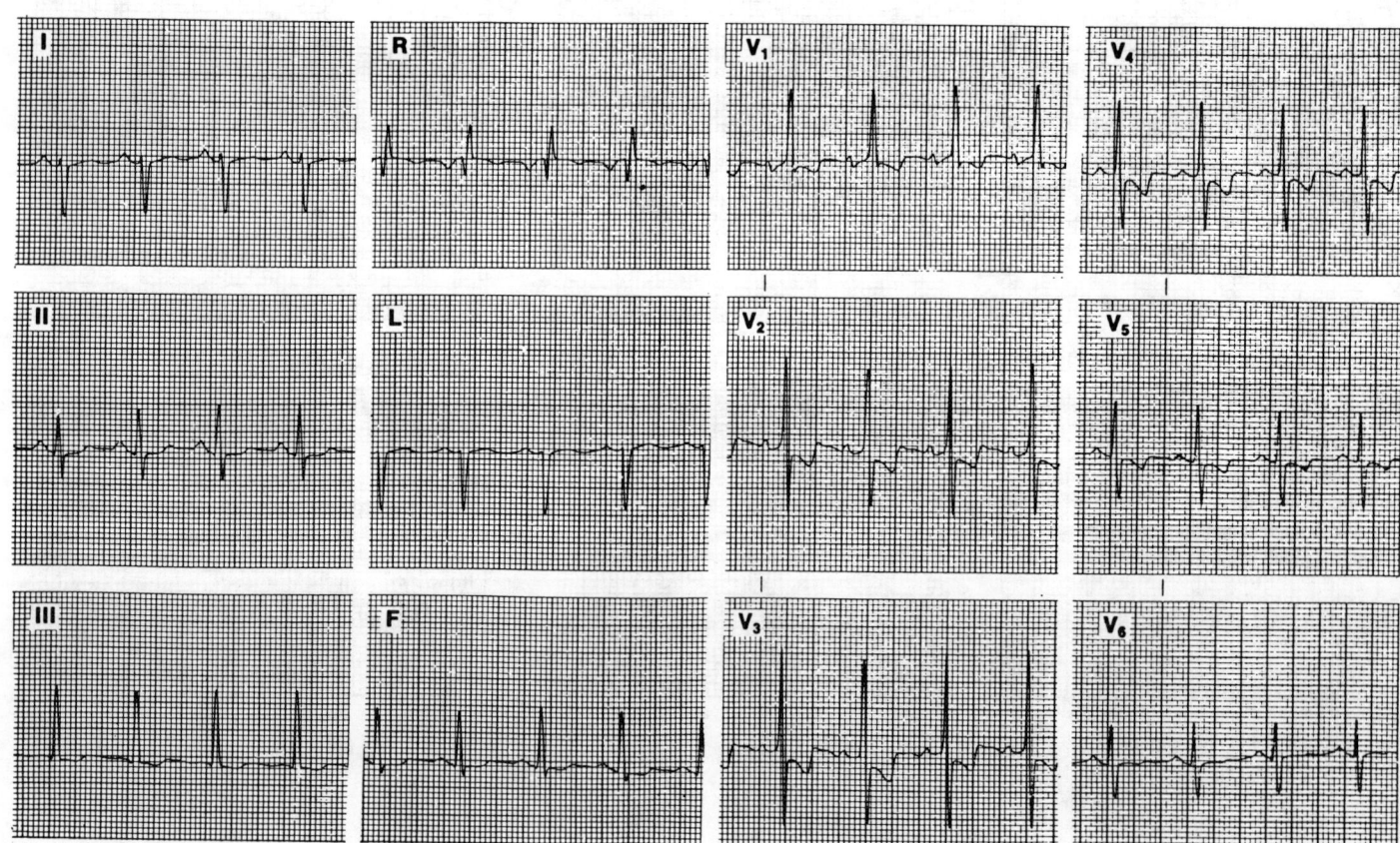

Figure 4.4. Right ventricular hypertrophy. Note the tall R wave in lead V1 and the deep S wave in V6. Note the right axis deviation. Note the strain pattern. Used with permission from N Laiken et al. *Interpretation of electrocardiograms.* New York: Raven Press, 1988, p 67.

3

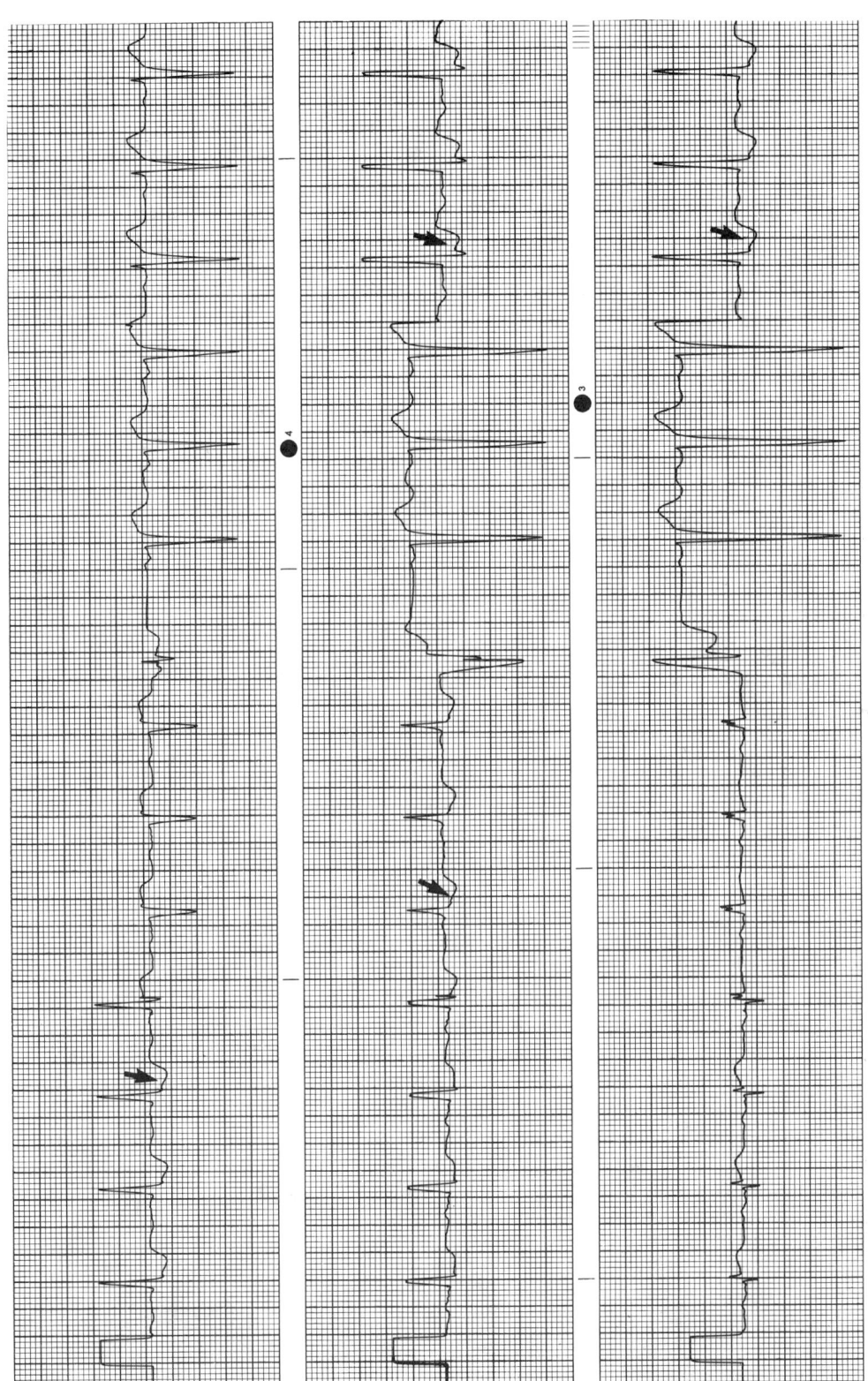

Figure 4.5. Left ventricular hypertrophy. Note voltage of QRS complexes in leads V1 and V6 and downward sagging ST segments and flipped T waves in leads with tall R waves. Note strain pattern in leads I, aVL, V5, and V6.

3

Table 4.2.
Features of Right and Left Ventricular Hypertrophies

	Right	Left
Leads V1/V2	R taller than S Strain pattern	S deeper than r No strain pattern

Leads V5/V6	Deep S wave
	No strain pattern
		Tall R wave
		Strain pattern
		Sum of S in V1
		  or V2 plus the R
		  in V5 or V6
		  ≥35 mm

CLINICAL SIGNIFICANCE

Clinically, right atrial abnormality is seen in any condition that creates a backup of volume or pressure. Conditions resulting from volume overload would be right-sided heart failure secondary to a right ventricular infarction or tricuspid regurgitation. A condition resulting from a backup of higher than normal pressures is pulmonary hypertension secondary to chronic obstructive pulmonary disease or pulmonary stenosis.

It is important to note that tall peaked P waves are not always indicative of right atrial chamber abnormality. They may also be seen whenever there is increased sympathetic nervous system activity and a resulting tachycardia.

Conditions causing a backup of volume or pressure on the left side of the heart will result in left atrial abnormality. Examples of those caused by volume overload are mitral regurgitation and left ventricular failure. Those caused by a backup of pressure are aortic stenosis and systemic hypertension.

Patients with an enlarged left atrium are more likely to develop atrial dysrhythmias, especially atrial fibrillation. Not only are atrial dysrhythmias more likely to occur, but they are also much more difficult to control in these individuals. If the atrial dysrhythmia is converted to a sinus rhythm, usually it will remain so only temporarily. Because it is so difficult to convert atrial fibrillation in these patients, often no attempt is made to do so. Instead emphasis is placed on keeping the ventricular response to this dysrhythmia controlled.

Right ventricular hypertrophy will accompany chronic obstructive pulmonary disease, pulmonary stenosis, and systemic hypertension. Left ventricular hypertrophy results from chronic systemic hypertension

and aortic stenosis. Individuals with LVH may be at increased risk for a myocardial infarction and/or sudden death. They are more apt to have ventricular ectopy, which is either difficult or impossible to suppress with medication.

Key questions to ask yourself when performing this step of the systematic process are:

Are the P waves in leads II and V1 normal, tall and peaked, notched, or widened?
- Assess for right, left, or bilateral atrial abnormalities.
- Assess for presence of atrial dysrhythmias.
- Assess for possibility of pulmonary embolism if changes are acute.
- Assess for signs and symptoms of acute volume overload.
- Prepare for treatment of acute volume overload, if present.

Are the QRS complexes in the V leads increased in amplitude?
- Assess for right, left, or bilateral ventricular hypertrophy.
- Assess for ventricular dysrhythmias.
- Prepare for treatment of ventricular dysrhythmias.

What is the significance of these P and QRS changes?
- Assess for history of chronic hypertension, chronic obstructive pulmonary disease (COPD), aortic stenosis, tricuspid regurgitation or stenosis.

SELF-ASSESSMENT EXERCISES 19–24

In the following six ECG examples complete the following steps:

Step One: Determination of Rhythm
Step Two: Determination of Axis
Step Three: Determination of Chamber Enlargement
         Atrial abnormality: Right___ Left___
         Ventricular hypertrophy: Right___ Left___

You must be able to perform these steps successfully before proceeding. When you have completed all of the exercises in this book, come back to this exercise and complete the remaining steps of the *systematic approach.*

Check your answers with the suggested interpretations found at the end of this chapter. Answers for remaining steps will be found in Appendix A.

3

Exercise 19. An 85-year-old man admitted after a cardiac arrest in the emergency department.

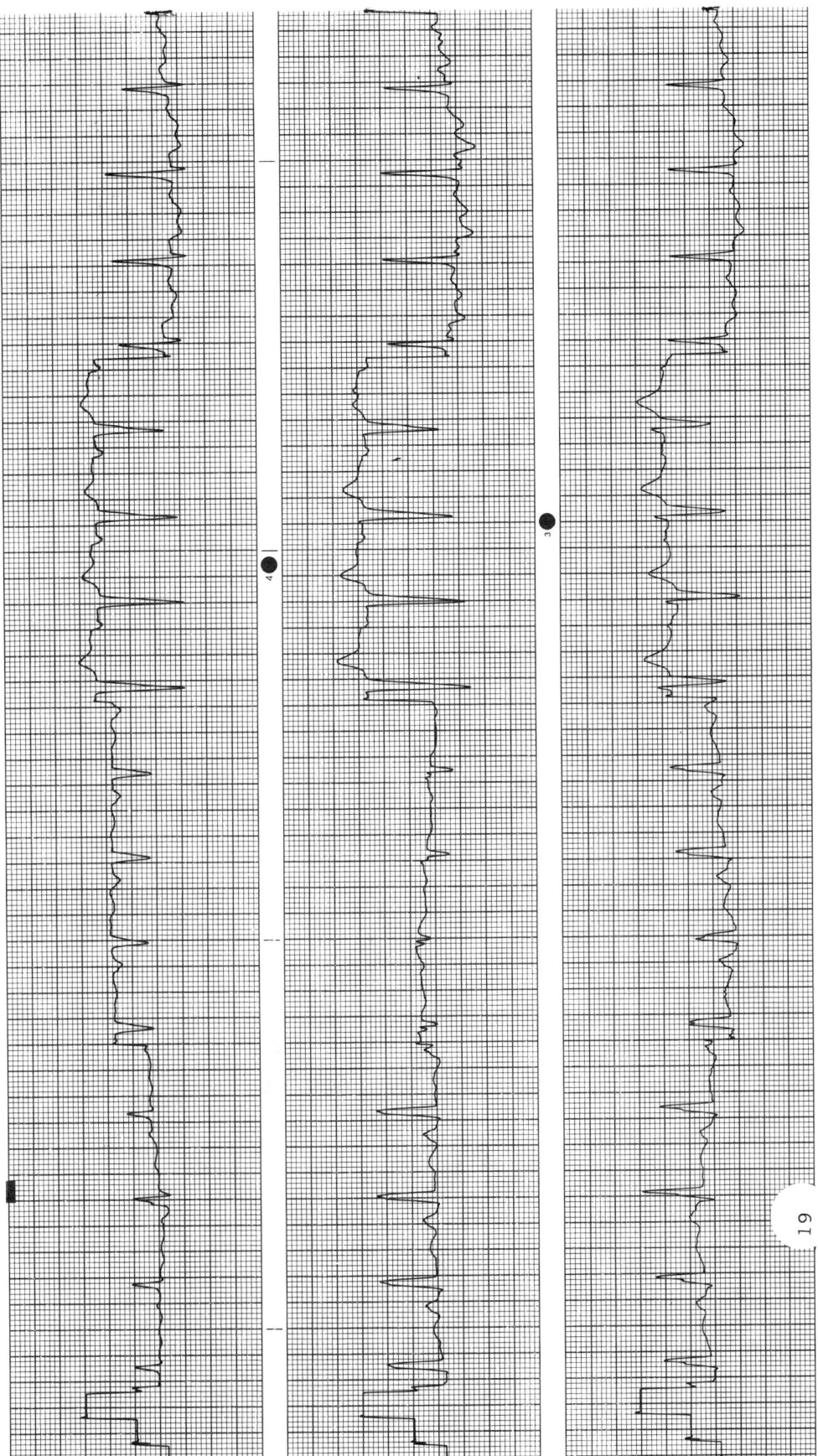

19

3

Exercise 20. An 83-year-old woman admitted from a nursing home complaining of weakness and a cough. History of congestive heart failure, aortic stenosis, and atrial tachycardia.

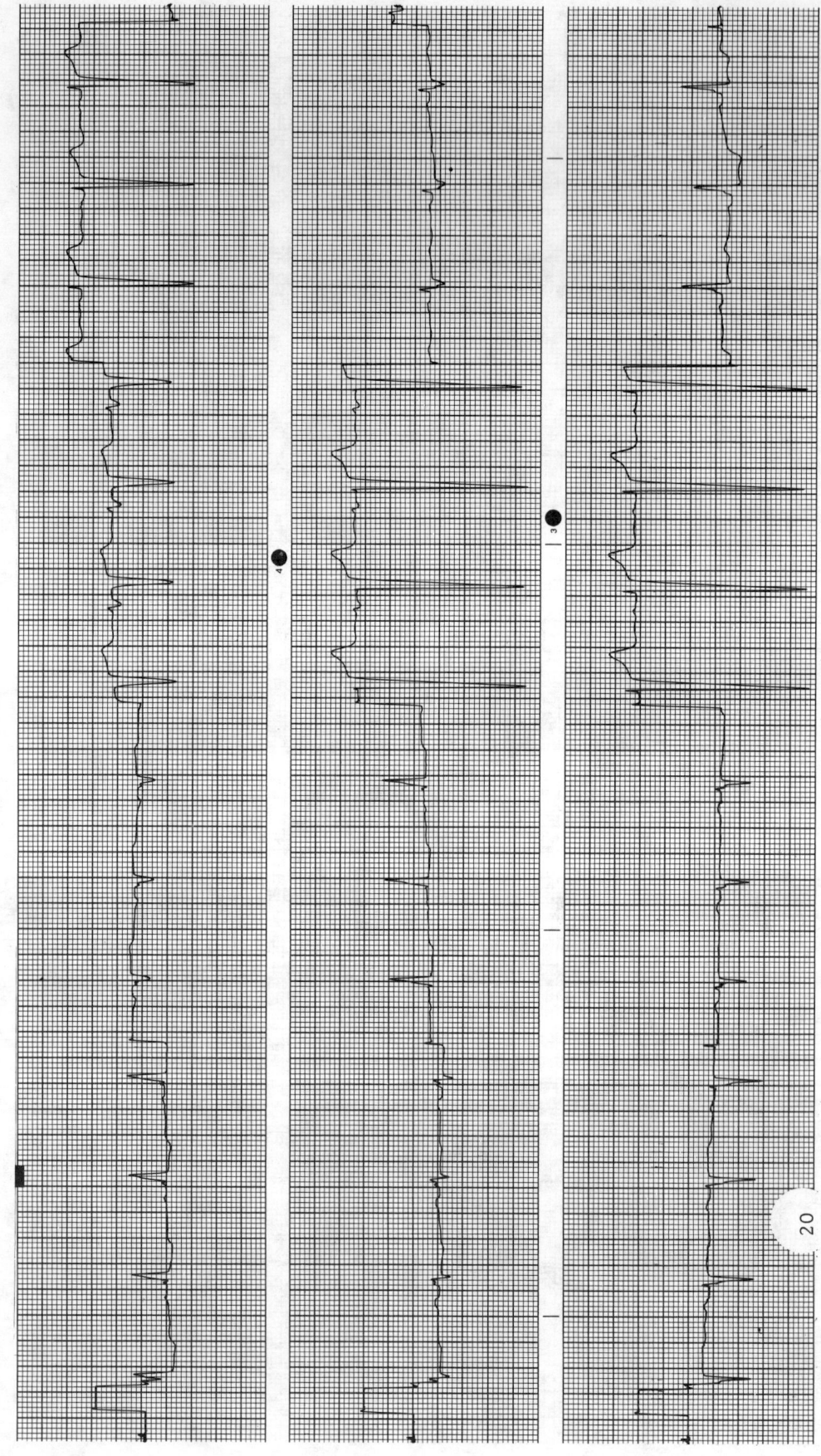

20

Exercise 21.   An 80-year-old man admitted with shortness of breath and chest pain.

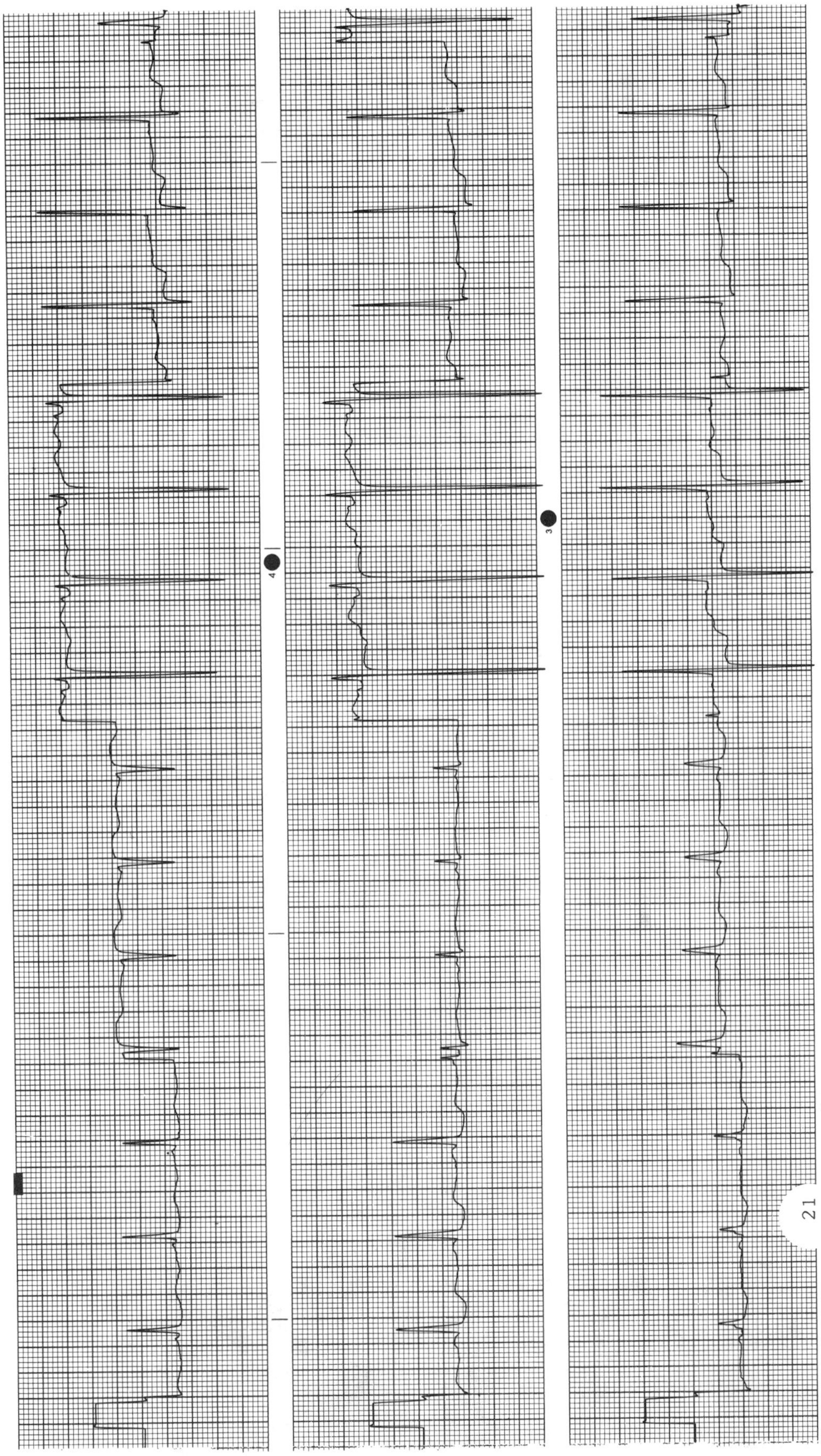

3

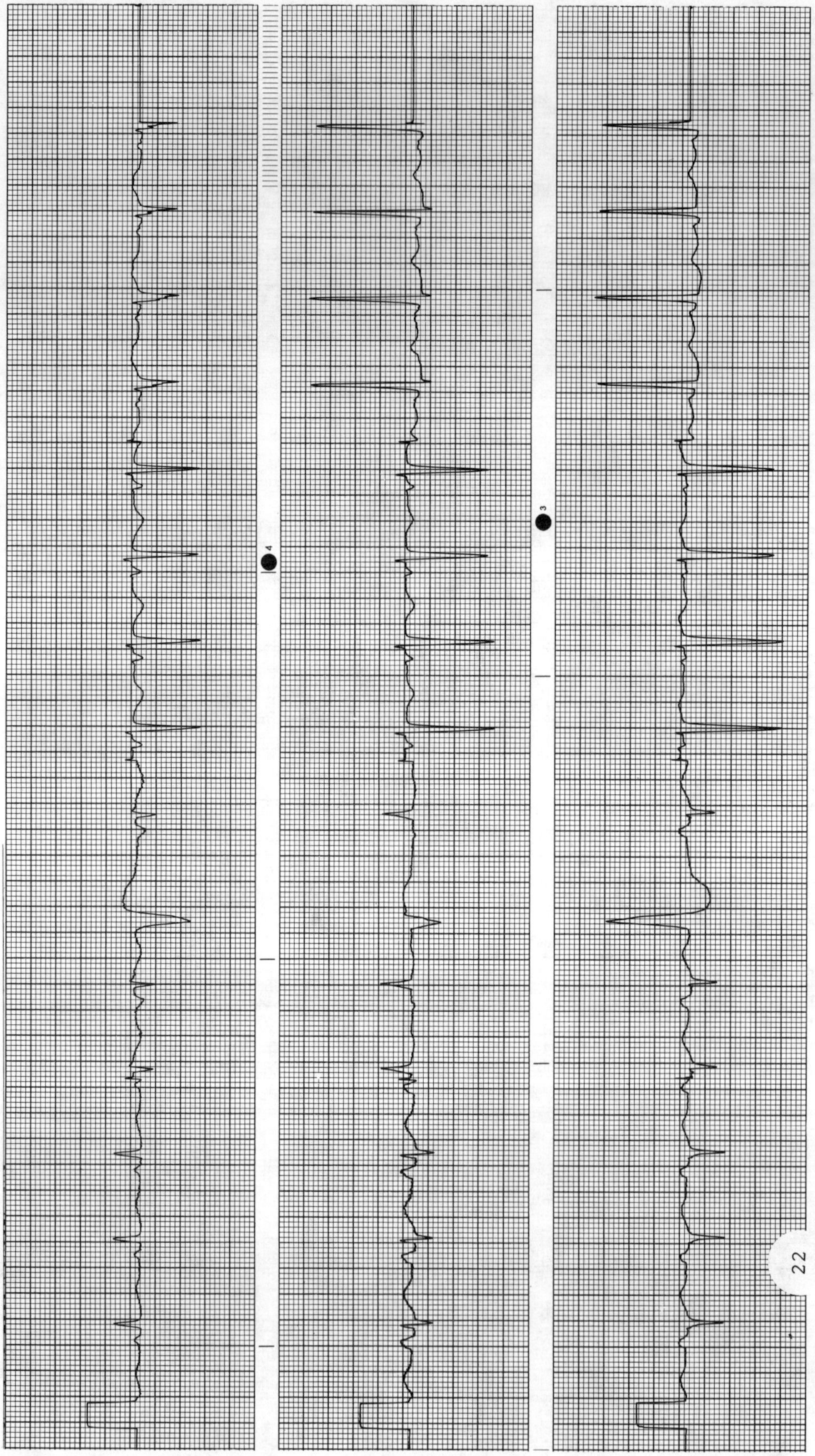

Exercise 22. A 61-year-old woman admitted with congestive heart failure.

22

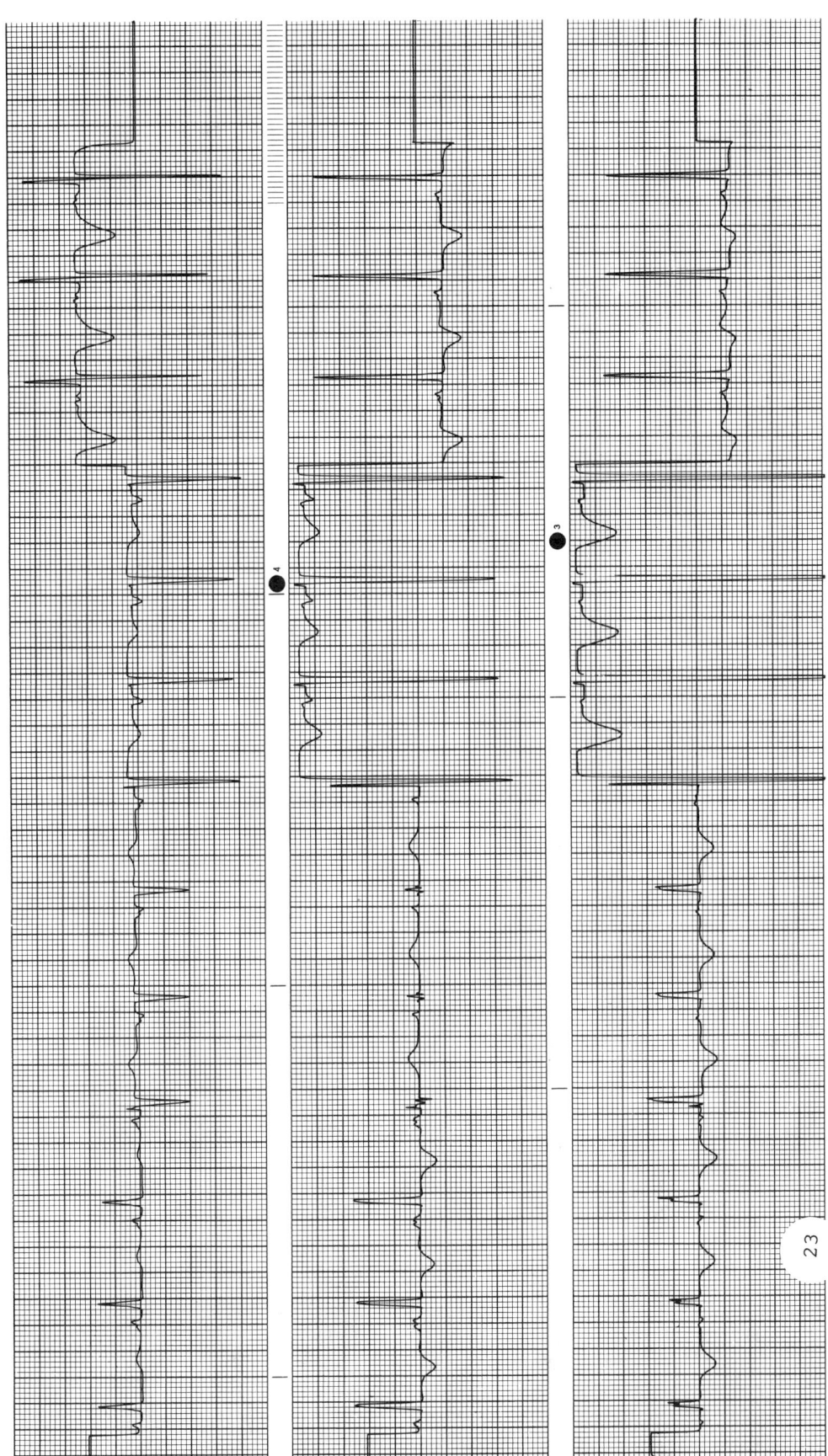

Exercise 23. A 25-year-old woman admitted with shortness of breath and chest pain. History of hypertension, cocaine abuse, and seizures.

3

23

3

Exercise 24. A 59-year-old man admitted to the hospital from the recovery room after having chest pain following ambulatory surgery. History of chronic obstructive pulmonary disease, congestive heart failure, and an old myocardial infarction.

24

SELF-ASSESSMENT ANSWERS TO EXERCISES 19–24

EXERCISE 19

STEP 1. Rhythm Determination

- Ventricular rate *90*
- QRS shape *Slightly widened*

- R-R rhythm *Regular*
- QRS interval *0.10*
- QT interval *0.36*

- Atrial rate *90*
- P wave shape *Positive except negative aVR, aVL, V1, and V2*
- P-P rhythm *Regular*
- P-R interval *0.18*
- P:R conduction ratio *1:1*

- Dominant pacemaker site *Sinus*
- Interpretation *NSR*

STEP 2. Axis Determination

Normal

STEP 3. Chamber Enlargement Determination

Right atrial abnormality. Borderline LVH.

EXERCISE 20

STEP 1. Rhythm Determination

- Ventricular rate *78*
- QRS shape *Normal*

- R-R rhythm *Regular*
- QRS interval *0.09*
- QT interval *0.36*

- Atrial rate *78*
- P wave shape *Positive except negative aVR, aVL, diphasic V1, and V2*
- P-P rhythm *Regular*
- P-R interval *0.18*
- P:R conduction ratio *1:1*

- Dominant pacemaker site *Sinus*
- Interpretation *NSR*

STEP 2. Axis Determination

Left axis

STEP 3. Chamber Enlargement Determination

Left atrial abnormality with LVH

EXERCISE 21

STEP 1. Rhythm Determination

- Ventricular rate *82*
- QRS shape *Normal*

- R-R rhythm *Regular*
- QRS interval *0.08*
- QT interval *0.36*

- Atrial rate *82*
- P wave shape *Positive except negative aVR, flat in V4–V6*
- P-P rhythm *Regular*
- P-R interval *0.12*
- P:R conduction ratio *1:1*

- Dominant pacemaker site *Sinus*
- Interpretation *NSR*

STEP 2. Axis Determination

Normal axis

STEP 3. Chamber Enlargement Determination

LVH

EXERCISE 22

STEP 1. Rhythm Determination

- Ventricular rate *90*
- QRS shape *Normal*

- R-R rhythm *Regular, occasional irregular beat*
- QRS interval *0.09*
- QT interval *0.36*

- Atrial rate *90*
- P wave shape *Tall and pointed II, diphasic V1–V2, negative in aVR and aVL*
- P-P rhythm *Regular*

- P-R interval *0.14*
- P:R conduction ratio *1:1*

- Dominant pacemaker site *Sinus*
- Interpretation *NSR with occasional PVC*

STEP 2. Axis Determination

Left axis

STEP 3. Chamber Enlargement Determination

Biatrial abnormality with LVH

3

EXERCISE 23

STEP 1. Rhythm Determination

- Ventricular rate *77*
- QRS shape *Normal, tall*

- Atrial rate *77*
- P wave shape *Notched I, II, aVF, V4–V5, diphasic III, V1 and V2, positive aVL and V3*

- R-R rhythm *Regular*
- QRS interval *0.08*
- QT interval *0.44*

- P-P rhythm *Regular*
- P-R interval *0.18*
- P:R conduction ratio *1:1*

- Dominant pacemaker site *Sinus*
- Interpretation *NSR*

STEP 2. Axis Determination

Normal axis

STEP 3. Chamber Enlargment Determination

Left atrial abnormality and LVH

EXERCISE 24

STEP 1. Rhythm Determination

- Ventricular rate *96*
- QRS shape *Small*

- Atrial rate *96*
- P wave shape *Positive and flat except negative in aVR and aVF*

- R-R rhythm *Regular*
- QRS interval *0.09*
- QT interval *0.32*

- P-P rhythm *Regular*
- P-R interval *0.18*
- P:R conduction ratio *1:1*

- Dominant pacemaker site *Sinus*
- Interpretation *NSR*

STEP 2. Axis Determination

Indeterminate axis

STEP 3. Chamber Enlargement Determination

None

5
Intraventricular Conduction Blocks Determination

STEP 4

Now that we have determined the rate, rhythm, axis, and presence or absence of a chamber enlargement, we should examine the electrocardiogram (ECG) for any intraventricular conduction blocks, the *fourth step* in the systematic process. In this step we are going to determine the presence of right and left bundle branch blocks, incomplete bundle branch blocks, intraventricular conduction delays (IVCD), and left anterior and posterior hemiblocks.

Before describing the ECG changes found with intraventricular conduction blocks, normal ventricular conduction in leads V1 and V6 will be reviewed (Figure 5.1). Remember that a positive deflection results when the impulse travels toward the positive electrode. In V1 the positive electrode is at the fourth intercostal space along the right sternal border over the area of the right ventricle. The left side of the septum will depolarize a split second before the right. Therefore, the impulse travels from left to right toward the V1 electrode producing a small r wave.

From the bundle of His the impulse travels down the left and right bundle branches. Because the left ventricle has greater muscle mass than the right, it exerts greater electrical force and causes a larger deflection. Right-sided electrical activity becomes buried in the deflection caused by the left. The wave that results on the ECG is a deep S wave.

Just the opposite will occur in lead V6. In this lead the positive electrode is at the fifth intercostal space midaxillary line. The area of the heart that lies under this electrode is the left ventricle.

The intraventricular septum depolarizes from left to right, or away from the positive electrode in V6. This results in a small q wave. Next, a large R wave occurs as the ventricles depolarize and the impulse travels toward the left.

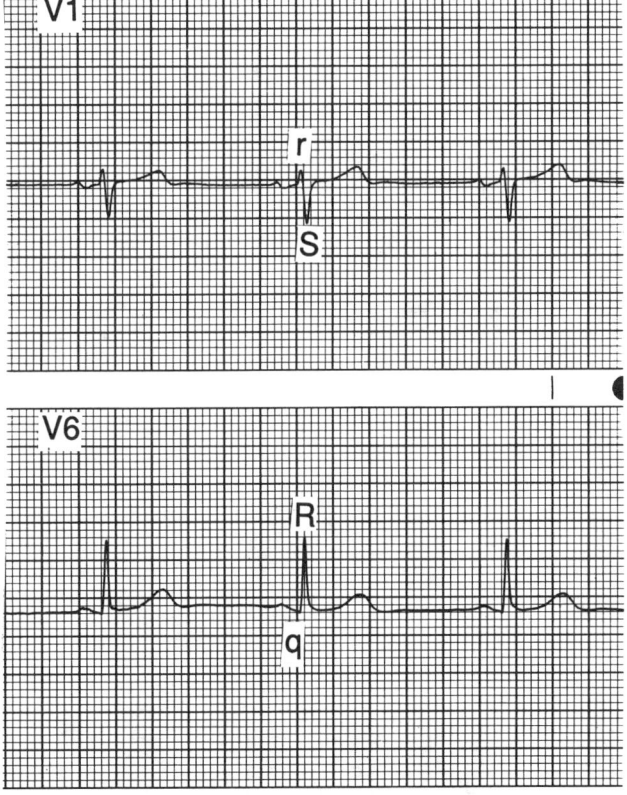

Figure 5.1. Normal ventricular depolarization. Note the small r wave and deep S wave in V1 and the small q wave and tall R wave in V6.

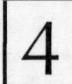

The first thing to look for when determining the presence of a bundle branch block is the *width of the QRS*. The QRS widens when conduction is delayed after the AV node. The normal width of the QRS complex is 0.06–0.09 seconds. A QRS with a width of 0.10–0.11 seconds represents an intraventricular conduction delay or an incomplete bundle branch block. If the width becomes ≥0.12 seconds, a bundle branch block is present. Once a bundle branch block is identified, *examine leads V1 and V6* to determine whether the blockage occurred in the right or the left bundle.

In addition to depolarization changes, repolarization changes occur with bundle branch blocks. Repolarization is represented by the ST segment and T wave. Whenever the QRS is widened, the T wave deflection will be opposite the terminal portion of the QRS.

RIGHT BUNDLE BRANCH BLOCK

A right bundle branch block (RBBB) causes the QRS to widen to ≥0.12 seconds and to change its configuration (Figure 5.2). In lead *V1* the configuration will change in the following manner. Septal depolarization is not affected so the initial small r wave remains. It is followed

by a deep S wave representing left ventricular depolarization and a tall R wave (R prime) representing late right ventricular depolarization.

In lead *V6*, just the opposite will occur. As stated above the initial portion of depolarization is not affected and is represented by a small q wave in this lead. Depolarization of the left bundle and ventricle produces a tall R wave. As the impulse spreads toward the right ventricle it depolarizes and a large S wave occurs.

Therefore, in RBBB the terminal portion of the QRS in lead V1 is positive so the T wave will be negative in this lead. In lead V6, the terminal portion of the QRS is negative, so the T wave should be positive. These changes are called secondary T wave changes and are of no clinical concern.

LEFT BUNDLE BRANCH BLOCK

When examining an ECG for left bundle branch block (LBBB), we examine the same two leads as for RBBB. The first sign is the same for both, a QRS that is 0.12 seconds or wider in width.

Once we have determined that a block exists, we should again examine the configuration of the QRS in lead V1 (Figure 5.3). In LBBB the initial portion of ven-

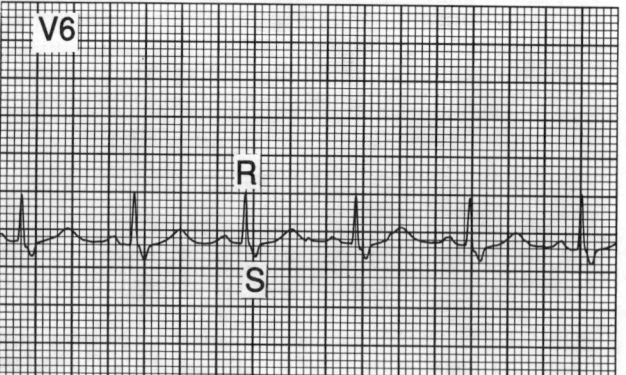

Figure 5.2.   Right bundle branch block. Note the width of the QRS complex and the rSR pattern in V1 and the broad S wave in V6.

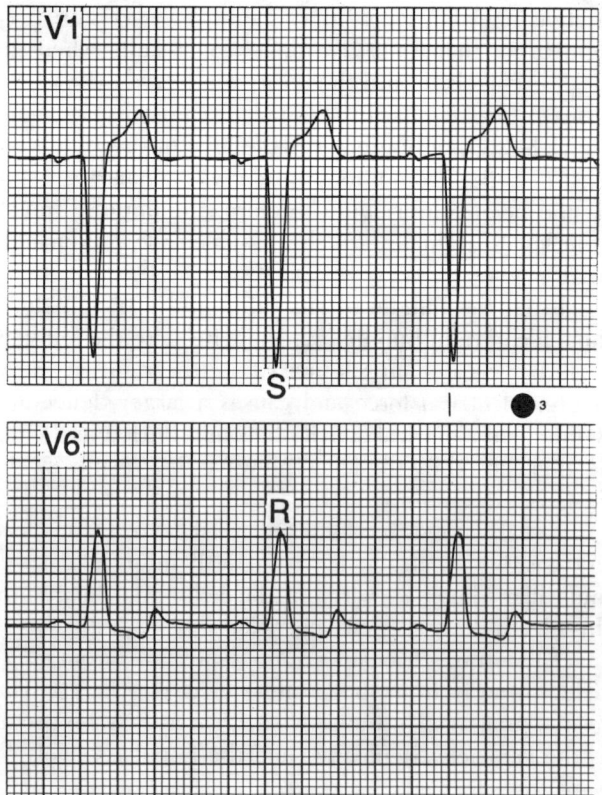

Figure 5.3.   Left bundle branch block. Note the width of the QRS complex and the broad S waves in V1 and broad R waves in V6.

Table 5.1.
Features of QRS Complex in Leads V1 and V6 in Normal Conduction and Bundle Branch Blocks

	Lead V1	Lead V6
Normal	Width 0.06–0.09 seconds rs	Width 0.06–0.09 seconds qRs
RBBB	Width ≥0.12 seconds rsR′ or rR′ Depressed ST seg with negative T wave	Width ≥0.12 seconds Broad S wave Slightly elevated ST with positive T wave
LBBB	Width ≥0.12 seconds Broad S wave May have rS Slightly elevated ST with positive T wave	Width ≥0.12 seconds Broad R wave Depressed ST segment with negative T wave

tricular depolarization remains undisturbed. From the right septum, depolarization continues down the right bundle and ventricle producing an R wave. As the wave of depolarization spreads from the right ventricle to the left, a deep S wave is produced.

In lead V6 we should expect to find just the opposite changes (Figure 5.3). Initially, we should see a Q wave as the right septum, bundle, and ventricle depolarize. Then a tall R wave will be produced as the impulse spreads to the left ventricle.

As in RBBB, secondary T wave changes also occur. In lead V1, the terminal portion of the QRS will be negative, so the T wave should be positive. In lead V6, the terminal portion of the QRS should be positive, so the T wave in that lead will be negative.

Table 5.1 summarizes the features of normal conduction and right and left bundle branch block in leads V1 and V6.

INCOMPLETE BUNDLE BRANCH BLOCKS

Bundle branch blocks can be either complete or incomplete. An incomplete bundle branch block has a QRS complex between 0.10 and 0.11 seconds. The configuration of the QRS must resemble that of either a RBBB or a LBBB. If the configuration resembles that of a RBBB, then it is called an incomplete RBBB. If it resembles that of a LBBB, it is called an incomplete LBBB. If the QRS is wide (0.10–0.11 seconds) but resembles neither a RBBB or a LBBB, then it is called an intraventricular conduction delay (IVCD).

HEMIBLOCKS

The right bundle consists of a single branch. A block that occurs along this branch affects the entire bundle.

The left bundle consists of two branches or fascicles, the left anterior fascicle and the left posterior fascicle. A block along the left bundle can affect one or both of its fascicles. If it affects both, then it is simply a LBBB. If it affects the left anterior fascicle alone, then it is a left anterior hemiblock (LAH). If it affects the left posterior fascicle alone, then it is a left posterior hemiblock (LPH).

Although a block affecting the entire bundle will widen the QRS, a hemiblock will not. In order to determine whether a hemiblock exists, we must examine the limb leads. The primary change that occurs is an *axis shift*. A left anterior hemiblock will cause a left axis deviation (Figure 5.4). A left posterior hemiblock will cause a right axis deviation (Figure 5.5).

In addition to a hemiblock, an axis shift can be caused by a myocardial infarction (MI). Therefore, before a hemiblock can be diagnosed, an MI must be ruled out as the cause of the axis shift. An inferior MI can cause a left axis deviation, and a lateral infarct can cause a right axis deviation. A simple method for determining the cause of the axis shift is to examine *leads I and III*. When a left axis deviation is caused by a left anterior hemiblock and not an inferior MI, there will be a Q wave in lead I and an S wave in lead III (Dubin, 1989). When a right axis deviation is caused by a left posterior hemiblock and not a lateral MI, there will be an S wave in lead I and a Q wave in lead III (Dubin, 1989). Table 5.2 summarizes the features of hemiblocks.

BIFASCICULAR BLOCKS

A bifascicular block is one which affects any two fascicles. Examples of bifascicular blocks would be a RBBB with a left anterior hemiblock (Figure 5.6), or a RBBB with a left posterior hemiblock, or a LBBB alone because the left bundle contains two fascicles.

CLINICAL SIGNIFICANCE

Whenever considering the clinical significance of a bundle branch block or hemiblock, it is important to know whether it has occurred acutely. All of these changes may occur as a result of the aging process and, if so, have no clinical significance. If they occur acutely, they may be a sign of an acute myocardial infarction.

Right bundle branch block can occur as a result of any number of conditions that affect the right side of the heart. It may be a result of chronic pulmonary disease, an atrial septal defect, or a pulmonary embolus. Right bundle branch block when it occurs alone requires no treatment and is often present in healthy individuals with no cardiac disease.

Left bundle branch block usually does not occur normally. It may be caused by conditions that affect the left side of the heart such as hypertensive heart disease,

4

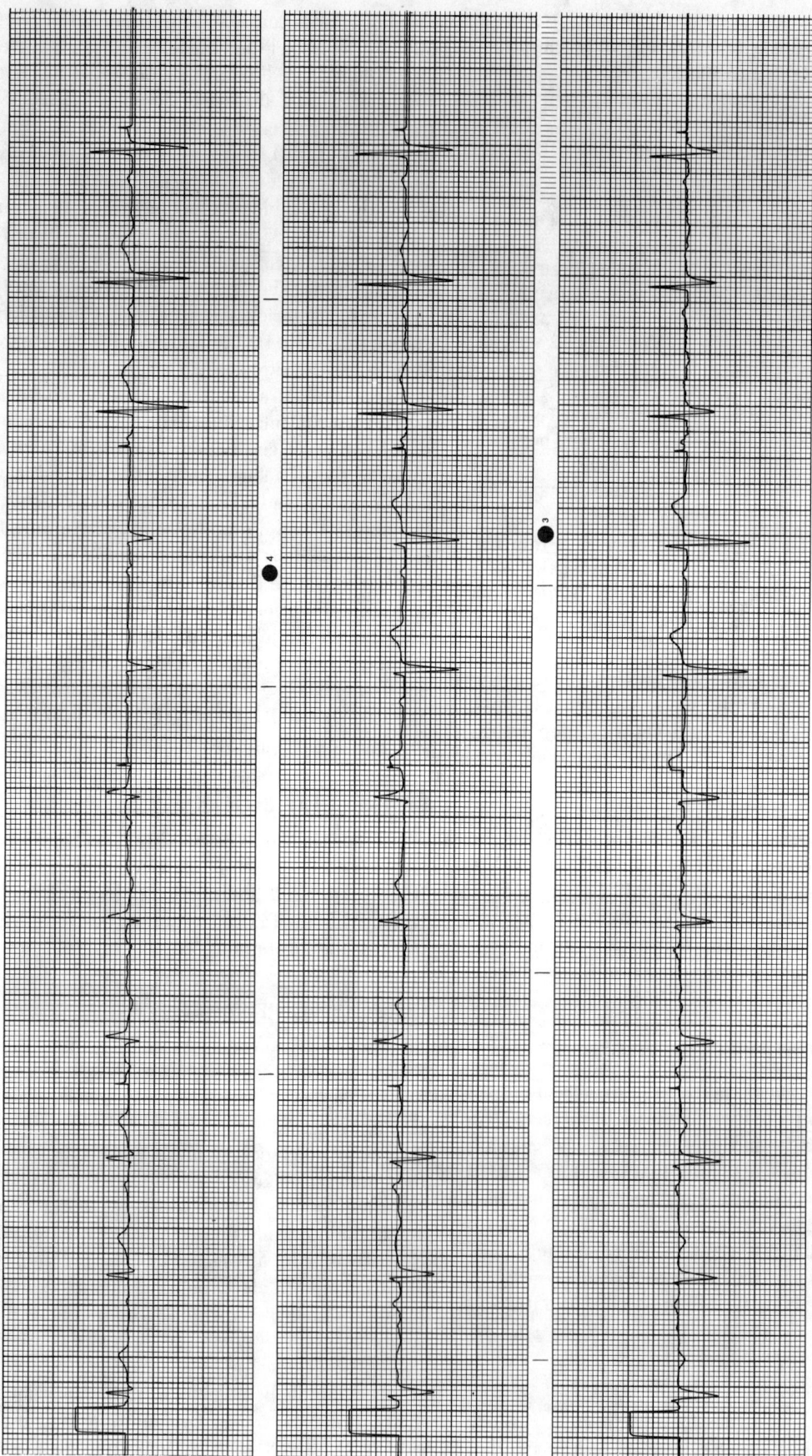

Figure 5.4. Left anterior hemiblock. Note the left axis shift with q in lead I and an S wave in lead III.

aortic stenosis, degenerative changes of the conduction system, or coronary artery disease. As with RBBB it does not require any treatment unless it is an acute change. When LBBB occurs in conjunction with an anterior myocardial infarction, it is serious and usually a forerunner of complete heart block. If an external pacemaker is available, it should be readied and applied until a transvenous pacemaker can be inserted.

Sometimes patients with chronic LBBB will have temporary pacemakers placed if they require a pulmonary artery catheter. If so, the physician may choose a paceport pulmonary artery catheter. The reason is that when the catheter is passed through the right ventricle, the right bundle branch can be traumatized. This may result in a temporary RBBB. If the patient already has a LBBB, complete heart block will result with the potential of a cardiac arrest. Once the catheter has been placed, there is little danger of its affecting the right bundle.

Both right and left bundle branch blocks may occur as a result of a rapid heart rate. In some individuals the bundles are unable to repolarize quickly enough to be prepared to depolarize when the heart rate is rapid. When the heart rate slows, normal conduction will resume and the bundle branch block will disappear. The bundle itself generally does not compromise the patient,

Table 5.2.
ECG Features of Hemiblocks

Left Anterior Hemiblock	Left Posterior Hemiblock
Left axis deviation	Right axis deviation
Q wave lead I	S wave lead I
S wave lead III	Q wave lead III

but the rapid heart rate may. Treatment is directed at slowing the heart rate.

A left anterior hemiblock occurs more commonly than a left posterior hemiblock for two reasons. The first reason is that the posterior fascicle is shorter and wider and is located in a segment of the left ventricle that undergoes lower pressures. The anterior fascicle is long and thin and located near the aortic ring, an area of higher pressures and therefore greater chance of injury. The other reason is that the posterior fascicle has a double blood supply, the right posterior descending artery and the circumflex artery. The anterior fascicle is supplied only by the left anterior descending artery. When either of these conditions occurs alone, it is usually of no clinical significance.

Hemiblocks do gain important clinical significance when they occur with a RBBB in the setting of an acute

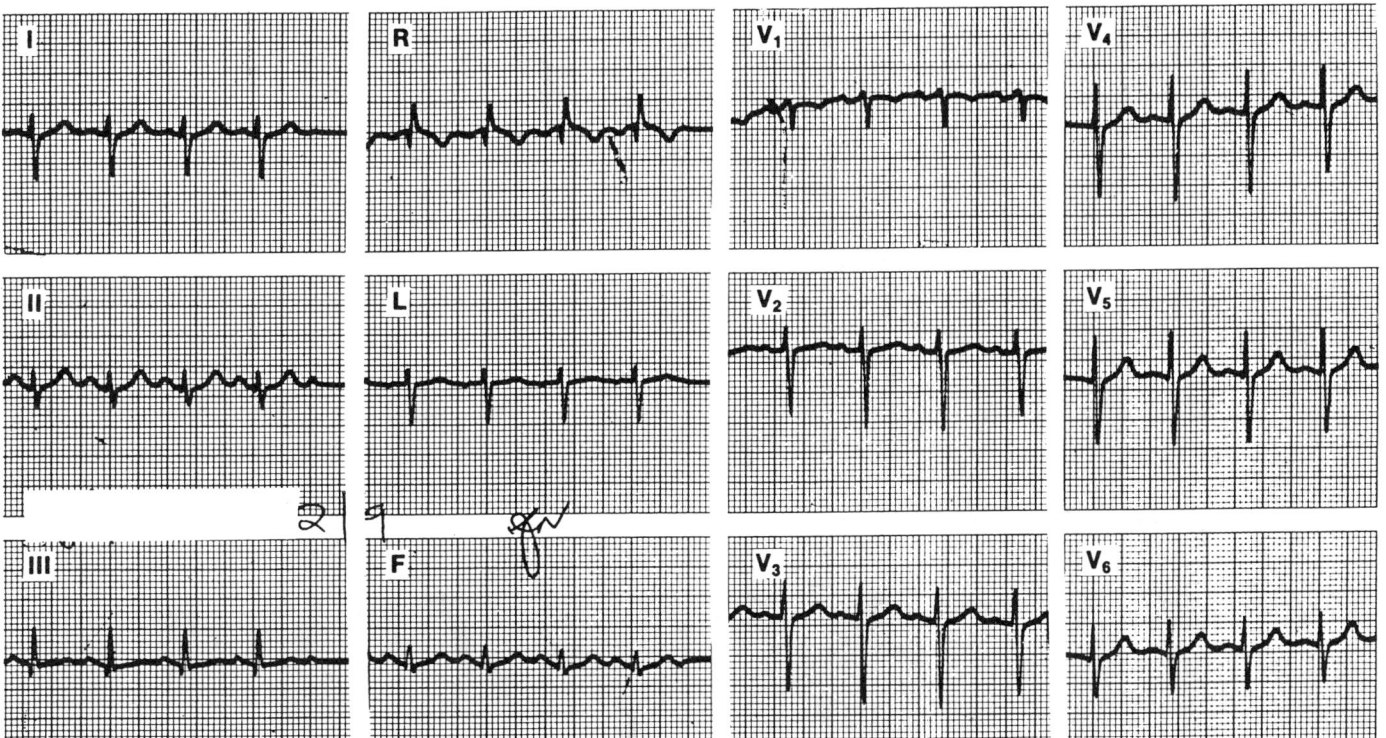

Figure 5.5. Left posterior hemiblock. Note the right axis shift with S wave in lead I and a Q in lead III. Used with permission frm N Laiken et al. *Interpretation of electrocardiograms.* New York: Raven Press, 1988, p. 106.

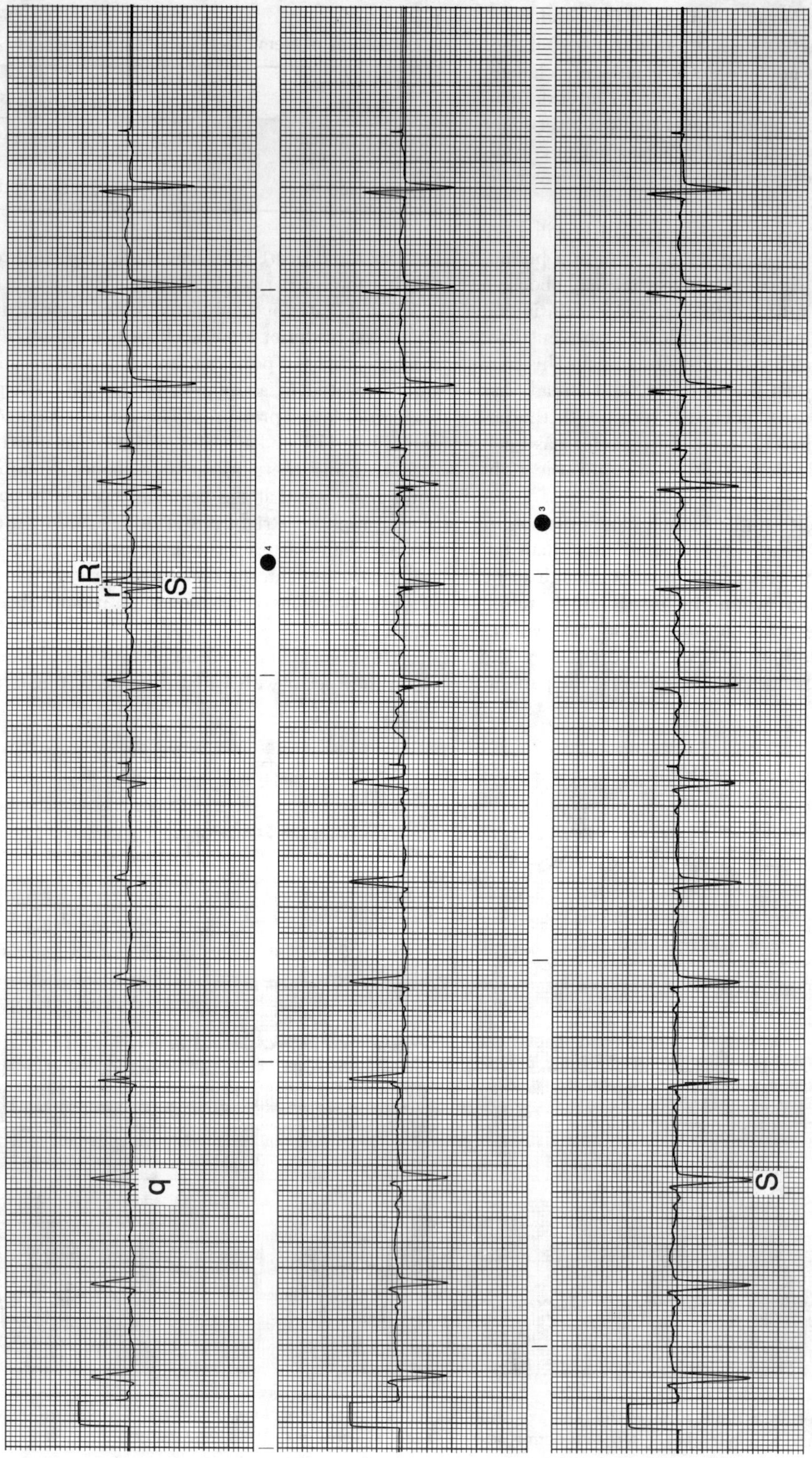

Figure 5.6. Left anterior hemiblock with right bundle branch block (bifascicular block). Note left axis shift with q wave in lead I and an S wave in lead III. Note rSR configuration and width of QRS complex in V1.

anterior myocardial infarction. Patients who have either a hemiblock or a RBBB must be monitored vigilantly for the development of the other. The development of a RBBB with a LAH may progress to complete heart block and cardiac arrest.

Key questions to ask yourself when performing this step of the systematic process are:

What monitoring lead should be used to determine the presence of a bundle branch block?
- Monitor on lead V1 or MCL1.

What should be assessed when monitoring lead V1 or MCL1?
- Assess for QRS complex that is ≥0.12 seconds.
- Assess for rSR′ or rR′ = RBBB.
- Assess for broad S wave or rS = LBBB.

What monitoring lead should be used to determine the presence of a hemiblock?
- Monitor on limb leads; if QRS morphology changes, do 12-lead ECG and determine axis.
- If LAD, look for Q wave in lead I and S wave in lead III = LAH.
- If RAD, look for S wave in lead I and Q wave in lead III = LPH.

What is the clinical situation in which the bundle or hemiblock is occurring?
- Assess patient for signs and symptoms of myocardial ischemia or infarction.
- Assess for presence of rate-related bundle branch block.
- Assess for change in QRS width and morphology. Perform 12-lead ECG; if new bundle or hemiblock, report findings to physician.
  If chronic, assess for progression of block to bifascicular and/or complete heart block.

What treatment should you prepare for or initiate in the presence of an intraventricular conduction block?
- If LBBB present and Swan Ganz catheter required, prepare for a transvenous pacemaker.
- If bifascicular block with an anterior MI, apply external pacemaker pads and prepare for insertion of transvenous pacemaker. Initiate external pacemaker as established by treatment protocols.
- Provide O_2, establish an IV, and be prepared for drug treatment (atropine).

SELF-ASSESSMENT EXERCISES 25–30

In the following six ECG examples, complete steps one through four in the systematic process:

Step One: Determination of Rhythm
Step Two: Determination of Axis
Step Three: Determination of Chamber Enlargement
Step Four: Determination of Intraventricular Conduction Blocks
            RBBB___ LBBB___
            Incomplete RBBB___ Incomplete LBBB___
            IVCD___ LAH___ LPH___

You must be able to perform these steps successfully before proceeding. When you have completed all of the exercises in this book, come back to this exercise and complete the remaining steps of the *systematic approach*.

Check your answers with the suggested interpretations found at the end of this chapter. Answers for remaining steps will be found in Appendix A.

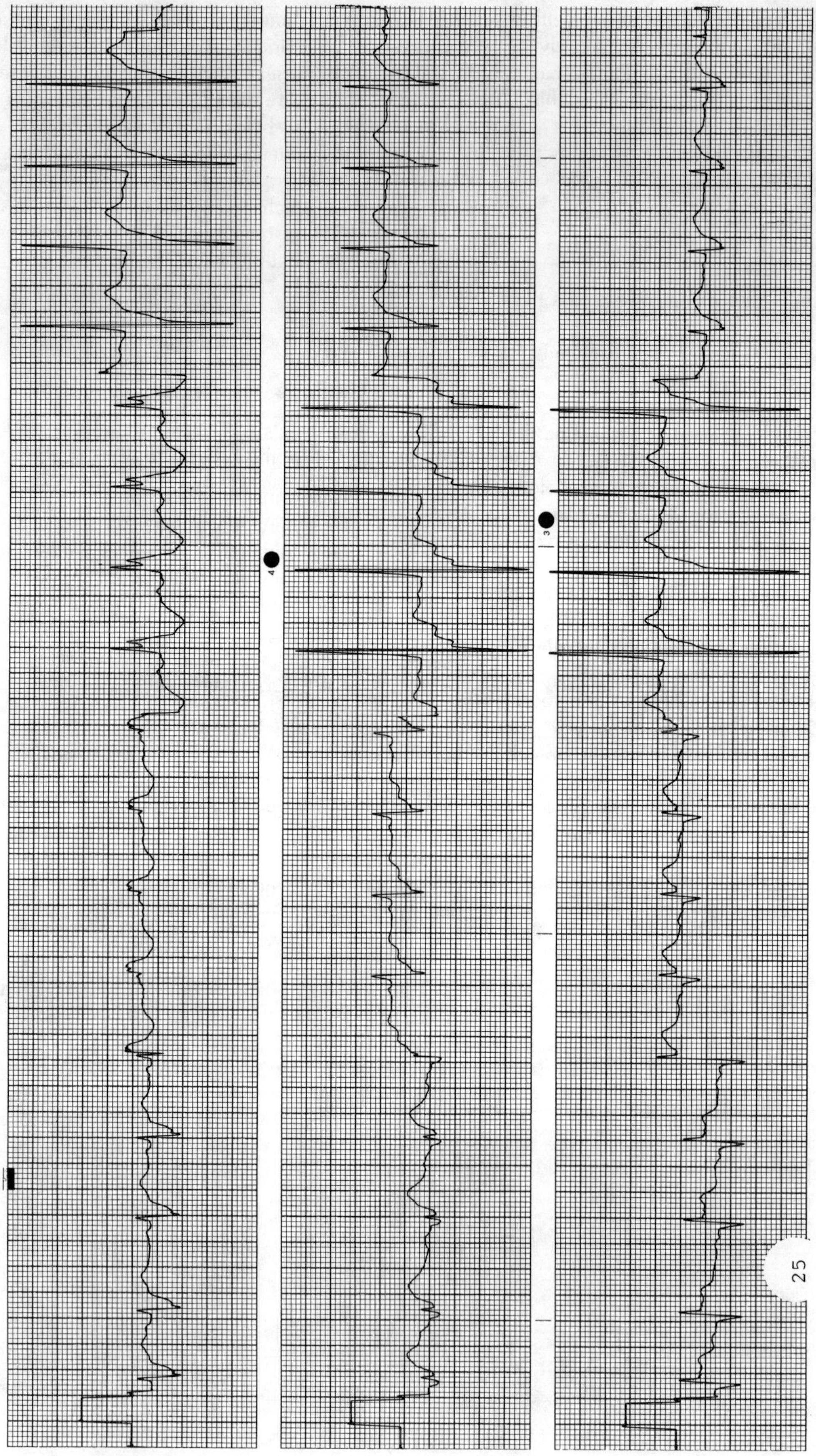

Exercise 25. A 55-year-old man complaining of midsternal chest pain.

4

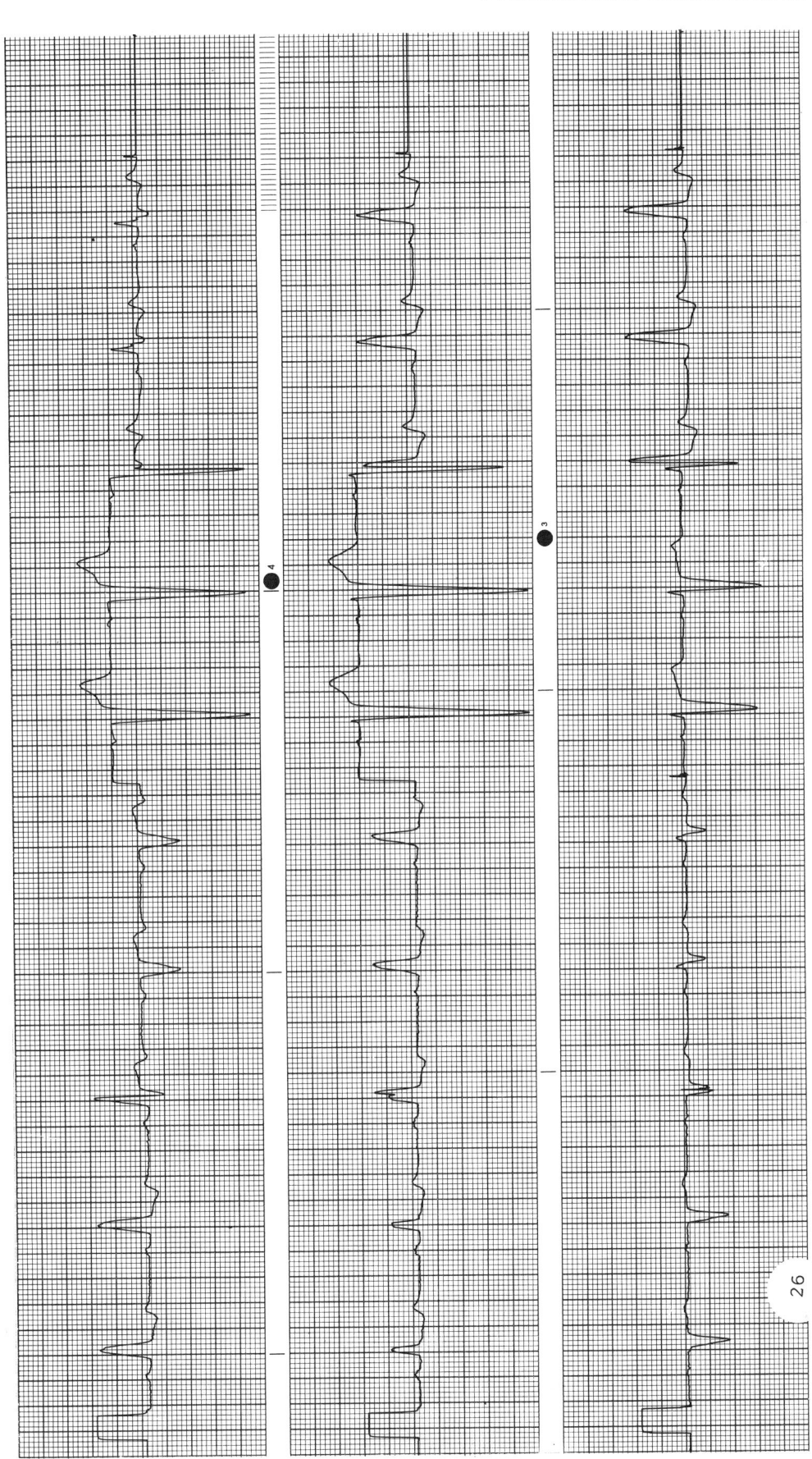

Exercise 26. An 87-year-old man admitted with chest pain.

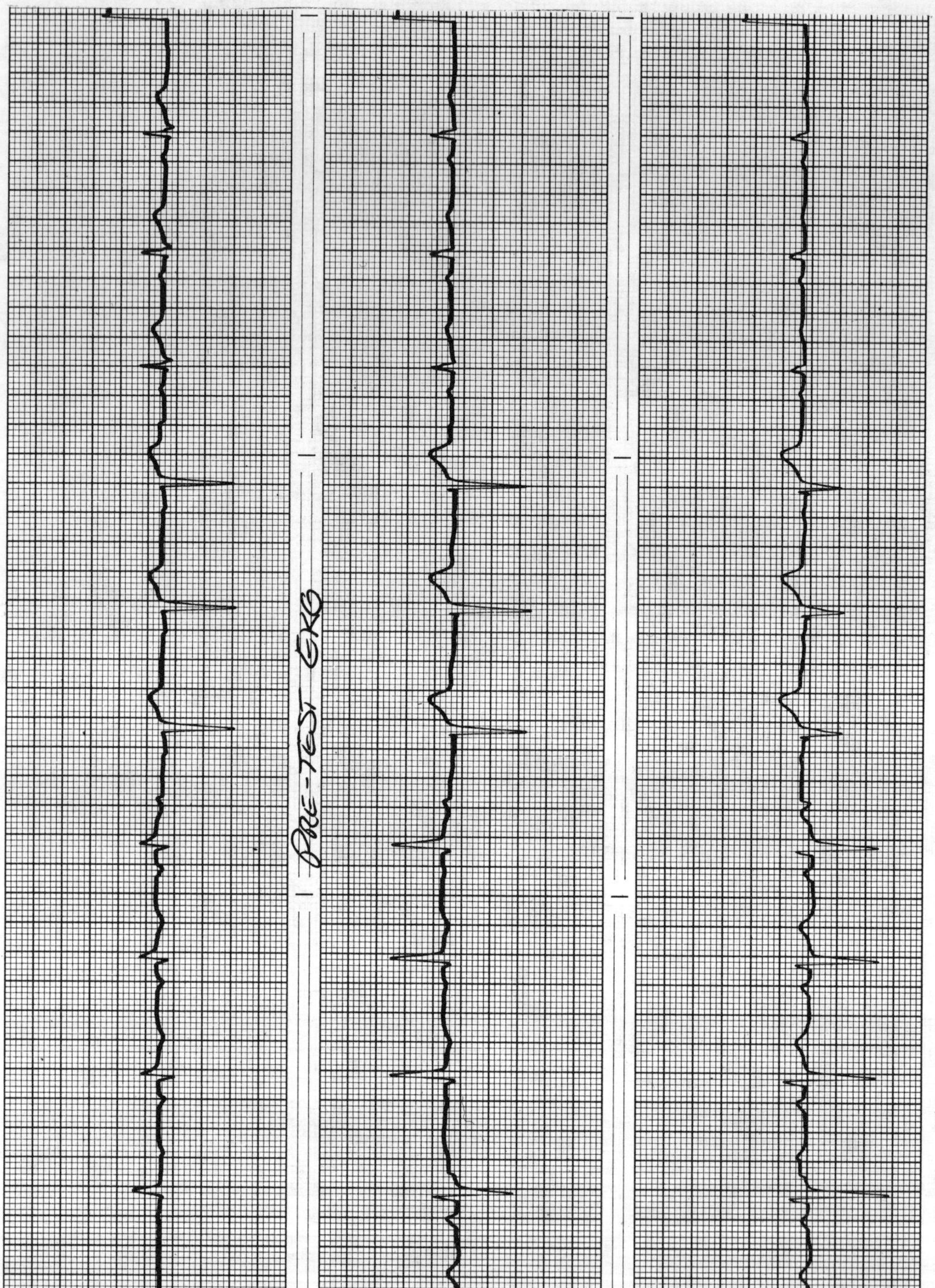

Exercise 27. A 58-year-old man experiencing substernal chest pain radiating to his left arm associated with diaphoresis.

PRE-TEST EKG

27

4

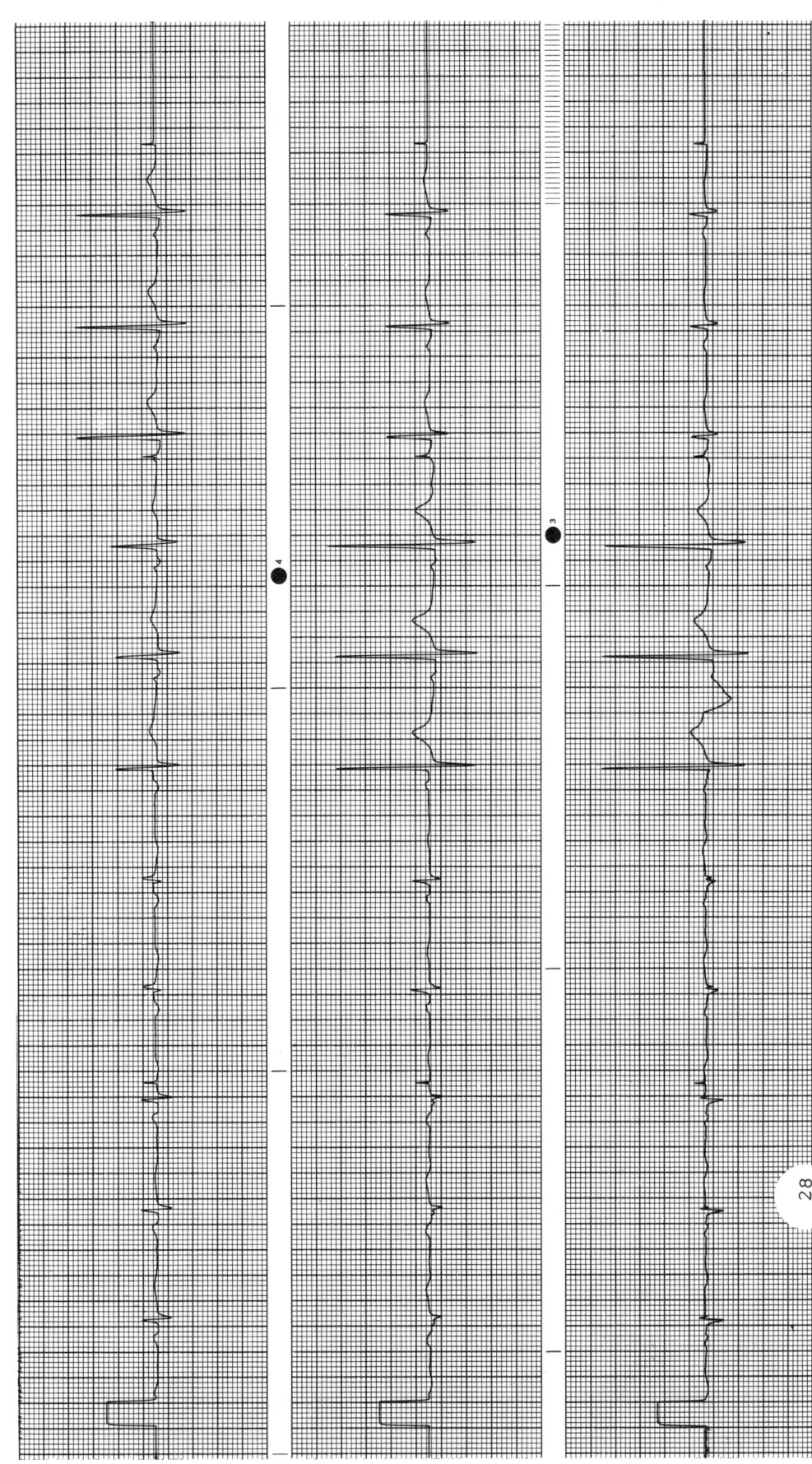

Exercise 28. A 59-year-old man with a history of myocardial infarction 2 years ago.

28

4

Exercise 29. A 66-year-old man admitted to the coronary care unit with recent onset angina. He awoke from sleep complaining of severe chest pain. ECG showed elevated ST segments and cardiac enzymes positive.

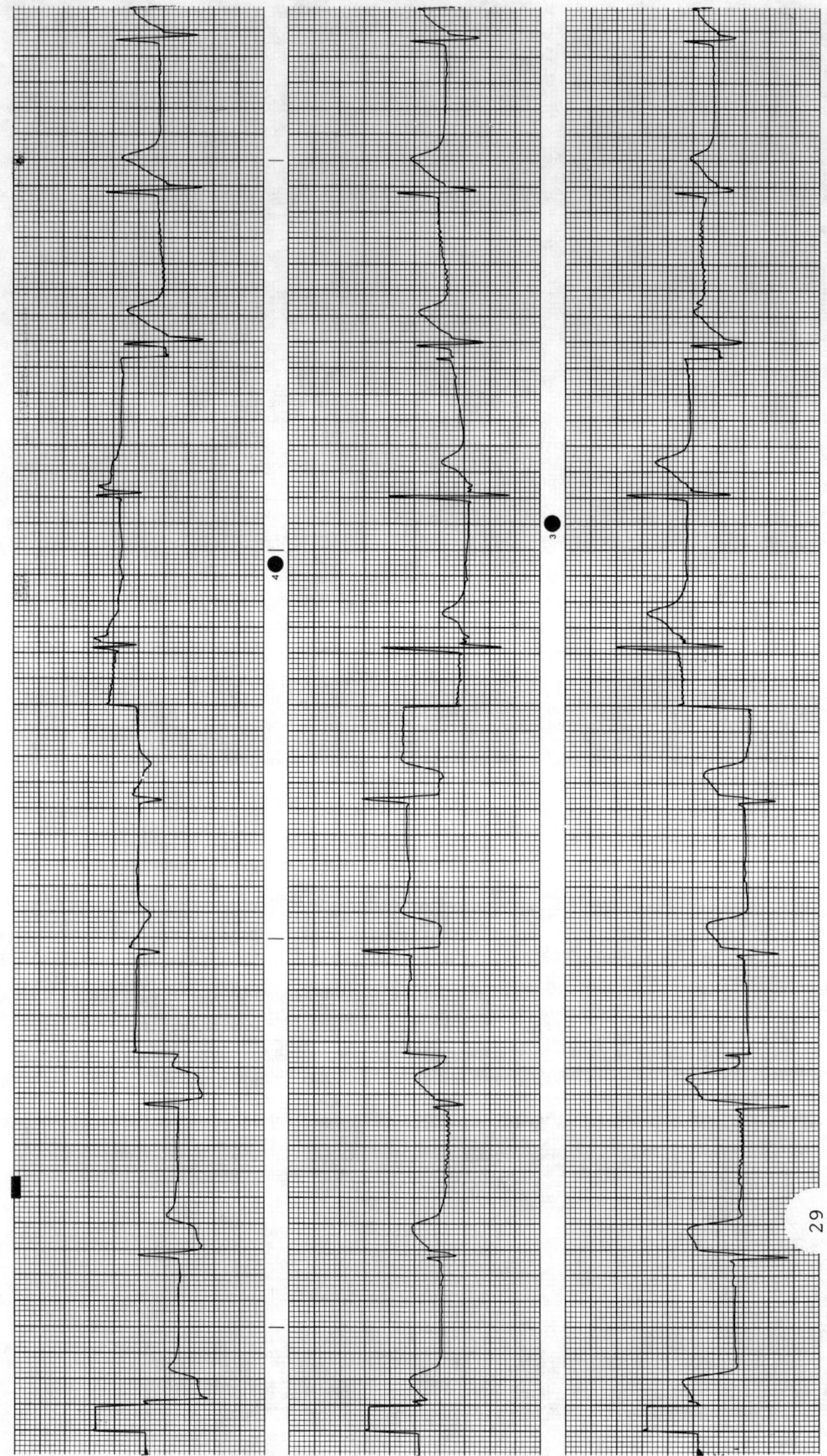

29

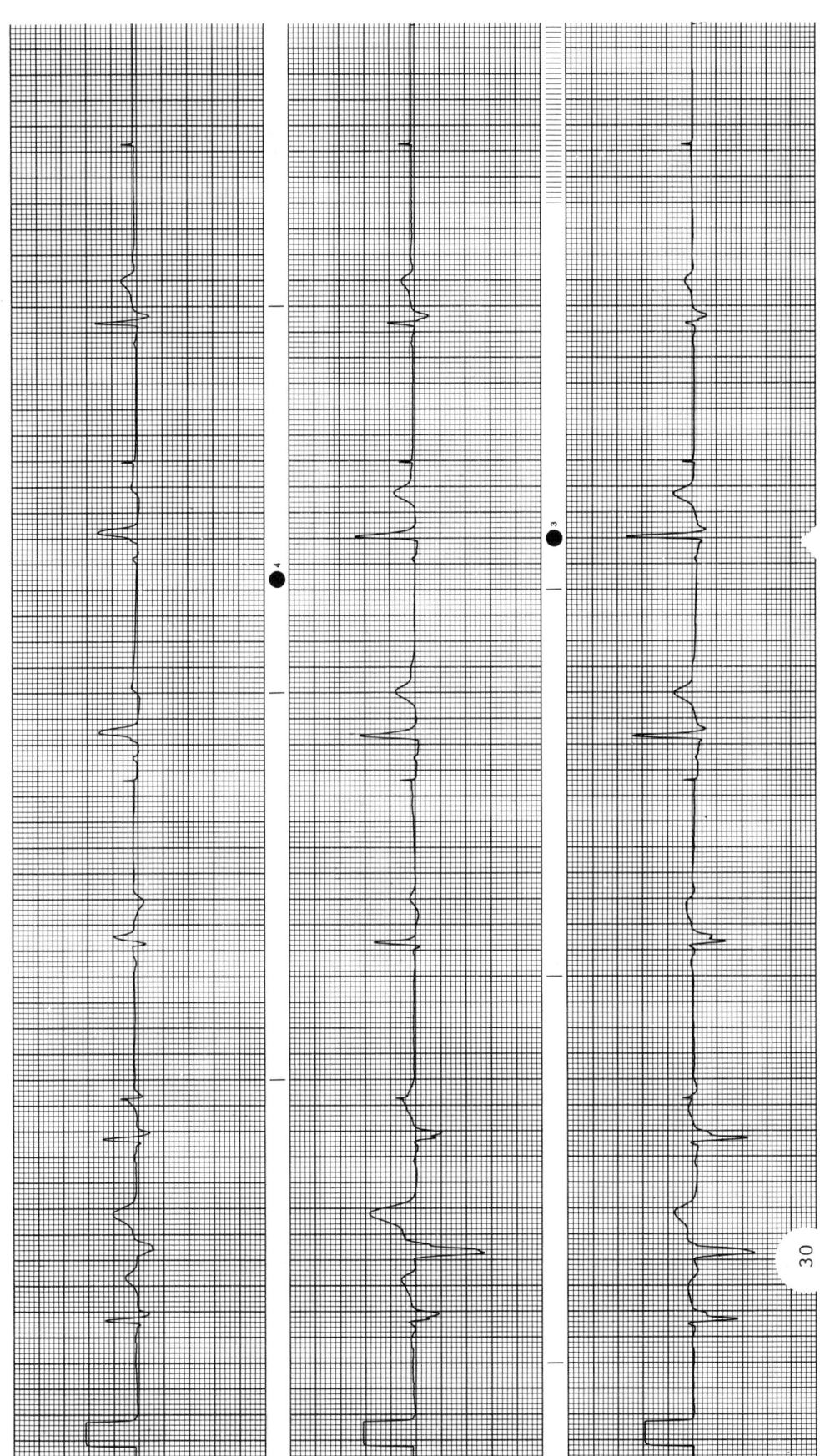

Exercise 30. An 80-year-old man admitted with new onset substernal chest pain that radiated down his left arm.

30

4

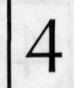

SELF-ASSESSMENT ANSWERS TO EXERCISES 25–30

EXERCISE 25

STEP 1. Rhythm Determination

- Ventricular rate 96
- QRS shape *Notched V1 widened*
- R-R rhythm *slightly irregular*
- QRS interval *0.16*
- QT interval *0.40*
- Dominant pacemaker site *Sinus*
- Interpretation *NSR with APB*

- Atrial rate 96
- P wave shape *Positive except negative in aVR and diphasic in V1*
- P-P rhythm *slightly irregular*
- P-R interval *0.18*
- P:R conduction ratio *1:1*

STEP 2. Axis Determination

Right axis

STEP 3. Chamber Enlargement Determination

None

STEP 4. Intraventricular Conduction Blocks Determination

RBBB with left posterior hemiblock

EXERCISE 26

STEP 1. Rhythm Determination

- Ventricular rate 60
- QRS shape *Widened*

- R-R rhythm *Regular*
- QRS interval *0.14*
- QT interval *0.44*
- Dominant pacemaker site *Sinus*
- Interpretation *Sinus bradycardia*

- Atrial rate 60
- P wave shape *Positive except negative in aVR, diphasic in V1*
- P-P rhythm *Regular*
- P-R interval *0.19*
- P:R conduction ratio *1:1*

STEP 2. Axis Determination

Borderline left axis

STEP 3. Chamber Enlargement Determination

None

STEP 4. Intraventricular Conduction Blocks Determination

LBBB

EXERCISE 27

STEP 1. Rhythm Determination

- Ventricular rate *75*
- QRS shape *Normal*

- R-R rhythm *Regular*
- QRS interval *0.08*
- QT interval *0.40*
- Dominant pacemaker site *Sinus*
- Interpretation *NSR*

- Atrial rate *75*
- P wave shape *Positive except negative aVR and aVL, diphasic in V1*
- P-P rhythm *Regular*
- P-R interval *0.19*
- P:R conduction ratio *1:1*

STEP 2. Axis Determination

Left axis

STEP 3. Chamber Enlargement Determination

None

STEP 4. Intraventricular Conduction Blocks Determination

LAH

EXERCISE 28

STEP 1. Rhythm Determination

- Ventricular rate 70
- QRS shape *Normal*

- R-R rhythm *Regular*
- QRS interval *0.08*
- QT interval *0.42*
- Dominant pacemaker site *Sinus*
- Interpretation *NSR*

- Atrial rate 70
- P wave shape *Positive except negative aVR, diphasic III, V1*
- P-P rhythm *Regular*
- P-R interval *0.19*
- P:R conduction ratio *1:1*

STEP 2. Axis Determination

Left axis

STEP 3. Chamber Enlargement Determination

None

STEP 4. Intraventricular Conduction Blocks Determination

Normal conduction. Even though there is a LAD, there is no LAH because there is no Q wave in I or an S wave in III.

EXERCISE 29

STEP 1. Rhythm Determination

- Ventricular rate *51*
- QRS shape *Notched V1*
- R-R rhythm *Regular*
- QRS interval *0.10*
- QT interval *0.40*
- Atrial rate *=*
- P wave shape *=*
- P-P rhythm *=*
- P-R interval *=*
- P:R conduction ratio *=*
- Dominant pacemaker site *AV node*
- Interpretation *Junctional rhythm*

STEP 2. Axis Determination

Left axis

STEP 3. Chamber Enlargement Determination

None

STEP 4. Intraventricular Conduction Blocks Determination

Incomplete RBBB

EXERCISE 30

STEP 1. Rhythm Determination

- Ventricular rate *38*
- QRS shape *Widened*

- R-R rhythm *Mostly regular*
- QRS interval *0.14*
- QT interval *0.48*
- Atrial rate *38*
- P wave shape *Positive but generally flattened, except negative aVR*
- P-P rhythm *Regular*
- P-R interval *0.16*
- P:R conduction ratio *1:1*
- Dominant pacemaker site *Sinus*
- Interpretation *Marked sinus bradycardia with PVC*

STEP 2. Axis Determination

Left axis

STEP 3. Chamber Enlargement Determination

None

STEP 4. Intraventricular Conduction Blocks Determination

RBBB with LAH

4

6
Ischemia, Injury, and Infarction Determination

STEP 5

The *fifth step* in the systematic process is to *determine the presence of myocardial ischemia, injury, or infarction.* This chapter will outline the fundamental concepts necessary to successfully complete this step.

What is the difference between ischemia, injury, and infarction? All are caused by insufficient or lack of oxygenated blood supply to the heart muscle via the coronary arteries. Ischemia is the first step in the process of decreased blood supply to the myocardium. It is manifested by a symmetrically inverted T wave or by ST segment depression (Davis, 1985). Injury is one step beyond ischemia, but it does not cause permanent muscle damage. Injury is evidenced by ST segment elevation. Both ischemia and injury are reversible. Infarction on the other hand causes necrosis or death of the myocardium. It follows the stages of ischemia and injury, and it is not reversible. Infarction is represented by the development of significant Q waves.

ECG CHANGES

The electrocardiogram (ECG) changes that are specific to myocardial ischemia, injury, and infarction are reflected in the ST segment, the T wave, and the Q wave. Before you proceed, review the information in Chapter 1 that defines and describes the normal ST segment, T wave, and Q wave found in all 12 leads.

ST Segment

The ST segment is normally isoelectric but may be elevated or depressed from the isoelectric baseline. An ST segment elevation greater than 1 mm above the baseline and an ST segment depression greater than 0.5 mm below the baseline are considered a significant ECG finding (Figure 6.1). *In this step, look for significant ST segment elevations or depressions, and note in which leads they occur.* Significant ST segment elevations may be described as concave or coved. Significant ST segment depressions may be described as horizontal or down-sloping. However, upsloping ST segment depression is considered a nonspecific finding but may indicate coronary artery disease (Thaler, 1988). Leads facing an injured area will have ST segment elevations whereas leads facing away from the injured area will display ST segment depressions.

Are the ST segment changes significant in Figure 6.2?

T Waves

A T wave is generally rounded and slightly asymmetrical with its upstroke longer than its downstroke (Frye & Lounsbury, 1988). An excessively tall, flat, or inverted T wave is considered abnormal depending on the lead (Figure 6.3). T waves are usually positive in leads I, II, V3–V6; inverted in lead aVR; variable in leads III, aVL, aVF, V1–V2. *In this step, also look for tall, flat, or inverted T waves, and note in which leads they occur.*

Are the T waves significant in Figure 6.4?

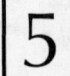

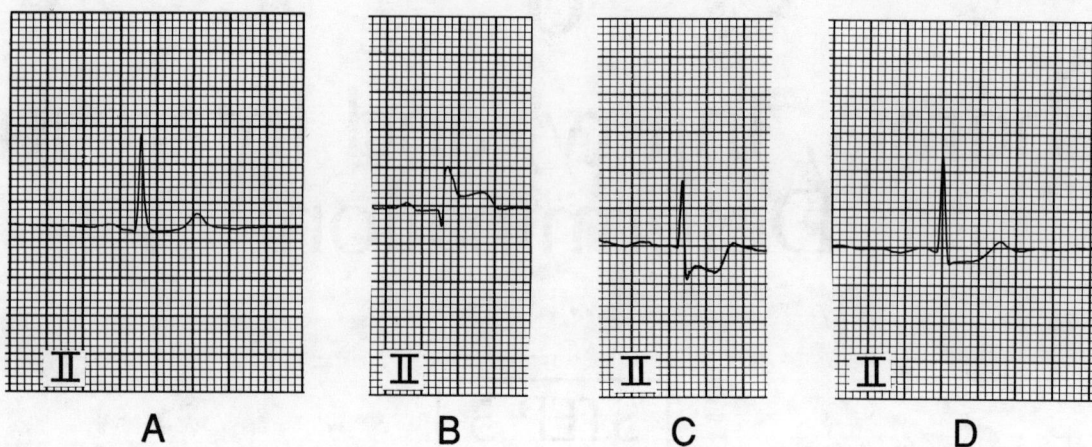

Figure 6.1. ST segment examples. *A,* normal isoelectric ST segment; *B,* elevated ST segment (coved shape); *C,* depressed ST segment (downsloping shape); *D,* depressed ST segment (horizontal shape).

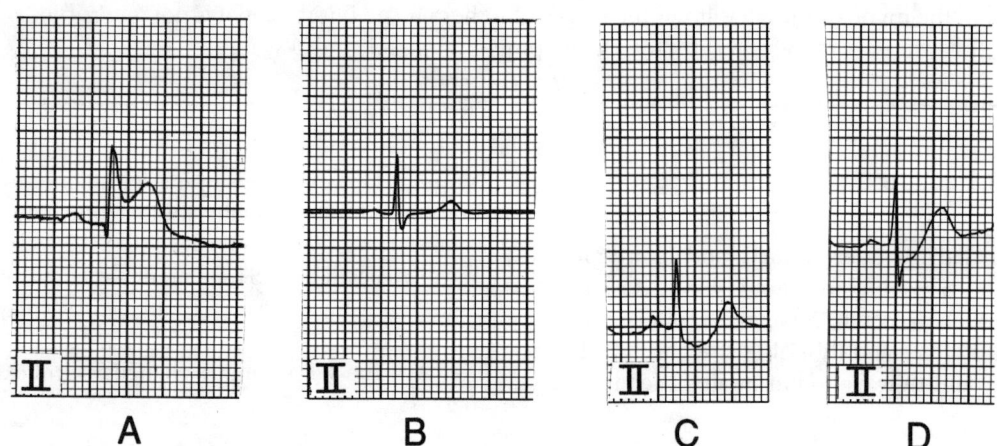

Figure 6.2. Are the following ST segment changes significant?

Answers: *A,* elevated coved shape; *B,* normal; *C,* depressed downsloping; *D,* nonspecific upsloping. All significant except *B* and *D.*

5

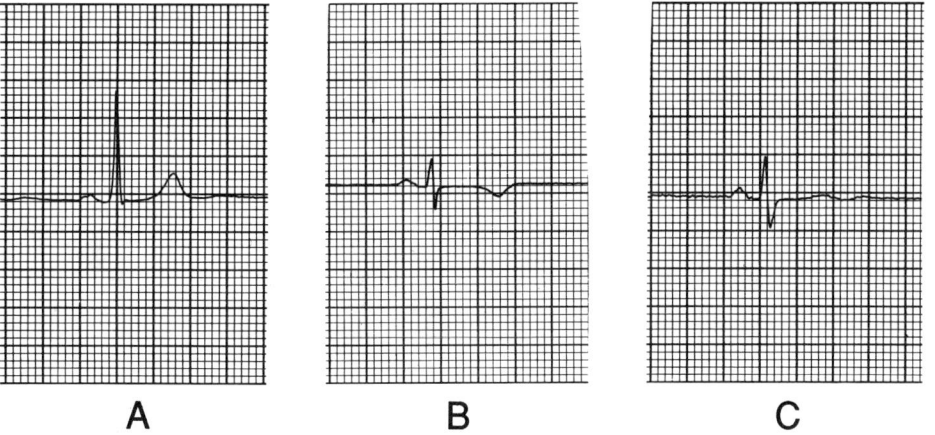

Figure 6.3. T wave examples. *A*, normal; *B* inverted and symmetrical; *C*, flat.

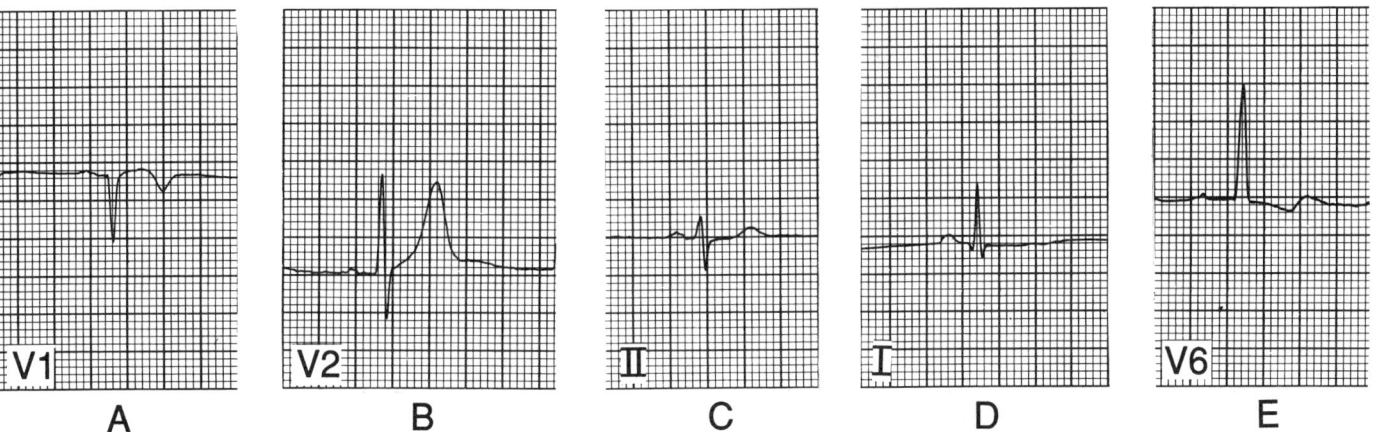

Figure 6.4. Are these T waves significant?

Answers: *A*, inverted and symmetrical; *B*, elevated; *C*, normal; *D*, flat; *E*, inverted and symmetrical. All significant except *C*.

Q Waves

A normal Q wave is generally less than 0.04 seconds in duration and height, and normally present in leads I, II, III, aVL, V5, and V6. A large significant or pathological Q wave is greater than 0.04 seconds in duration, or 4 mm or greater in depth, or one-third the height of the R wave (Figure 6.5). The significant Q waves will appear in leads that normally do not have Q waves. New Q waves frequently are associated with the loss of R waves in the same lead (Purcell & Haynes, 1984). Reminder: aVR has a normally large Q wave and should not be considered when assessing for significant Q waves.

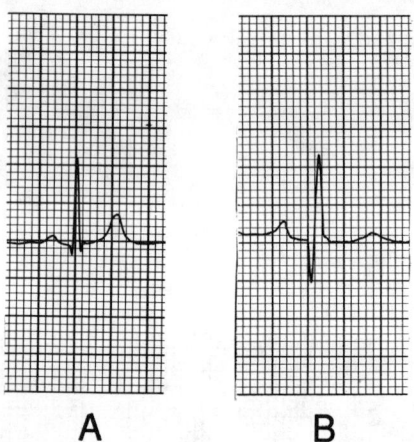

Figure 6.5.   Q wave examples using lead II. *A*, normal Q wave = less than 0.04 seconds in duration and height. *B*, significant Q wave = width >0.04 seconds in duration and height 1/3 the height of the R wave.

In this step, look for significant Q waves, and note in which leads they are present.

Are the Q waves significant in Figure 6.6?

LOCALIZATION

Localization of ischemia, injury, and infarction is the process of determining in which leads the significant ST segment, T wave, and Q wave changes occurred. This will isolate the specific area or surface of the left ventricle affected. The left ventricle is divided into several general anatomical areas: the inferior, anterior, lateral, and posterior surfaces. Combinations can be made from these general anatomical areas, most commonly anterolateral and anteroseptal. The leads representing each area of the left ventricle are vital to memorize. Leads V1–V6 represent the anterior surface. Leads II, III, and aVF represent the inferior wall. Leads I, aVL, V5, and V6 represent the lateral area. Leads V1–V4 represent the anteroseptal area. Because no leads are placed directly over the posterior wall of the left ventricle, only reciprocal ECG changes such as ST segment depression can be observed in V1 and V2.

It is necessary to determine whether the ECG changes are localized changes or diffuse changes. Diffuse changes are found in all or multiple leads and indicate generalized ischemia or infarction. The presence of localized or diffuse changes assist in determining the differential ECG diagnosis.

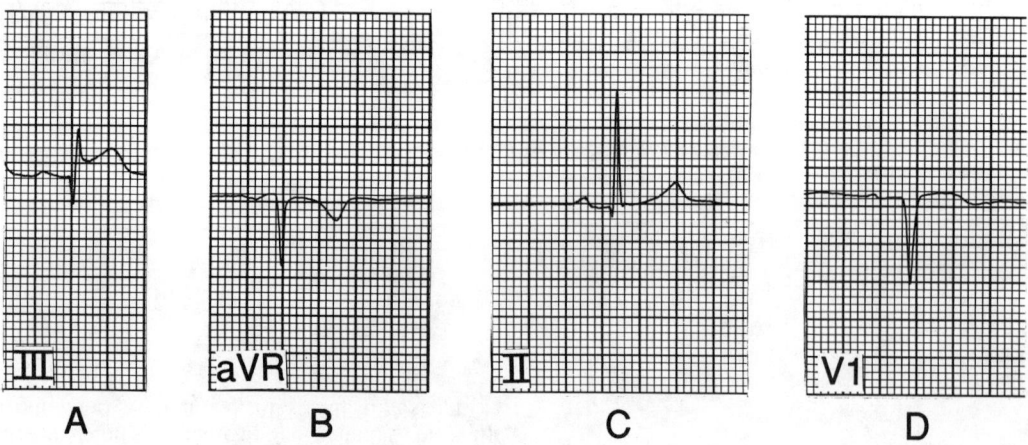

Figure 6.6.   Are these Q waves significant?

SPECIFIC ISCHEMIC AND INFARCTION ECG DIAGNOSES

The diversity of ECG changes as described above provide the elements for the following ECG diagnoses:

1. Q wave infarction (transmural)
2. Non-Q wave infarction (subendocardial)
3. Classic angina
4. Variant (Prinzmetal) angina

After determining whether the ECG changes are localized or diffuse, it is important *to determine the age* of these changes. Are they acute, evolving, or indeterminate? Then analyze the ST segment, T wave, and/or Q wave findings and *decide on an ECG diagnosis.*

Q Wave Infarction

A Q wave infarction involves the entire thickness of the left ventricular myocardial wall and is often called a myocardial infarction (MI). ECG changes indicative of an MI are *significant Q waves, loss of R waves in the chest leads, ST segment elevations, and T wave inversions in specific leads.* Axis shifts often accompany an MI. The axis generally deviates away from the site of the infarction.

Evolutionary Changes

The evolution of a Q wave MI usually proceeds as follows (Davis, 1985) (Figures 6.7 and 6.8):

1. *T wave peaking then inversion*
   With the onset of the infarction, the T wave becomes tall and narrow, or peaks. Often these are called *hyperacute T waves.* This is followed usually within a few hours by T wave inversion. T waves diagnostic of an MI usually *invert symmetrically with a gentle downslope* and *a rapid upslope,* and *are sharply pointed* (Thaler, 1988).
2. *ST segment elevation*
   ST segment elevation indicates myocardial injury and is a reliable sign that an MI has occurred. It usually

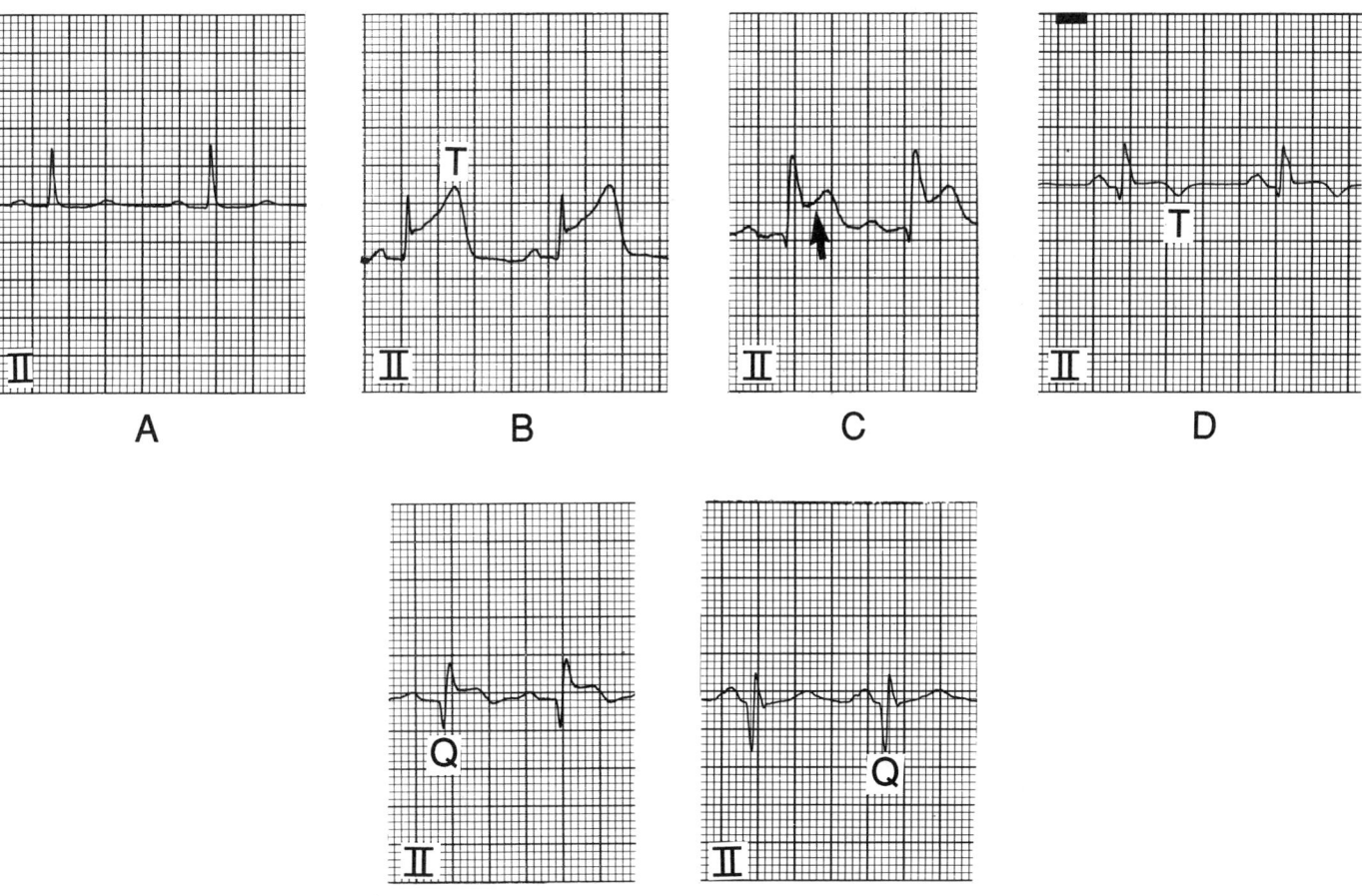

Figure 6.7. Evolutionary changes of a Q wave infarction as seen from lead II. Note examples above not necessarily from the same patient. *A,* normal; *B,* T wave becomes tall, then *D,* inverts symmetrically; *C,* ST segment elevates; *E,* significant Q waves develop; *F,* healed infarction. Q waves persist while ST segment and T wave return to normal.

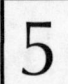

returns to baseline within a few days. The degree of elevation is determined by calculating the number of millimeters or small squares it deviates from the baseline. ST elevation indicative of myocardial injury is *bowed upward* and *tends to merge* with the *T wave* (Thaler, 1988). Its shape is often described as *convex* or *coved*.

3. *New significant Q waves*

The presence of significant Q waves is diagnostic of a Q wave infarction and appears within hours to days of the event. The presence of Q waves indicates necrosis. Q waves will persist on the ECG indefinitely. Q waves are seen only in the leads that face the infarcted area. See the beginning of this chapter for a description of significant Q waves.

Age of Infarction

Age can be determined by examining the ST segments and T waves and looking for the presence of significant Q waves.

Acute infarction	= Elevated ST segment
Evolving infarction	= ST segment at or returning to baseline and T waves inverted
Indeterminate infarction	= Normal ST segment and T waves but presence of significant Q waves or loss of R wave progression in chest leads

Reciprocal Changes

In electrocardiography, reciprocal is defined as the opposite, whether configurations or leads. In a Q wave infarction reciprocal changes are represented by ST segment depressions in the leads opposite the infarcted area. The presence of reciprocal changes confirms the existence of an MI.

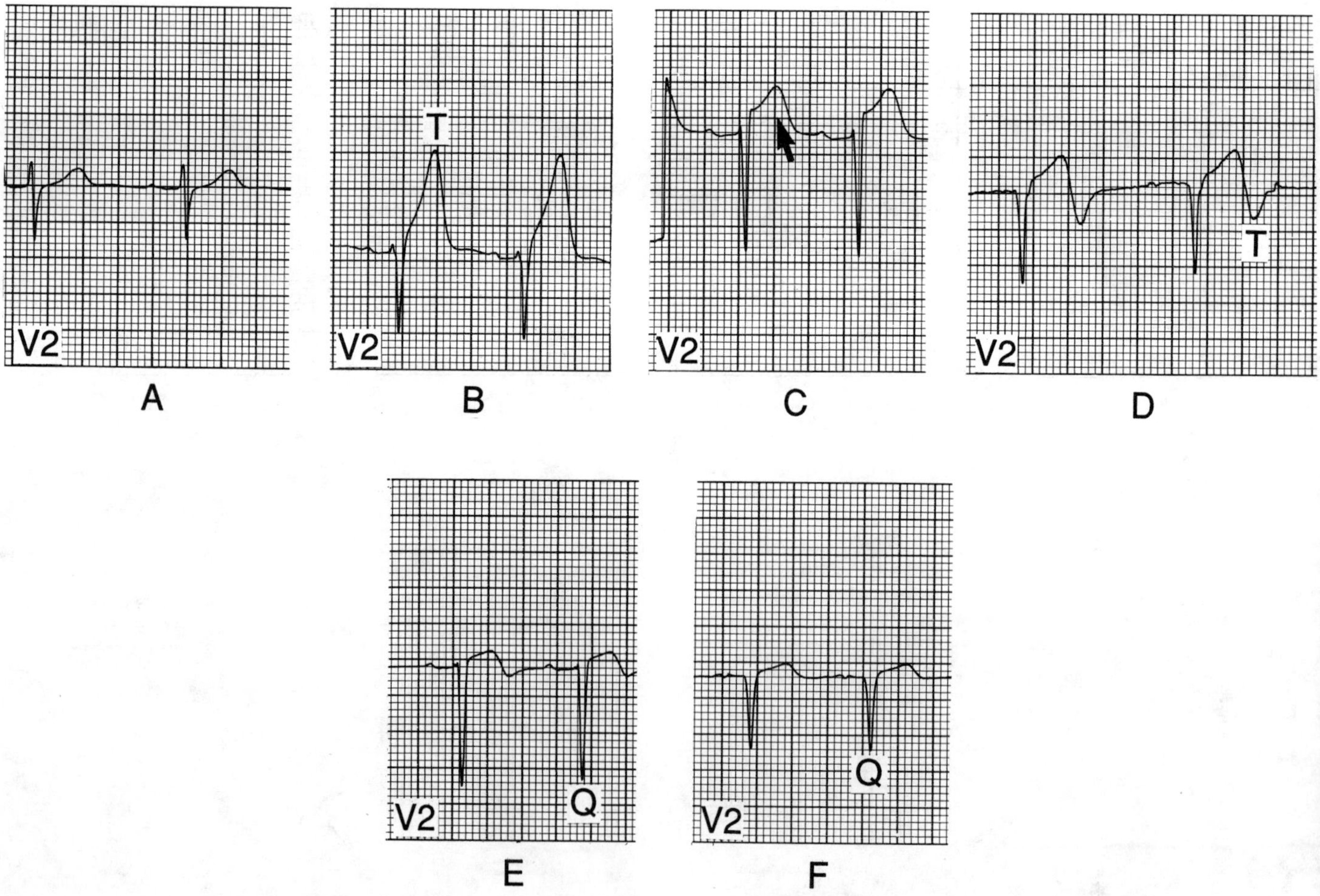

Figure 6.8. Evolutionary changes of a Q wave infarction as seen in lead V2. Note examples above not necessarily from the same patient. *A*, normal; *B*, T wave becomes tall and peaks, then *D*, inverts symmetrically; *C*, ST segment elevates; *D* and *E*, significant Q waves or loss of R wave; *F*, healed infarction. Q waves and loss of R waves persist while ST segment and T wave return to normal.

Location of Infarction

The characteristic ECG changes described are localized to the leads overlying the site of the infarction. An inferior infarction is usually caused by occlusion of the right coronary artery and produces indicative ECG changes in the inferior leads II, III, and aVF and reciprocal changes in the lateral leads I and aVL. An anterior infarction is generally caused by occlusion of the left anterior descending artery and causes indicative ECG changes in the anterior leads V1–V6 but mostly in V3–V5. The reciprocal leads for the anterior wall are the inferior leads. A lateral wall infarction is generally due to a blockage in the left circumflex artery and shows indicative changes in the left lateral leads I, aVL, V5, and V6. The reciprocal leads for a lateral wall infarction are V1–V3. A posterior infarction involves occlusion of either the right coronary or left circumflex arteries and produces reciprocal changes instead of indicative changes. The changes are tall R waves, ST segment depressions, and upright T waves. Posterior infarctions generally do not occur alone but accompany inferior infarctions.

Localization of an MI is important as it determines the therapeutic intervention and assists in predicting complications (Thaler, 1988). Table 6.1 summarizes the common types of myocardial (Q wave) infarctions, the coronary artery involved, the leads reflecting the indicative changes, the specific ECG changes, and the reciprocal leads.

Non-Q Wave Infarction

A non-Q wave infarction involves only the inner layer of the myocardium, the subendocardium. The ECG characteristics suggestive of a non-Q wave infarction are T wave inversions and/or ST segment depressions, without significant Q waves. The ST segment depression shape is described as *squared off* (Figure 6.9). The ST segment changes are often transient and often only the

Table 6.1.
Localization of Q Wave Infarctions[a]

Type of Infarction	Coronary Arteries Involved	Indicative Leads	ECG Changes	Reciprocal Leads
Inferior	RCA	II, III, aVF	ST elevation T wave inversion Path. Q waves Left axis deviation	I, aVL, V1–V6
Anterior	LCA	V1–V6, Mostly V3–V5	ST elevation T wave inversion Path. Q waves Loss of R wave progression	II, III, aVF
Lateral	Circumflex	I, aVL, V5, V6	ST elevation T wave inversion Path. Q waves Right axis deviation	V1, V3
Posterior	RCA or Circumflex	V1, V2	Reciprocal changes R > S ST depression Elevated T waves	
Anteroseptal	LAD	V1–V4	ST elevation T wave inversion Path. Q waves Loss of septal R in V1 Left axis deviation	
Anterolateral	LAD or Circumflex	I, aVL, V4–V6	ST elevation T wave inversion Path. Q waves Right axis deviation	II, III, aVF

[a]RCA = right coronary artery; LCA = left coronary artery; LAD = left anterior descending artery; Path. = pathological; ST = ST segment.

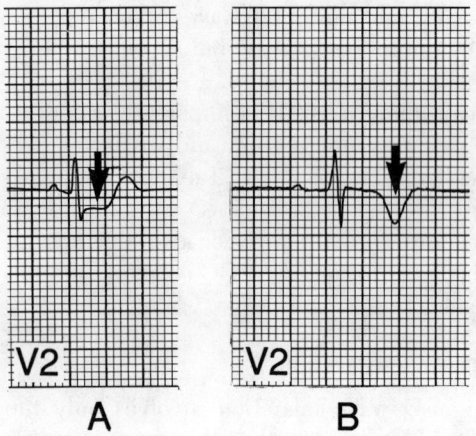

Figure 6.9. Non-Q wave infarction ECG characteristics. *A*, ST segment depression (squared off shape); *B*, deeply inverted symmetrical T wave inversion.

T wave inversion is present. T waves will appear *symmetrical* and *deeply inverted.*

Just as Q wave infarctions can be localized to a specific surface of the heart, so can non-Q wave infarctions. Because the ST segment and T wave changes are transient, localization of non-Q wave infarctions can only be done at the time of infarction. Because these transient changes may have already resolved and may reflect other problems, it is important to verify the ECG evidence with a positive patient history and cardiac enzymes.

Classic Angina

Classic angina is the typical chest pain which is relieved by nitroglycerin (NTG) or rest. The ECG characteristics present during an anginal attack are *ST segment depression* and/or *T wave inversion.* The ST segment depression is described as *downsloping* or *hor-*

izontal (Figure 6.10). The ST segment depression must be distinguished from nonischemic causes such as drug effect. These changes will display in the leads facing away from the event. In angina, the ST segment changes are localized to specific leads.

Variant Angina

Variant, often called Prinzmetal, angina differs from classic angina. It is chest pain that can occur at any time, even at rest, and is often related to coronary artery spasm. The ECG changes with it are *ST segment elevations* (Figure 6.11). The ST elevation returns to baseline as soon as the pain/spasm is relieved. The ST segment elevation seen *localizes* to specific leads similar to the ST segment changes seen in Q wave infarctions. Thus variant angina can be localized to the inferior wall, anterior wall, and so forth, similar to Q wave infarctions.

Table 6.2 summarizes the ECG and related findings

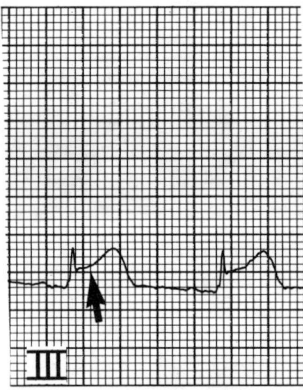

Figure 6.11. Variant angina ECG characteristics. ST segment elevations that resolve to baseline as pain or spasm is relieved.

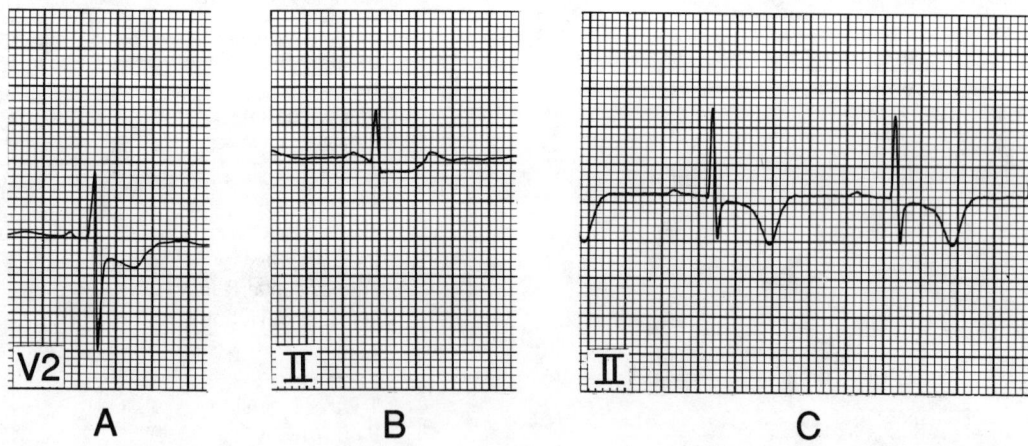

Figure 6.10. Classic angina ECG characteristics. *A*, ST segment depression (downsloping); *B*, ST segment depression (horizontal); *C*, T wave inversion (symmetrical).

Table 6.2.
Differentiating between Ischemia and Infarction Diagnoses

Diagnosis	ECG Changes[a]	Localization	Related Findings
Q Wave infarction	ST elevation (coved shape) T wave inversion (symmetrical; pointed) Pathological Q waves Loss of R wave progression in anterior leads	Localizes to specific leads	Chest pain Positive cardiac enzymes Axis deviation (away from site of infarction)
Non Q wave infarction	ST depressions (squared shape) T wave inversion (symmetrical)	Localizes to specific leads	Chest pain Positive cardiac enzymes ST changes transient, lasting 48 hours
Classic angina	ST depressions, (horizontal or downsloping) T wave inversion	Localizes to specific leads	Chest pain Negative cardiac enzymes ST changes return to normal with pain relief
Variant	ST elevation	Localizes to specific leads	Chest pain Negative cardiac enzymes ST changes to normal with pain relief

[a]ST = ST segment.

essential to identifying the specific ischemia or infarction diagnosis described above.

CLINICAL SIGNIFICANCE

It is clinically important to determine the etiology of the ST segment, T wave, and the Q wave findings. Is it due to ischemia, injury, or infarction? What type of ischemia is it, classic or variant? What type of infarction is it, Q wave or non-Q wave? Are the changes localized to specific leads or are the changes in all leads? The etiology and the location of these findings predict what symptoms, treatment, and complications to prepare for and anticipate.

ST segment elevations may be a normal variant but most often are indicative of myocardial transmural injury that can be either a Q wave infarction or variant angina (Thaler, 1988). The clinical situation, the accompanying ECG findings, and the cardiac enzyme results assist in differentiating between the causes. In a myocardial infarction, the ST segment elevations are in selected leads. ST segment elevations are also associated with the diagnosis of ventricular aneurysm, or pericarditis, and often accompany a LBBB (Frye & Lounsbury, 1988). In ventricular aneurysm the ST segment elevations are described as persistent.

ST segment depression is reflective of myocardial subendocardial injury that could be caused by either a non-Q wave infarction or classic angina (Thaler, 1988).

The clinical situation, other ECG findings, and the cardiac enzyme report are required to differentiate between them. ST segment depression might also indicate progressive hypokalemia, the presence of a bundle branch block, and the use of digoxin. Depressed ST segments may represent the reciprocal changes that accompany an MI.

T wave changes are a nonspecific finding. To determine their meaning consider the clinical situation, the patient's drug history, and the other ECG findings found. Increased height can indicate hyperkalemia, myocardial infarction, or ischemia. Flat or inverted T waves reflect hypokalemia, myocardial ischemia, or possibly a normal variant. Ventricular hypertrophy with strain and a bundle branch block can cause T waves to invert.

The appearance of *significant Q waves* especially in leads that normally do not have Q waves is indicative of myocardial necrosis. The main etiology is a Q wave myocardial infarction. The development of pathological Q waves in the anterior leads can lead to the development of poor R wave progression. Poor R wave progression may be a sign of an MI but may also be seen with LVH, COPD, and LBBB (Goldberger & Goldberger, 1986).

If an MI is diagnosed, the location of the infarction is important to determine as it can predict the clinical course and outcome for the patient. For example, an anterior wall MI is usually more serious and has a higher death rate. A patient with an inferior wall MI is more

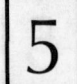

Table 6.3.
Comparison of Different MI Locations[a]

Location of MI	Electrical Complications	Mechanical Complications	Nursing Considerations[b]
Inferior	PVC SB ST JR APB Atrial fibrillation 1st° AV block Wenckebach	Right ventricular infarction Papillary muscle rupture Mitral insufficiency Atrial infarction	Monitor for dysrhythmias, systolic murmurs, large V waves on PCWP Assess for S+S of decreased CO and heart failure: chest pain, low BP, high PCWP, crackles, and S3 Assess for jugular venous distention Monitor for extension to posterior wall
Anterior	PVC SVT 2nd° AV block, (Type II) CHB BBB Hemiblocks	Ventricular aneurysm Heart failure Cardiogenic shock	Monitor for dysrhythmias, BBB If normal QRS, monitor on lead V1 to detect development BBB If BBB present, monitor for axis change to detect hemiblocks (Use leads I, aVF, or II) Assess for S+S of decreased CO and heart failure Monitor for extension to lateral/septal wall
Lateral	PVC SB ST APB Atrial fibrillation	Ventricular hypertrophy	Monitor for dysrhythmia, emboli Monitor for S+S of decreased CO and heart failure
Septal	Same as Anterior	Septal rupture	Same as anterior Monitor for systolic murmur
Posterior	Same as Inferior		

[a]S+S = signs and symptoms; BP = blood pressure; CO = cardiac output; PCWP = pulmonary capillary wedge pressure.
[b]Medicate for chest pain immediately in all locations.

likely to develop sinus bradycardia. Table 6.3 outlines the typical electrical and mechanical complications and nursing considerations based on the MI location. It is extremely important to identify the development of an MI in its early stages so the patient can receive treatment with a thrombolytic agent such as tissue plasminogen activator (TPA) to minimize the infarct size.

A non-Q wave infarction diagnosis puts the patient at high risk for a Q wave infarction and for developing a serious dysrhythmia such as ventricular tachycardia. A large percentage of these patients will develop unstable angina as a complication.

Classic angina and variant angina have normal cardiac enzymes. Classic angina may progress to variant or unstable angina. Variant leads to serious dysrhythmias, especially PVCs, heart blocks, VT, or VF, and serious hemodynamic changes that lead to decreased cardiac output.

There are limitations in using the ECG changes to diagnose an MI. An MI cannot be diagnosed in the presence of a LBBB, and it is difficult to determine in a patient with a pacemaker. To diagnose an MI in a pacemaker patient requires ST segment and T wave changes in serial ECGs with nonpaced rhythm, clinical signs, and positive cardiac enzyme studies. Because RVH and RBBB also present with large R waves in V1 and V2, it is difficult to diagnose a posterior wall MI unless the inferior wall is also involved and has a normal QRS interval.

Key questions to ask yourself in completing this step of the systematic process are as follows:

Are there ST segment elevations or depressions?
■ Assess shape of ST segment change.
  Convex or coved ST segment elevations?
  Horizontal or downsloping ST segment depressions?
Are there T wave inversions?
■ Assess shape of T wave change.
  Symmetrically or asymmetrically inverted?
Are there significant Q waves?
■ Assess leads for presence of Q waves.

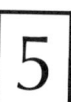

What combination of the above findings are present?

- Monitor for ST segment elevations, T wave inversions, and Q wave combination.
- Monitor for ST segment elevations only.
- Monitor for ST segment depressions only.
- Monitor for significant Q waves only.

In which leads are the above findings identified?

- Assess for localized or diffuse changes.
- Monitor for changes in inferior, anterior, etc. locations.

Are these changes acute (new) or chronic (old)?

- Notify physician of new changes.
- Determine the age, if possible (acute, evolving, indeterminate).
- Compare these changes with the patient's baseline or other serial ECGs.

What is the patient's clinical and drug history?

- Assess current drug therapy.
- Monitor serum drug levels and electrolyte levels, especially digoxin and potassium.
- Assess for history of past MI or angina.
- Monitor for positive cardiac enzymes.
- Assess patient for symptoms of chest pain.
- Assess patient's vital signs.

Does the ECG show signs of an MI?

- Monitor for coved ST segment elevations, symmetrical T wave inversions, and pathological Q waves.
- Assess for axis changes.
- Assess for location of infarction.
- Prepare for thrombolytic therapy.
- Monitor and prepare for potential complications (see Table 6.3).
- Select appropriate monitor or rhythm lead.
- Evaluate patient's response to therapy.
- Provide patient education.

Does the ECG show signs of non-Q wave infarction?

- Monitor for square-shaped ST segment elevations in specific leads.
- Assess for positive history of chest pain and cardiac enzymes.
- Prepare for potential complications.

Does the ECG show signs of classic angina?

- Monitor for ST segment depressions.
- Assess for positive history of chest pain.
- Monitor for negative cardiac enzymes.

Does the ECG show signs of variant angina?

- Monitor for ST segment elevations in specific leads.
- Assess for positive history of chest pain.
- Monitor for negative cardiac enzymes.
- Prepare for potential complications, especially ventricular dysrhythmias.

What other reasons could cause these findings?

- Correlate the patient's clinical and drug history.
- Monitor for drug or electrolyte causes.
- Assess for signs and symptoms of pericarditis.
- Assess for asymmetrical T wave inversion i.e., LVH with strain.

SELF-ASSESSMENT EXERCISES 31–36

In the following six ECG examples, complete the following steps:

Step One: Determination of Rhythm
Step Two: Determination of Axis
Step Three: Determination of Chamber Enlargement
Step Four: Determination of Intraventricular Conduction Blocks
Step Five: Determination of Ischemia, Injury, or Infarction
   Inferior leads (II, III, aVF): _____
   Anterior leads (V1–V6): _____
   Lateral leads (I, aVL, V5–V6): _____
   Anteroseptal leads (V1–V4): _____
   Posterior leads (V1–V2 reciprocal): _____
   Diffuse _____

You must be able to perform these steps successfully before you proceed. When you have completed all of the exercises in this book, come back to this exercise and complete the remaining steps.

Check your answers with the suggested interpretations found at the end of this chapter. Answers for remaining steps will be found in Appendix A.

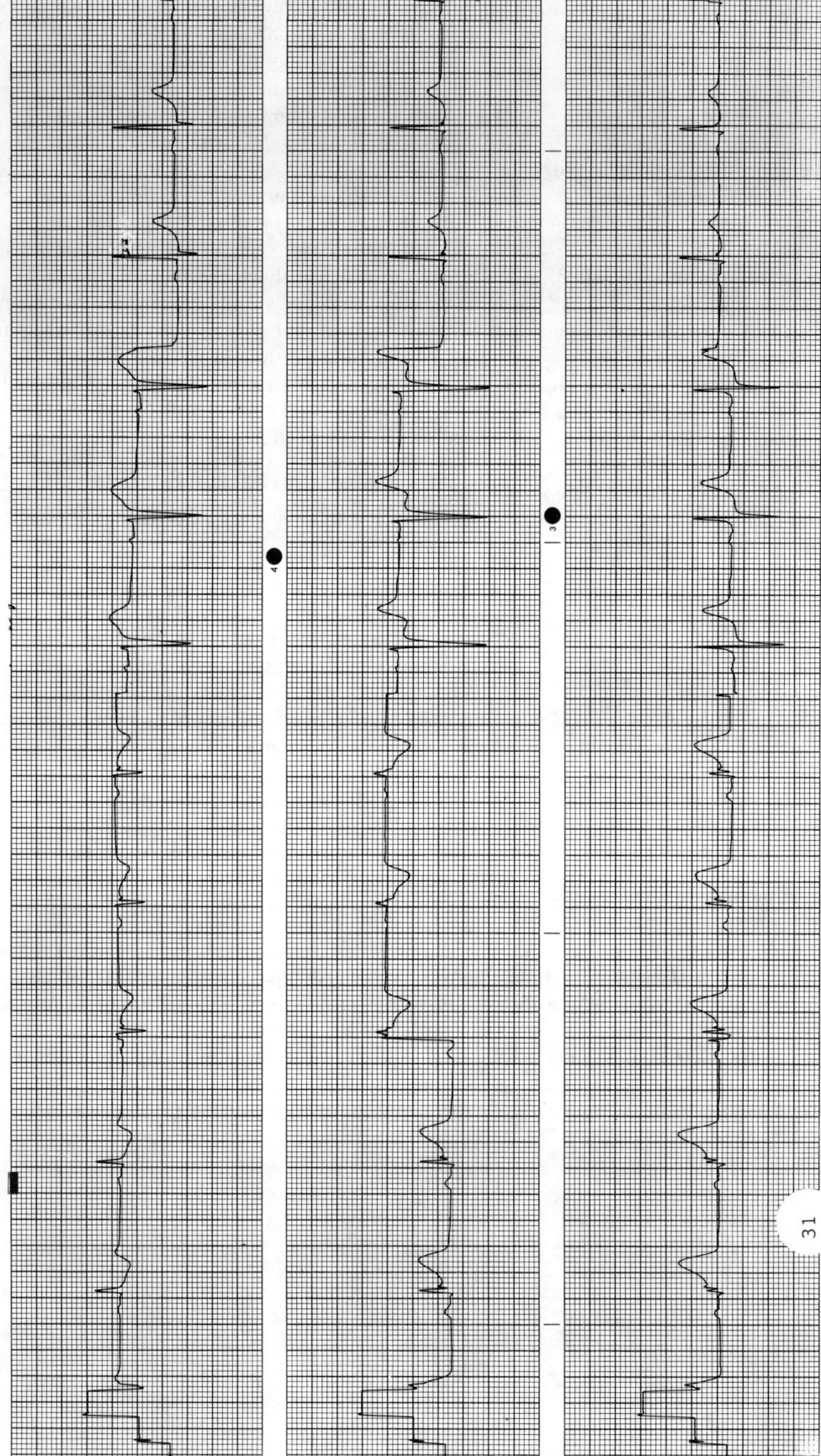

Exercise 31. A 62-year-old admitted with severe chest pain. History of angioplasty of right coronary artery.

5

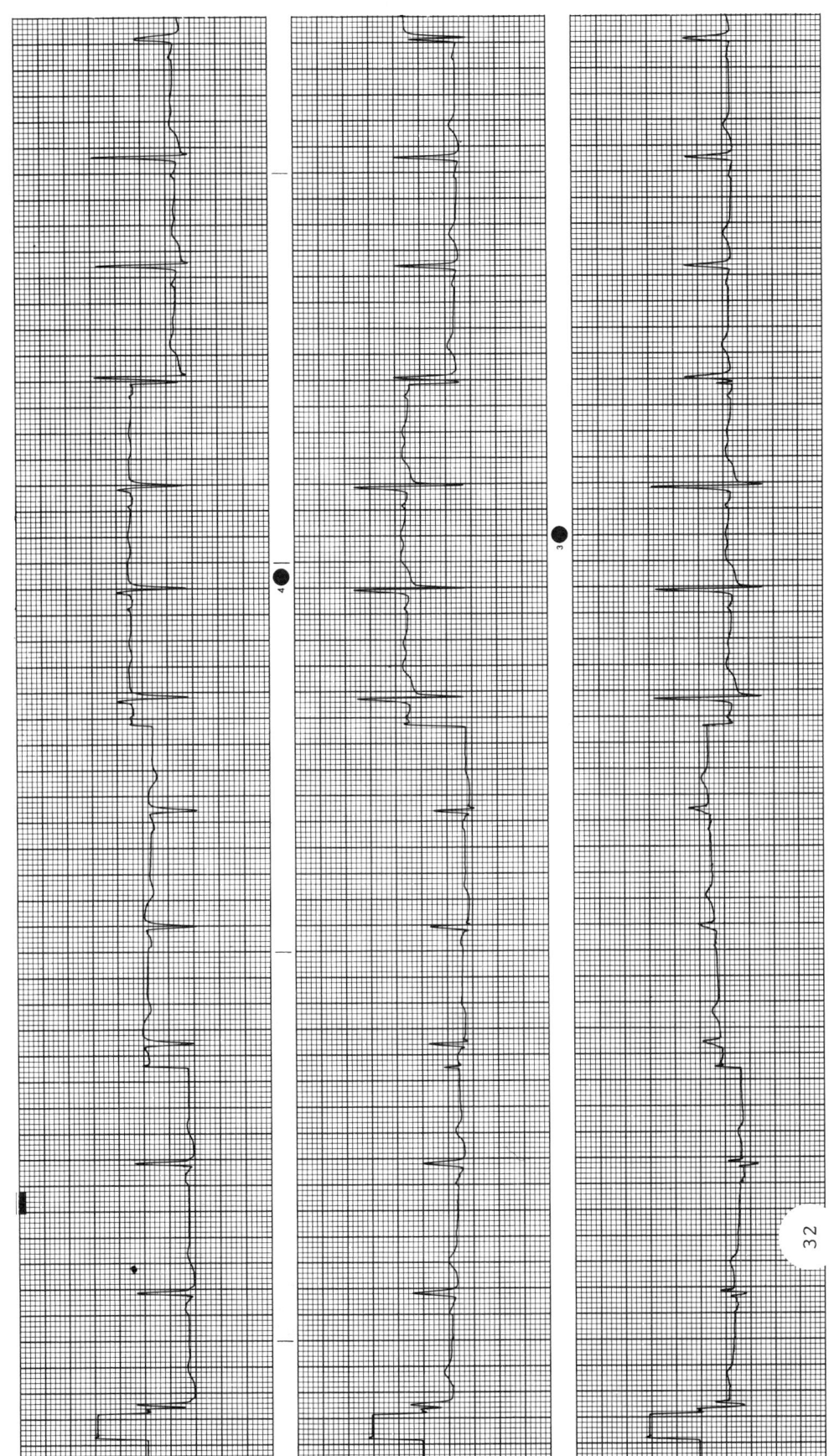

Exercise 32. A 59-year-old man admitted with acute chest pain and abnormal ECG. History of cigarette abuse.

32

5

Exercise 33. A 44-year-old man without cardiac history until admission when he developed substernal chest pressure with some shortness of breath.

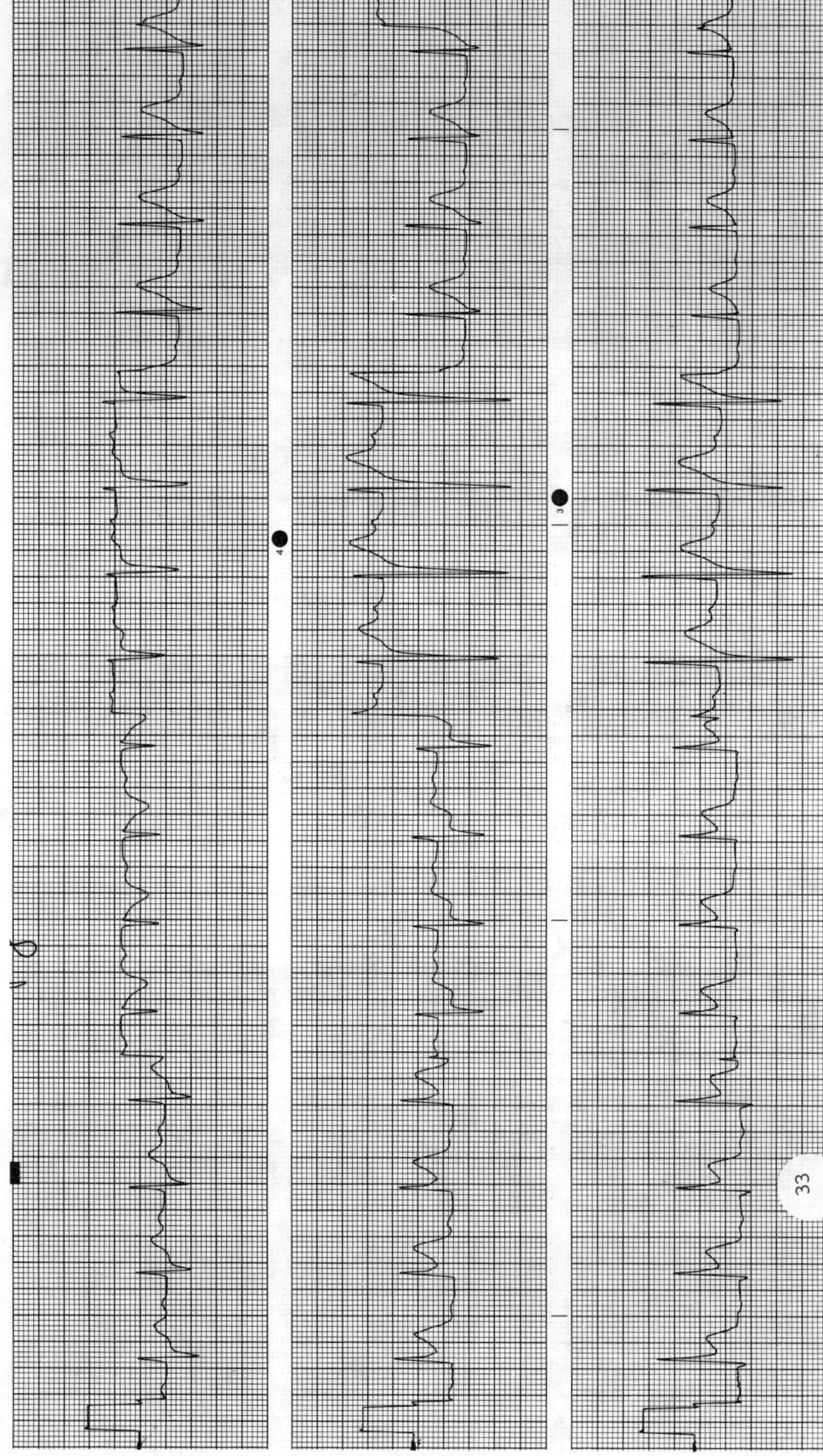

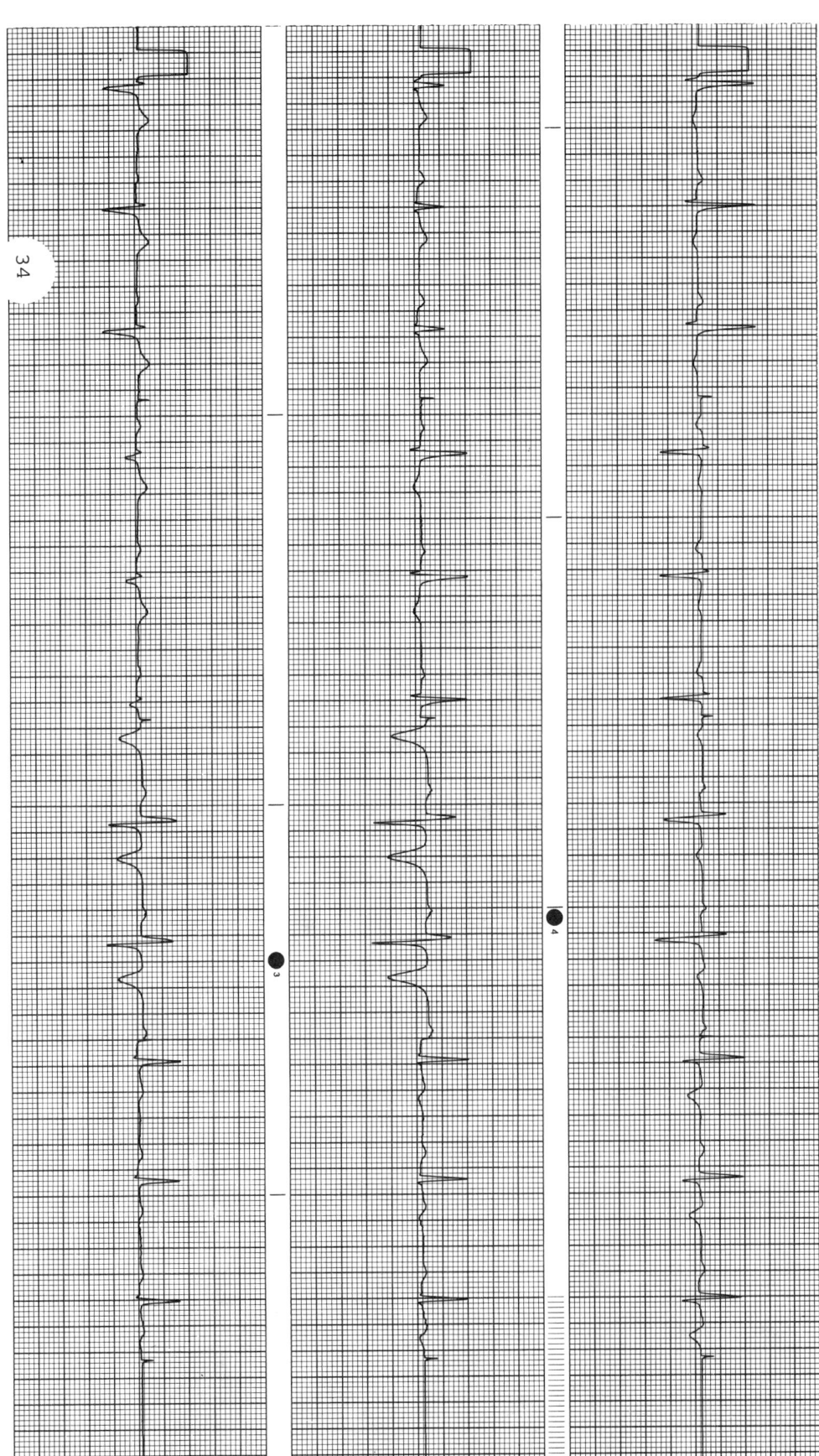

Exercise 34. A 54-year-old man admitted with prolonged angina. History of double coronary bypass surgery and angioplasty.

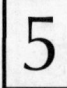

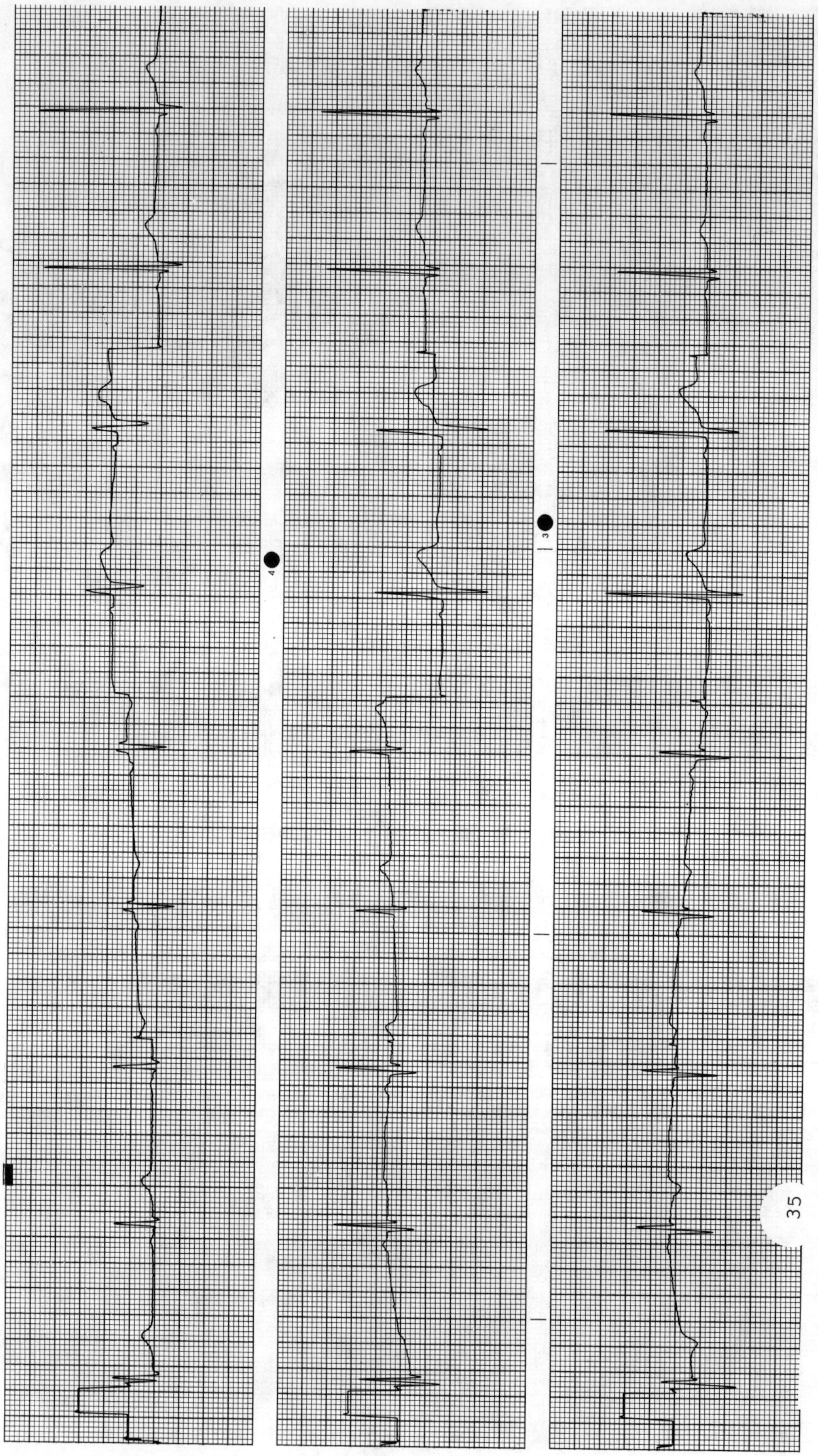

Exercise 35. A 65-year-old man admitted with chest discomfort of 1-hour duration.

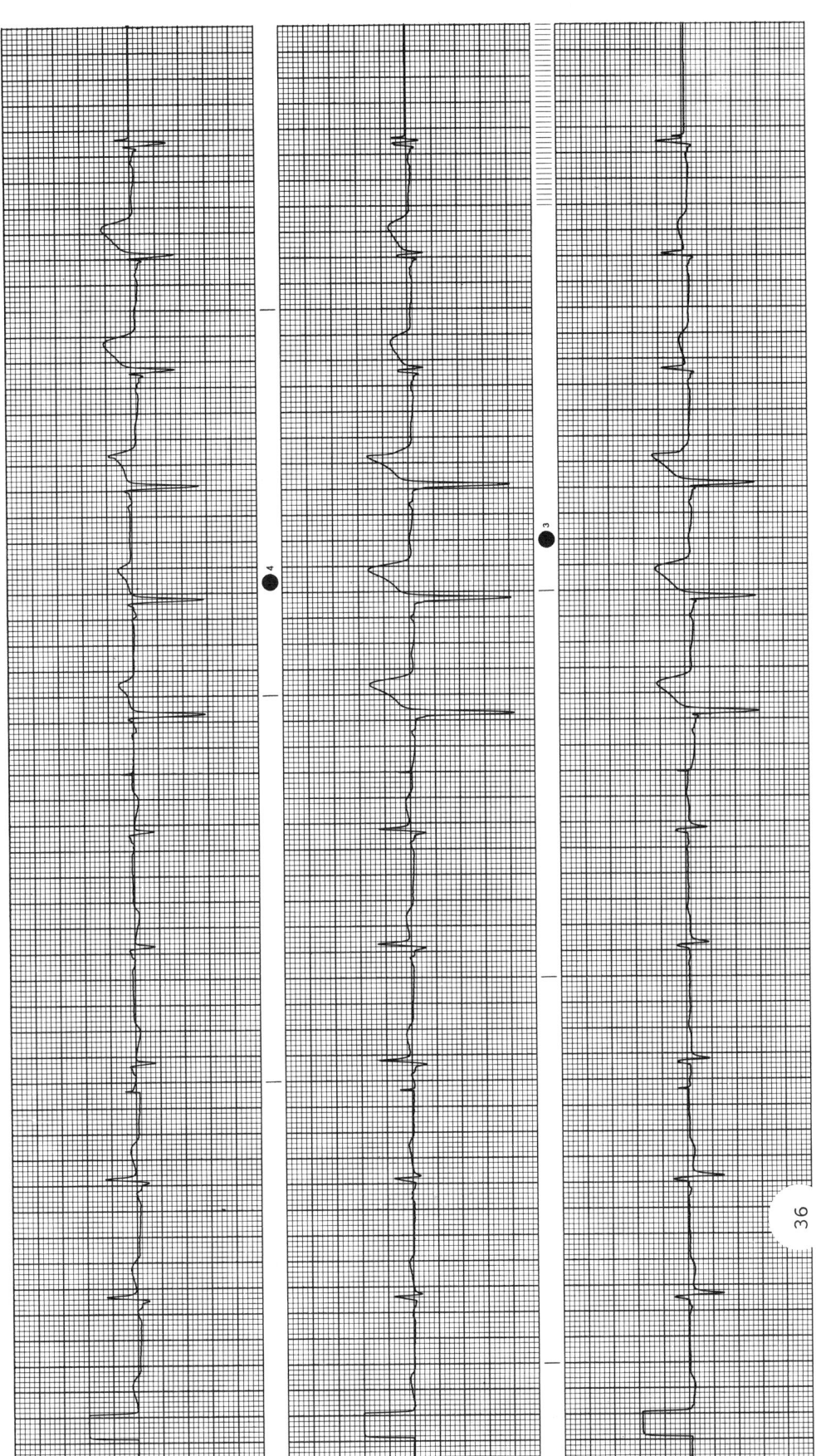

Exercise 36. A 64-year-old man admitted with substernal chest pain of 2-hour duration.

SELF-ASSESSMENT ANSWERS TO EXERCISES 31–36

EXERCISE 31

STEP 1. Rhythm Determination

- Ventricular rate *61*
- QRS shape *Normal*

- Atrial rate *61*
- P wave shape *Positive except negative aVR and aVL*

- R-R rhythm *Regular*
- QRS interval *0.08*
- QT interval *0.38*

- P-P rhythm *Regular*
- P-R interval *0.16*
- P:R conduction ratio *1:1*

- Dominant pacemaker site *Sinus*
- Interpretation *NSR*

STEP 2. Axis Determination

Normal axis

STEP 3. Chamber Enlargement Determination

None

STEP 4. Intraventricular Conduction Blocks Determination

Normal conduction

STEP 5. Ischemia, Injury, and Infarction Determination

ST segment elevations leads II, III, and aVF with reciprocal depressions and T wave inversions in leads I and aVL. ST segments depressed in leads V2–V3. T waves negative in aVR. Normal R wave progression. Q waves evolving in leads II, III, and aVF.

EXERCISE 32

STEP 1. Rhythm Determination

- Ventricular rate *67*
- QRS shape *Normal*

- Atrial rate *67*
- P wave shape *Positive except negative III, aVR and flattened in aVF*

- R-R rhythm *Regular*
- QRS interval *0.09*
- QT interval *0.38*

- P-P rhythm *Regular*
- P-R interval *0.14*
- P:R conduction ratio *1:1*

- Dominant pacemaker site *Sinus*
- Interpretation *NSR*

STEP 2. Axis Determination

Normal axis

STEP 3. Chamber Enlargement Determination

None

STEP 4. Intraventricular Conduction Blocks Determination

Normal conduction

STEP 5. Ischemia, Injury, and Infarction Determination

ST segments depressed leads I, aVL, and squared off and depressed in leads V2–V4. T waves positive in all leads except negative in aVR. R wave progression normal.

EXERCISE 33

STEP 1. Rhythm Determination

- Ventricular rate *92*
- QRS shape *Normal*

- R-R rhythm *Regular*
- QRS interval *0.10*
- QT interval *0.36*

- Atrial rate *92*
- P wave shape *Positive except negative III and aVR, and flat in aVF*
- P-P rhythm *Regular*
- P-R interval *0.28*
- P:R conduction ratio *1:1*

- Dominant pacemaker site *Sinus*
- Interpretation *NSR with 1st degree AV block*

STEP 2. Axis Determination

Normal axis

STEP 3. Chamber Enlargement Determination

None

STEP 4. Intraventricular Conduction Blocks Determination

IVCD

STEP 5. Ischemia, Injury, and Infarction Determination

ST segment elevations in leads II, III, and aVF with reciprocal depressions in leads I, aVL, and V1. T waves positive in all leads except aVR. Normal R wave progression.

EXERCISE 34

STEP 1. Rhythm Determination

- Ventricular rate *65*
- QRS shape *Slightly widened*

- R-R rhythm *Regular*
- QRS interval *0.10*
- QT interval *0.36*

- Atrial rate *65*
- P wave shape *Positive except negative in aVR*
- P-P rhythm *Regular*
- P-R interval *0.24*
- P:R conduction ratio *1:1*

- Dominant pacemaker site *Sinus*
- Interpretation *NSR with 1st degree AV block*

STEP 2. Axis Determination

Normal axis. Use null plane method.

STEP 3. Chamber Enlargement Determination

None

STEP 4. Intraventricular Conduction Blocks Determination

IVCD

STEP 5. Ischemia, Injury, and Infarction Determination

ST segments isoelectric. T waves positive in all leads except negative in leads I, aVR, aVL and V1–V4, and diphasic in V5–V6. Normal R wave progression.

EXERCISE 35

STEP 1. Rhythm Determination

- Ventricular rate *49*
- QRS shape *Normal*

- Atrial rate *49*
- P wave shape *Positive except negative in aVR, and flattened in III and aVL*

- R-R rhythm *Regular*
- QRS interval *0.10*
- QT interval *0.44*

- P-P rhythm *Regular*
- P-R interval *0.16*
- P:R conduction ratio *1:1*

- Dominant pacemaker site *Sinus*
- Interpretation *Sinus bradycardia*

STEP 2. Axis Determination

Normal axis

STEP 3. Chamber Enlargement Determination

None

STEP 4. Intraventricular Conduction Blocks Determination

IVCD

STEP 5. Ischemia, Injury, and Infarction Determination

ST segments isoelectric except J point ST elevations in leads V2–V3. T waves positive in all leads except negative in leads III, aVR, aVF. Tall R waves in leads V1–V2. Significant Q waves in leads II, III, and aVF.

EXERCISE 36

STEP 1. Rhythm Determination

- Ventricular rate *68*
- QRS shape *Normal*

- Atrial rate *68*
- P wave shape *Positive except negative in leads III and aVR and diphasic in V1*

- R-R rhythm *Regular*
- QRS interval *0.09*
- QT interval *0.36*

- P-P rhythm *Regular*
- P-R interval *0.14*
- P:R conduction ratio *1:1*

- Dominant pacemaker site *Sinus*
- Interpretation *NSR*

STEP 2. Axis Determination

Left axis. Use null plane method.

STEP 3. Chamber Enlargement Determination

None

STEP 4. Intraventricular Conduction Blocks Determination

Normal conduction

STEP 5. Ischemia, Injury, and Infarction Determination

ST segment elevations in leads I, aVL, V2–V6. T waves positive in all leads except negative in leads III and aVR and flattened in lead aVF. Poor R wave progression. Significant Q waves in leads I and aVL.

7

Miscellaneous ECG Changes

STEP 6

The *sixth step* in the systematic process is to examine the electrocardiogram for other conditions that may affect it. This chapter contains a potpourri of conditions that may cause changes in the ECG.

ELECTROLYTES

Hypokalemia

Hypokalemia is a serum potassium level less than 3.5 mEq/L. Look for the following ECG changes in all 12 leads (Figure 7.1) when assessing a patient for hypokalemia (Marriott, 1988):

Mild Hypokalemia
- ST segment depression
- Flattening of T wave
- Prominent U wave
- P wave increases in size
- P-R interval lengthens

Severe Hypokalemia
- ST segment becomes more depressed
- T wave inverts
- U wave taller than T wave
- QRS widens uniformly

Some of the above ECG changes will not be as apparent in all leads. The magnitude of the changes are dependent on the potassium level.

Hyperkalemia

Hyperkalemia is a serum potassium level greater than 5.0 mEq/L. Look for the following distinctive ECG changes (Figure 7.2) when assessing a patient for hyperkalemia (Surawicz, 1967):

Serum Potassium
- >5.5 mEq/L
- >6.5 mEq/L
- >7.0 mEq/L

ECG Change
- Peaking of T wave
- Widened QRS
- P wave amplitude decreases
- Duration of P wave increases
- P-R interval frequently prolonged

Serum Potassium
- >8.8 mEq/L
- 12–14 mEq/L

ECG Change
- P wave frequently invisible
- Ventricular asystole or fibrillation

Hypocalcemia

Hypocalcemia occurs when the serum calcium level falls below 8.6 mg/dl. Hypocalcemia causes lengthening of the QT interval by causing the ST segment to lengthen. The T wave generally is unaffected but may become diphasic with a terminal negative deflection (Marriott, 1988).

Hypercalcemia

Hypercalcemia occurs when the serum calcium level rises above 10.4 mg/dl. Hypercalcemia causes shortening of the QT interval. The shortening occurs between the beginning of the QRS to the beginning of the T wave (Figure 7.3). The most characteristic change in the T wave is that its initial portion rapidly upslopes to its peak (Marriott, 1988).

CLINICAL SIGNIFICANCE

Fluctuations in potassium and calcium levels affect the electrical activity and therefore normal function of myocardial cells. Their serum levels must be monitored carefully. This is especially important in the patient who is ischemic because unless replaced, low serum potassium and calcium levels will increase the likelihood of

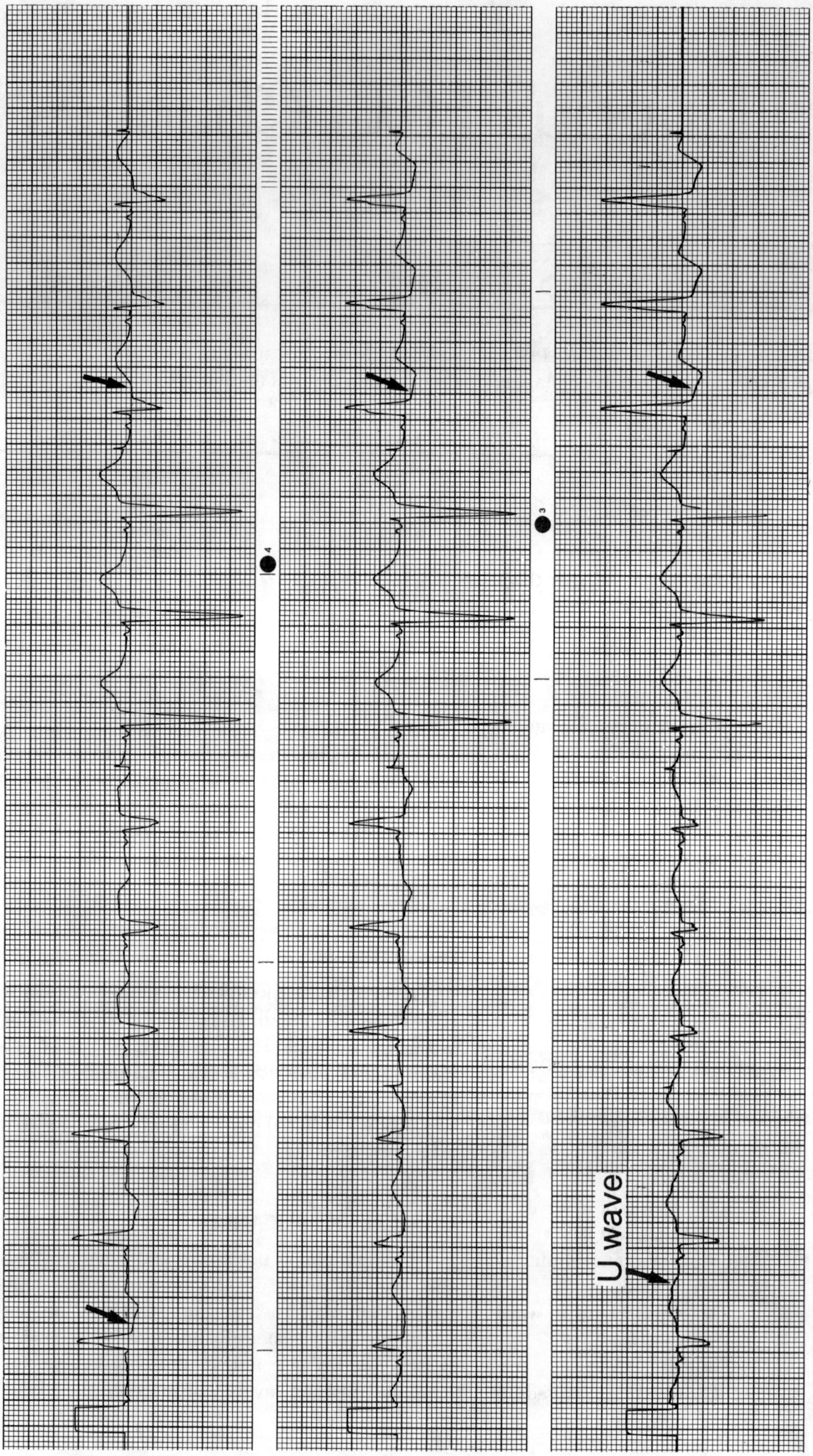

Figure 7.1. Hypokalemia. Note the depressed ST segments. Note U waves. Potassium level = 2.1.

U wave

6

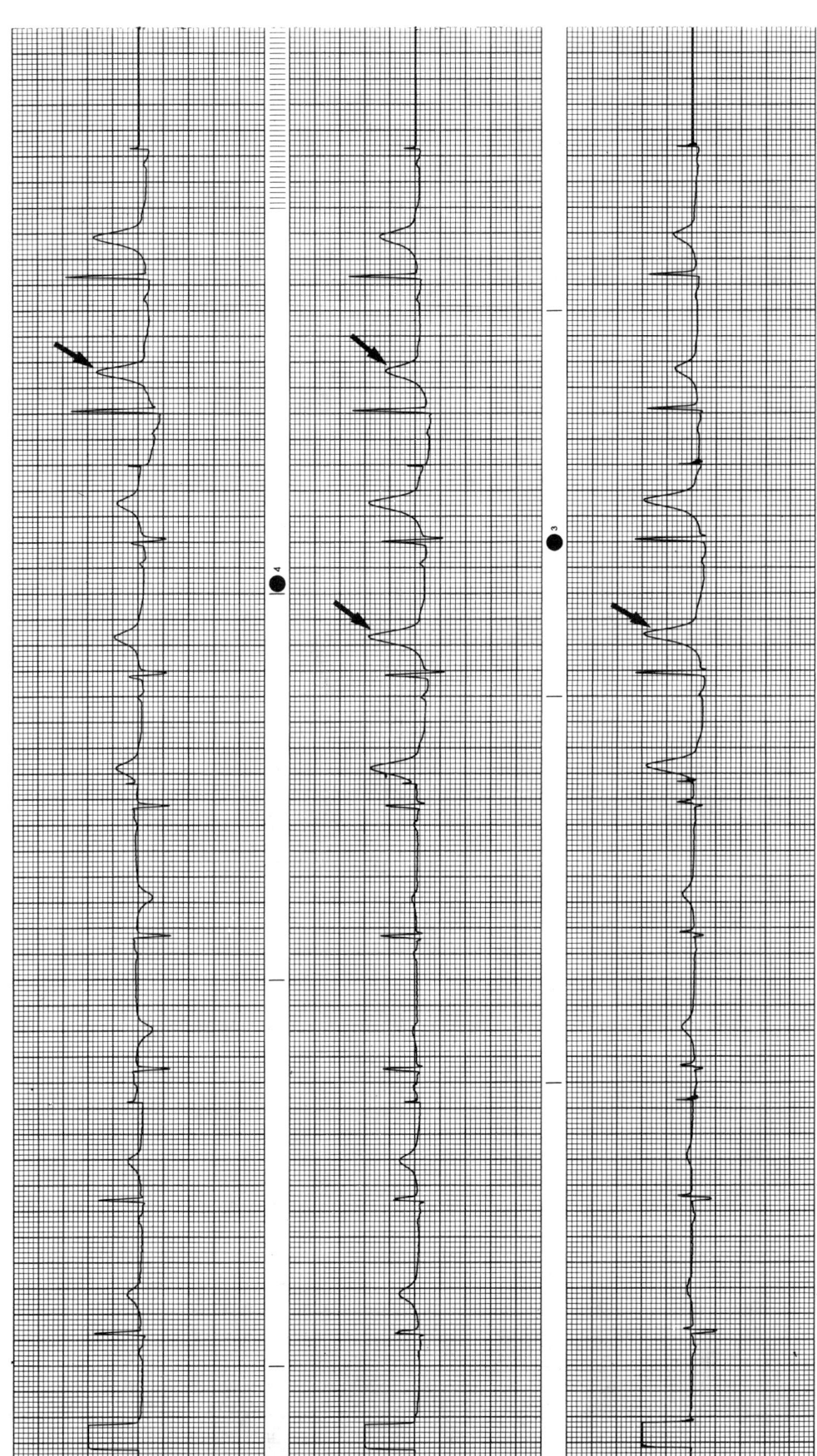

Figure 7.2. Hyperkalemia. Note the peaking of T waves, especially in leads V2–V5. Potassium level = 6.3.

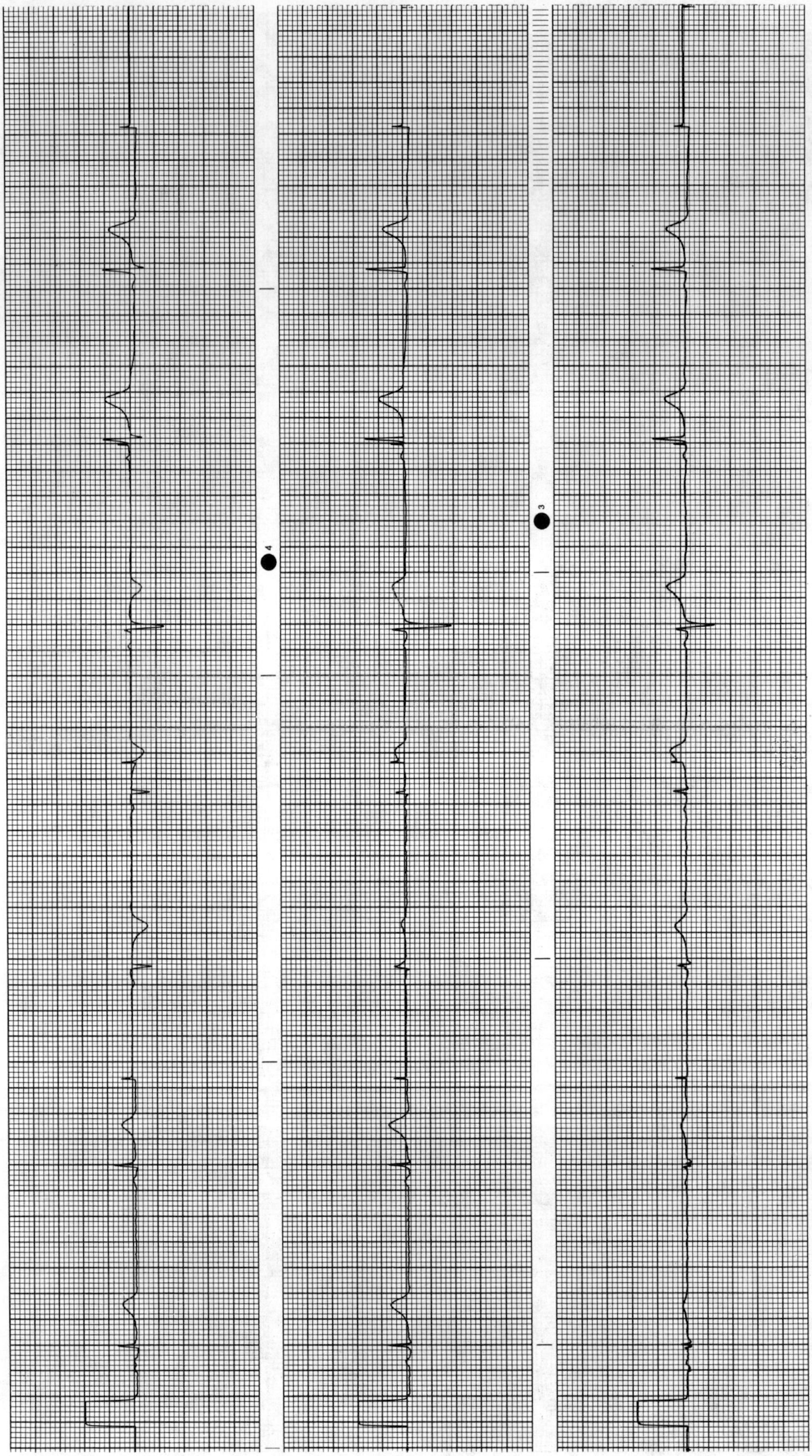

Figure 7.3. Hypercalcemia. Note the shortening of QT interval and the rapid initial upstroke to T wave peaks. QT interval = 0.41; corrected QT interval = 0.53; calcium level = 15.

ventricular dysrhythmias. A low serum potassium level will also potentiate the toxic effects of a high serum digoxin level and increase the likelihood of death in the unmonitored patient (Marriott, 1988).

A low serum calcium level will affect contractility of heart muscle. As the serum calcium level falls, the contractile force of the myocardium will decrease. If the calcium level falls far enough, cardiac arrest will occur (Berne and Levy, 1986).

Clinically, patients with high potassium and calcium levels have increased ventricular irritability and increased incidence of sudden cardiac death. It is especially important to monitor the ECG when rapidly replacing potassium intravenously. Shifts in serum levels can happen quickly, especially in critically ill patients with shifting acid-base balances.

A high serum calcium level will also enhance myocardial contractile force. As contractility increases, so does myocardial demand. In patients with already compromised myocardial blood flow, this increased demand can cause ischemia. If calcium levels continue to rise, cardiac arrest can occur as a result of tetany of the heart muscle (Berne and Levy, 1986).

DRUG EFFECTS

Two drugs will be discussed in this section, digitalis and quinidine. Both produce global or diffuse ECG changes. The most obvious change produced by digitalis is in the ST segment (Figure 7.4). Therapeutic levels of this drug will produce globally sagging ST segments. Marriott (1988) describes them as having the appearance of being pulled down by a hooked finger. Dubin (1989) likens them to Salvador Dali's moustache. At the same time the ST segments are sagging, the T waves will be either flattened or inverted. Both of these changes typically occur in leads with tall R waves.

The other segment of the ECG that will be affected is the P-R interval. The P-R will lengthen in individuals receiving digitalis preparations. Some may even develop first degree AV block.

Unlike digitalis, quinidine affects only the ventricular portion of the ECG. It may cause T waves to be depressed, widened, notched, or inverted. The QT interval will lengthen due to widening of the QRS. In this step, measure the QT interval and remember to correct it for heart rate.

CLINICAL SIGNIFICANCE

Digitalis slows the transmission of the atrial impulse through the AV node. It is frequently used to slow the ventricular rate in atrial fibrillation. Individuals receiving digitalis therapy may develop a first degree AV block.

The development of a first degree block is not cause for stopping the drug unless it is markedly prolonged. Clinically, the most important aspect of the nursing care of these patients is to monitor their ECG for progression of a block. If the patient develops a prolonged first degree, second degree, or third degree AV block, the drug should be held and the rhythm reported to the physician.

The diffuse ST and T wave changes are of no clinical significance. They are due to the drug effect alone. The important point is to recognize them and not to mistake them for ischemic changes. It is also important to realize that when they are present, the ECG cannot be used to diagnose ischemia.

When a patient is receiving quinidine therapy, it is very important to monitor the QT interval. One of the most serious problems that can be caused by quinidine therapy is torsades de pointes. Briefly, this is a type of ventricular tachycardia, usually with a rate greater than 250, that generally degenerates into ventricular fibrillation. The warning sign that this may be developing is a lengthening QT interval. Because quinidine is known to lengthen the QT interval, it is important to monitor QT intervals in these patients for prolongation. If the width of the QRS complex lengthens to 50% or more of its baseline value, the drug should be held and the physician notified.

PERICARDITIS

The last condition of the potpourri discussed in this chapter is pericarditis. Pericarditis is a condition caused by inflammation of the pericardial sac, which is a membranous sac surrounding the heart. The inflammation may be caused by a bacterial or viral infection, some chemotherapy drugs such as adriamycin, and radiation therapy to the chest wall. It can also be secondary to a myocardial infarction and commonly occurs with inferior infarctions.

The ECG changes that occur with pericarditis are diffuse. In the acute stage, which lasts from 10 days to 2 weeks, the ST segments will appear *concave* and be *elevated* globally with upright T waves. P-R intervals will appear depressed except in lead aVR, where the P-R interval will be elevated and the ST segment will be depressed (Figure 7.5). In the later stage, from 2 weeks to 4 weeks, the ST segments will return to baseline and the T waves will invert or may just flatten (Marriott, 1988). Therefore, in this step look for ST segment and T wave changes.

CLINICAL SIGNIFICANCE

Because patients with pericarditis may also have acute chest pain and their ECG may appear like that of

6

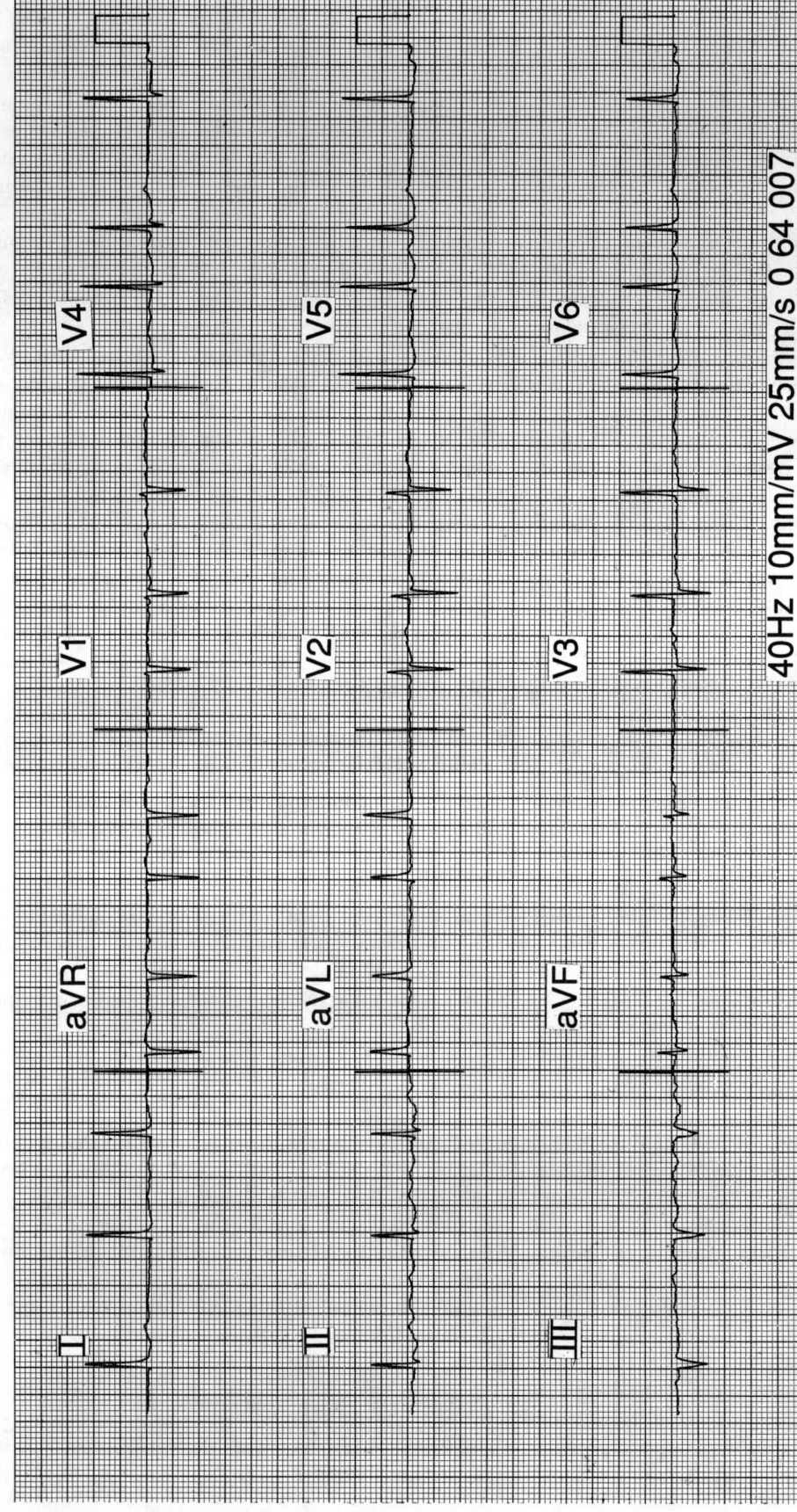

Figure 7.4.   Digitalis effect. Note the global sagging of ST segments and the flattening of T waves.

6

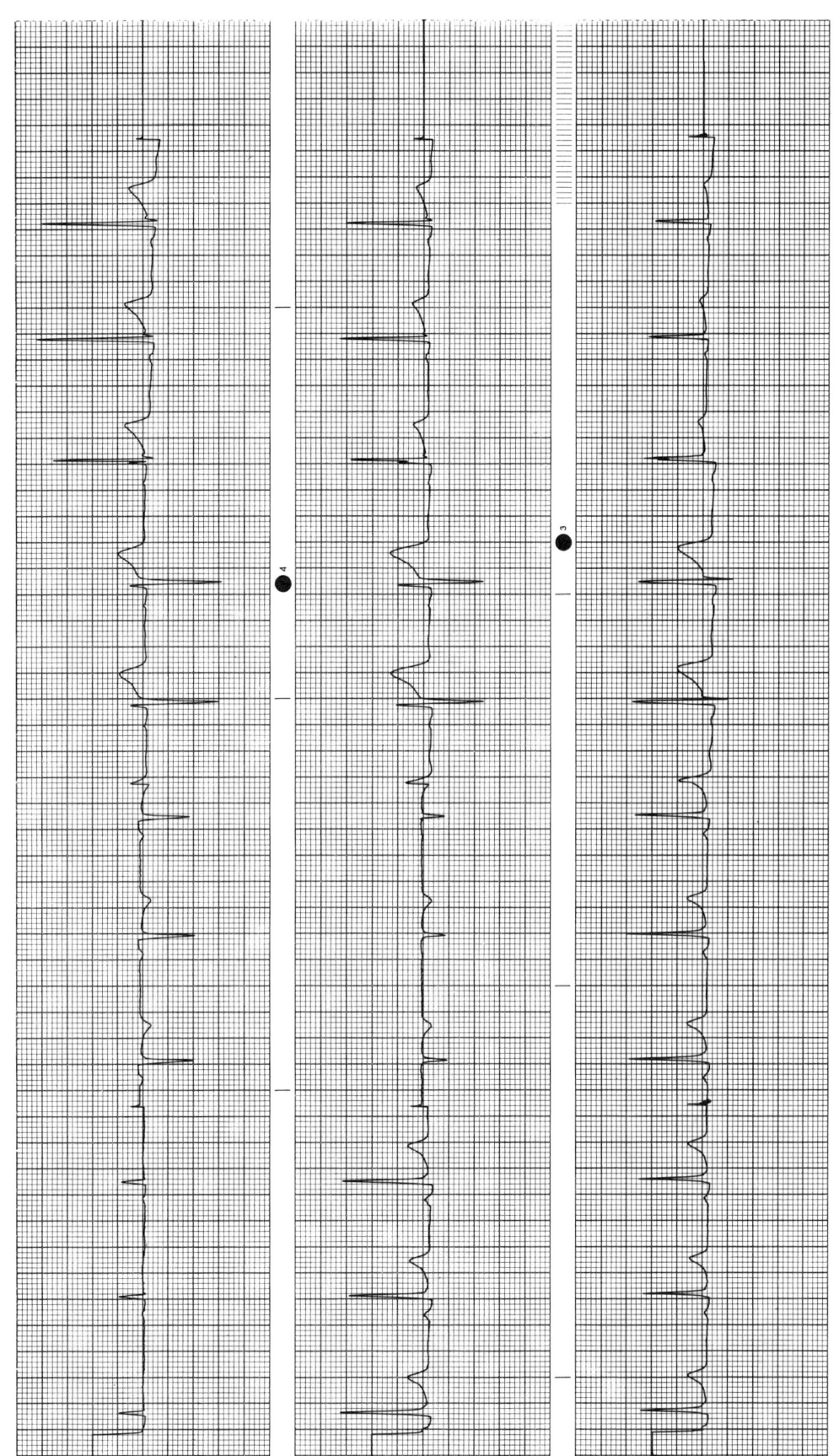

Figure 7.5. Pericarditis. Note the elevated ST segments that are concave in appearance globally. In aVR note the elevated P-R interval and the depressed ST segment.

MAR

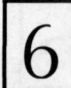

someone having an infarct, it is important to be able to differentiate between the two. The most important clue is that the ST segment elevations in pericarditis appear in most of the 12 leads and have a concave shape rather than the convex shape of an infarction. Another clue is the quality of the pain. Pericardial pain is pleuritic in nature and usually positional. When positional, it will intensify when the patient's position causes the heart to come closer to the chest wall, such as sitting up and leaning forward or lying in the left lateral position.

Key questions to ask yourself when performing this step of the systematic process are:

Are ST segment changes present?
- Assess the shape and direction of the ST segment change
  Are they diffusely concave and elevated = acute pericarditis
  Are they sagging in all leads with a tall R wave = digitalis effect
  Are they diffusely depressed with flattened T waves = hypokalemia
- Assess the length of the ST segment
  Are they lengthened = hypocalcemia
  Are they shortened with rapidly upsloping T waves = hypercalcemia

Are T wave changes present?
- Assess the shape and direction of the T waves
  Are they flattened = hypokalemia (mild)
  Are they inverted = severe hypokalemia
  Are they tall and peaked = hyperkalemia
  Are the initial segments rapidly upsloping = hypercalcemia

What is the QT interval?
- Measure the QT interval and correct it for heart rate
  Is it shortened = hypercalcemia
  It is lengthened = hypocalcemia or quinidine effect

What is the patient's clinical and drug history?
- Assess current drug therapy
- Monitor drug and electrolyte levels
- Correlate with any rhythm disturbances

Does the patient have signs and symptoms of pericarditis?
- Assess vital signs
- Assess quality of chest pain:
  Does it have a pleuritic nature?
  Does it intensify or improve with position changes?
- Assess ECG for diffuse concave elevations of ST segments
- Assess for atrial dysrhythmias such as PACs, atrial fibrillation, and atrial flutter

SELF-ASSESSMENT EXERCISES 37–42

In the following six ECG examples complete the following steps:

Step one:	Determination of Rhythm
Step two:	Determination of Axis
Step three:	Determination of Chamber Enlargement
Step four:	Determination of Intraventricular Conduction Blocks
Step five:	Determination of Ischemia, Injury, or Infarction
Step six:	Miscellaneous ECG changes
	Electrolytes ___Drugs ___Pericarditis ___ Other ___

You must be able to perform these steps successfully before proceeding. When you have completed all of the exercises in this book, come back to this exercise and complete the remaining step of the *systematic approach*.

Check your answers with the suggested interpretations found at the end of this chapter. Answers for the remaining step will be found in Appendix A.

6

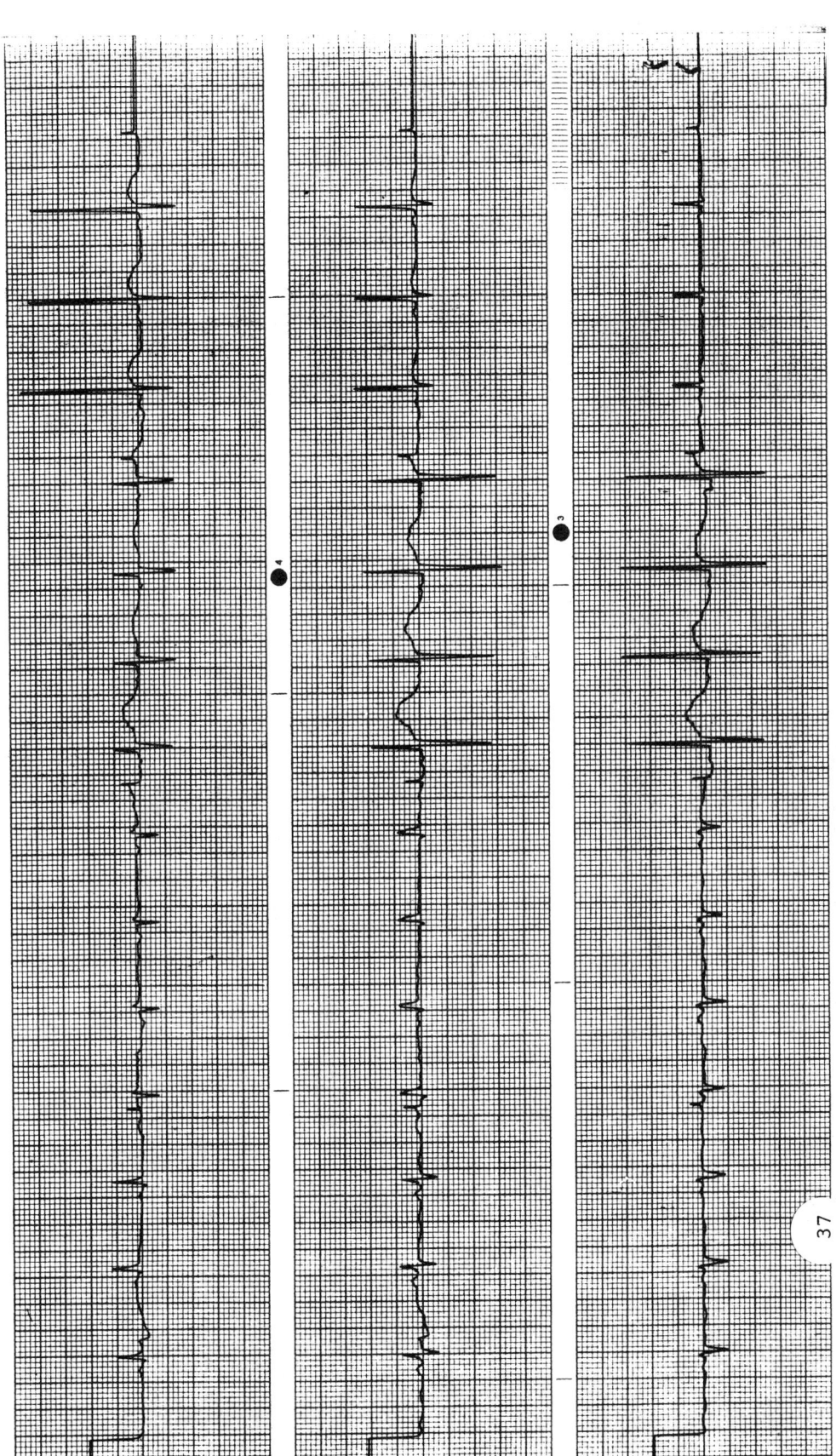

Exercise 37. A 26-year-old man admitted in acute diabetic ketoacidosis. Potassium levels were drawn and were abnormal.

37

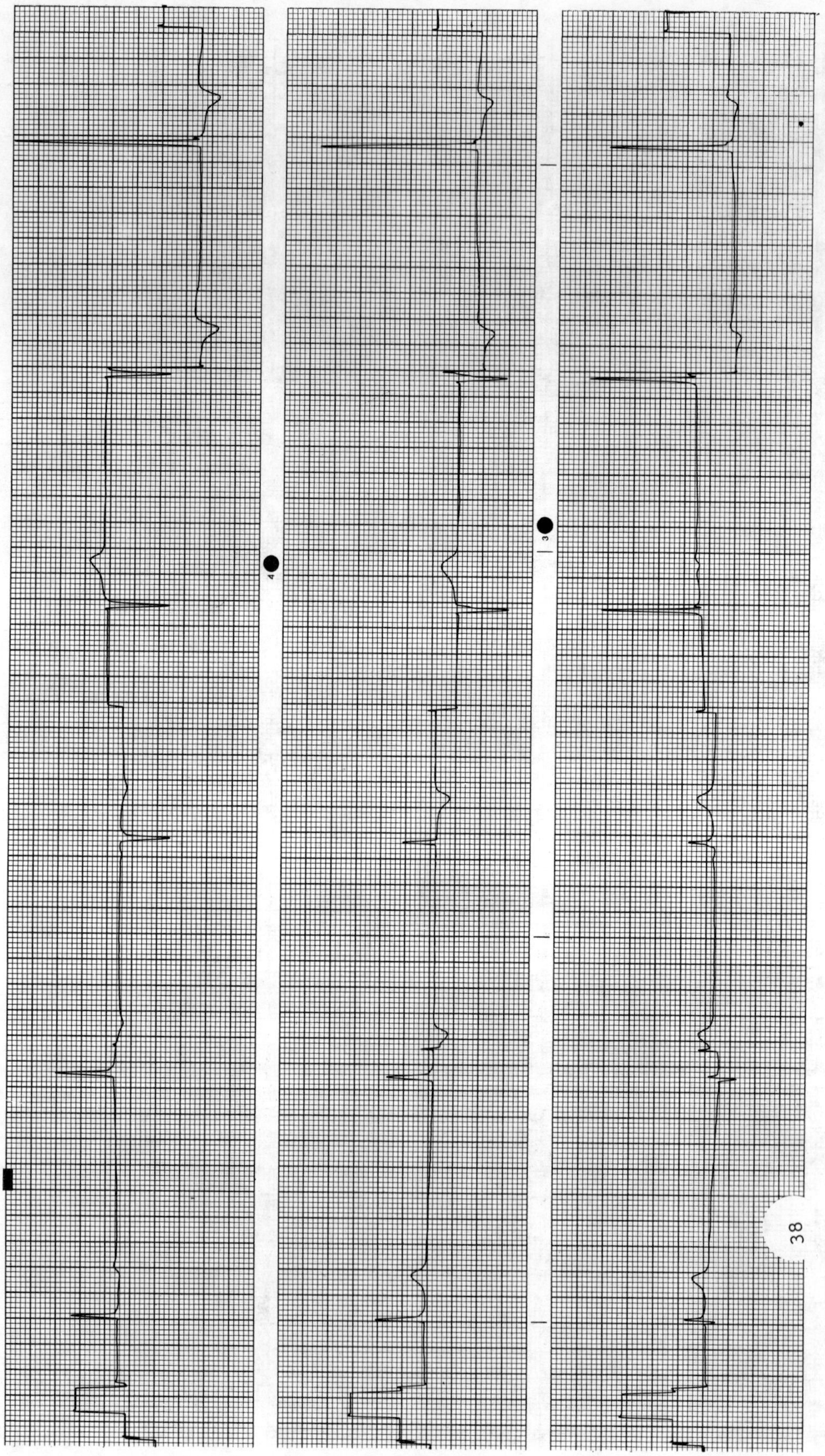

Exercise 38. A 72-year-old woman admitted with severe shortness of breath. History of chronic congestive heart failure. Presently on digoxin daily.

38

6

Exercise 39. A 55-year-old woman admitted with upper right quadrant abdominal pain. Calcium levels were drawn and were abnormal.

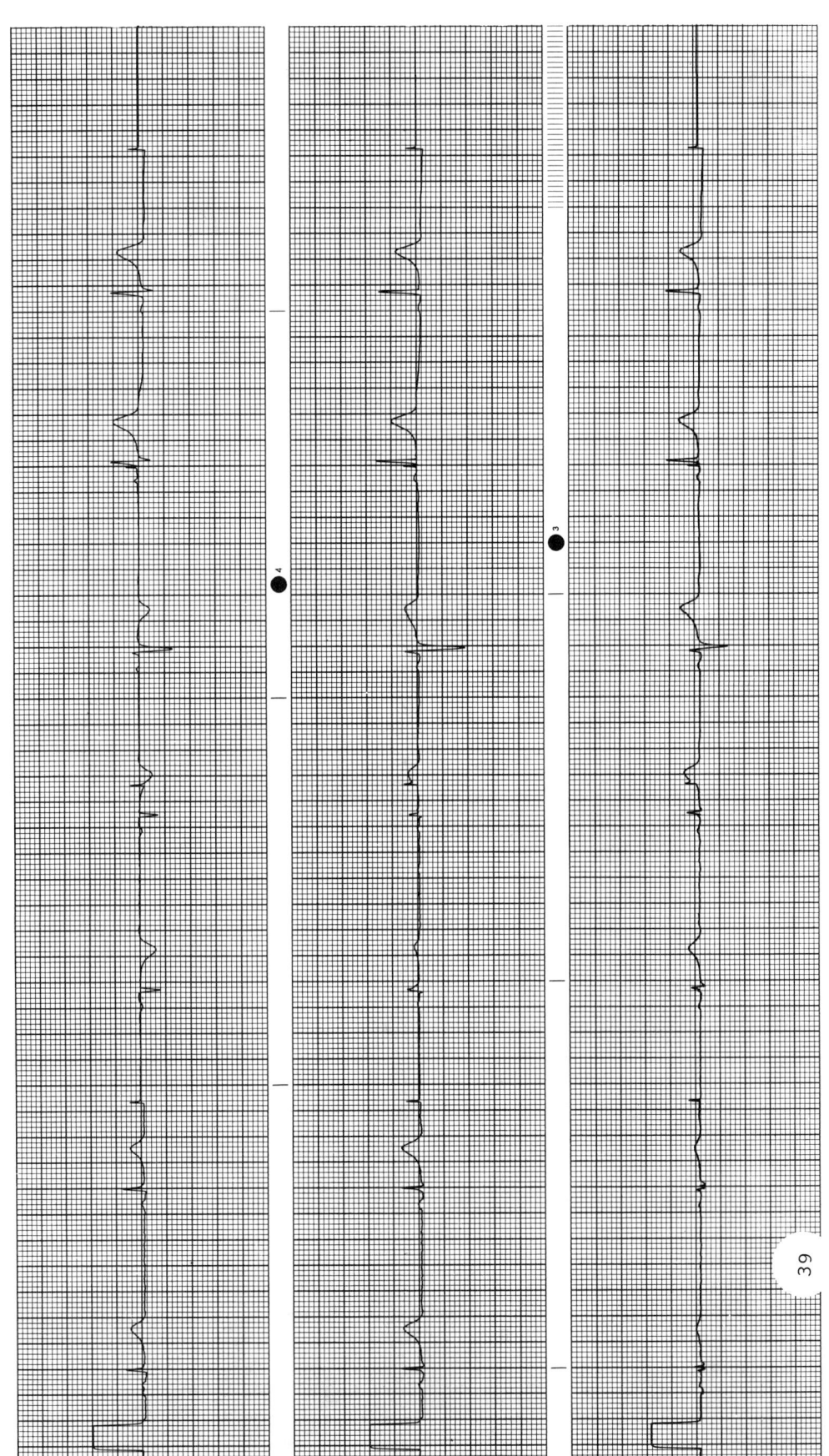

39

6

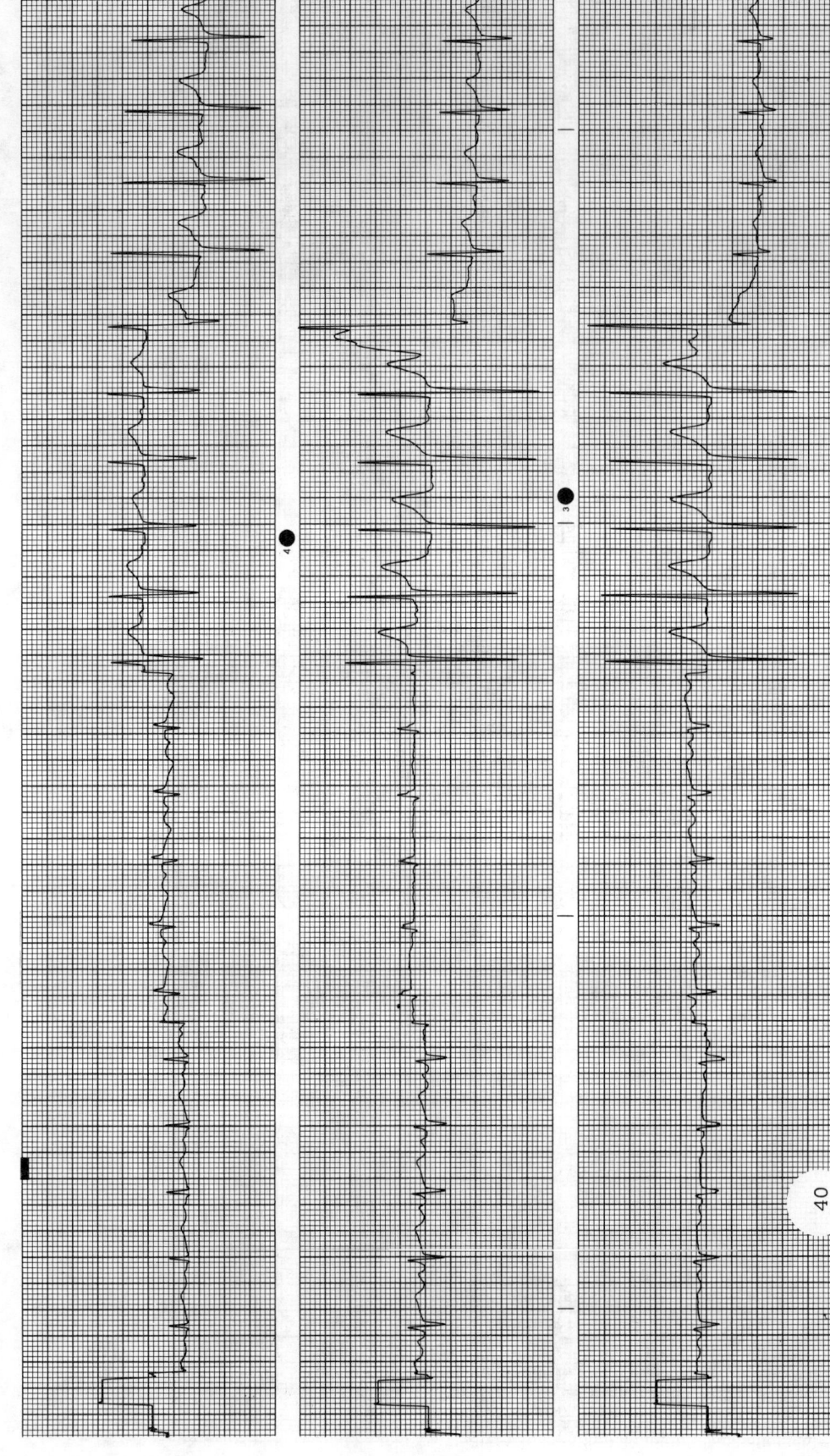

Exercise 40. A 26-year-old man admitted in acute diabetic ketoacidosis. Potassium levels were abnormal.

40

6

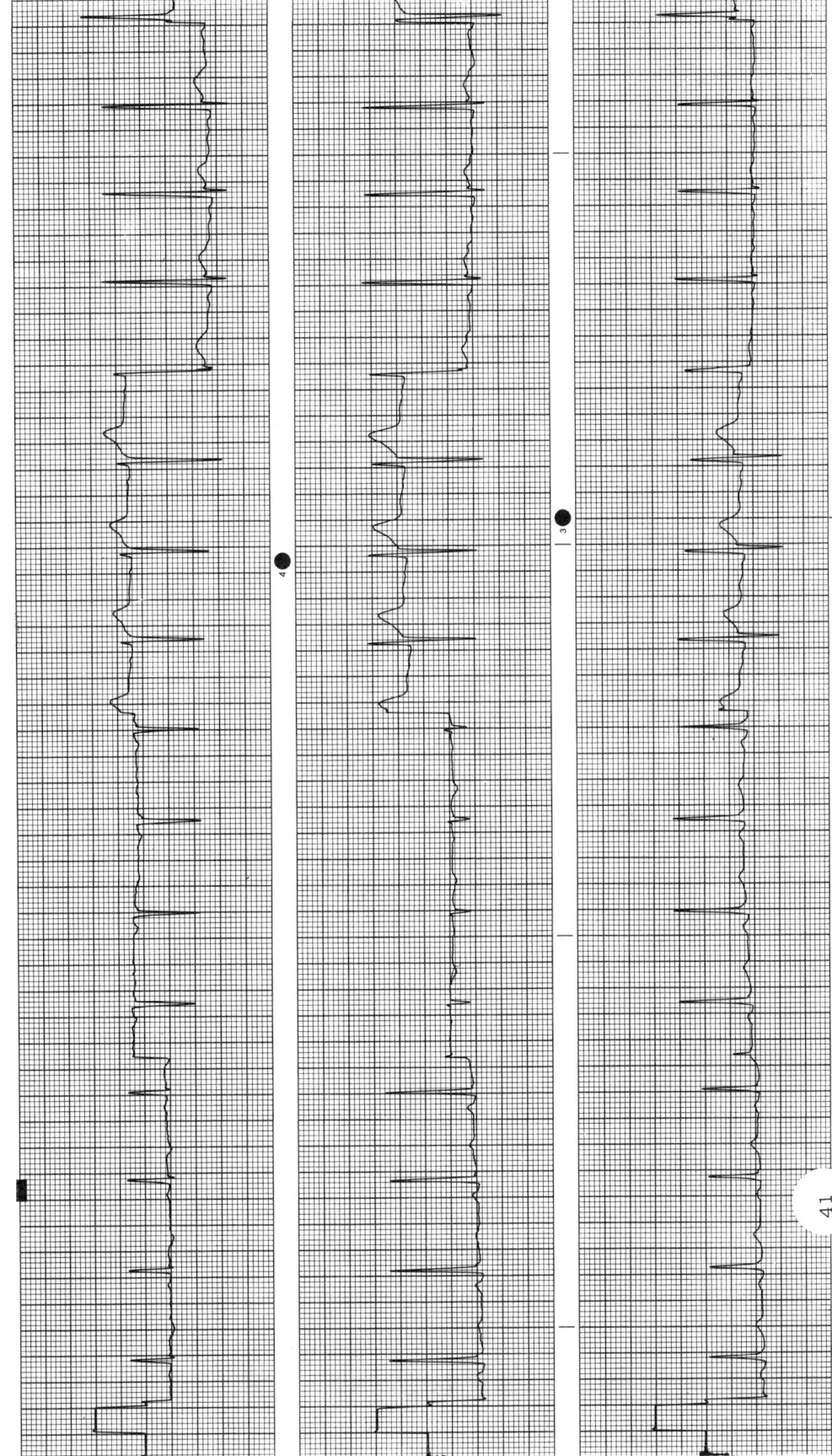

Exercise 41. A 45-year-old man admitted with unstable angina. Negative cardiac enzymes.

41

6

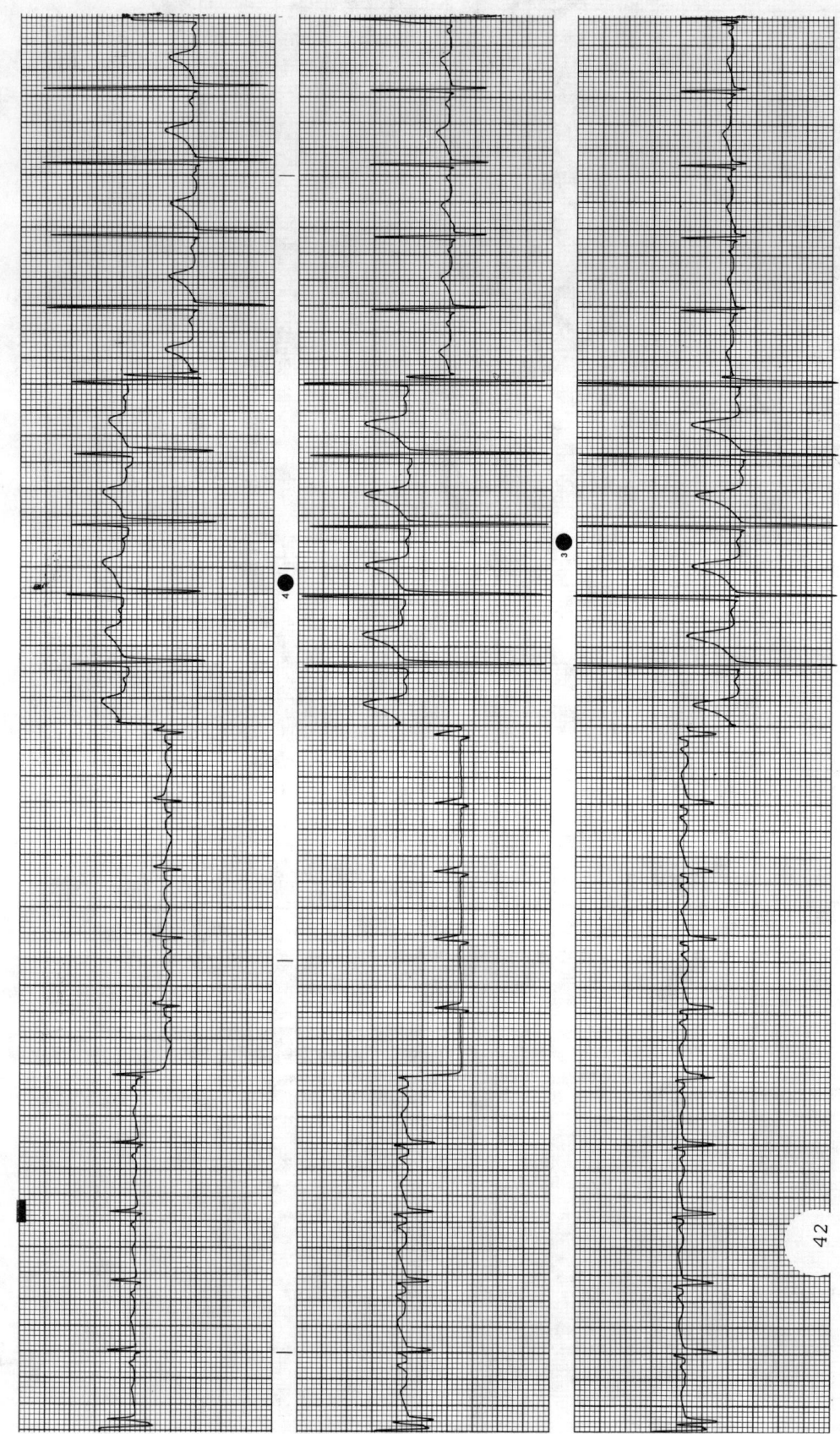

Exercise 42.   A 38-year-old man admitted with acute pancreatitis. Electrolytes were drawn.

SELF-ASSESSMENT ANSWERS TO EXERCISES 37–42

6

EXERCISE 37

STEP 1. Rhythm Determination

- Ventricular rate *90*
- QRS shape *Normal*

- Atrial rate *90*
- P wave shape *Positive except negative in aVR, flattened in aVL, and diphasic in V1*

- R-R rhythm *Regular*
- QRS interval *0.08*
- QT interval *0.36*

- P-P rhythm *Regular*
- P-R interval *0.12*
- P:R conduction ratio *1:1*

- Dominant pacemaker site *Sinus*
- Interpretation *NSR*

STEP 2. Axis Determination

Left axis

STEP 3. Chamber Enlargement Determination

None

STEP 4. Intraventricular Conduction Blocks Determination

LAH

STEP 5. Ischemia, Injury, and Infarction Determination

ST segments isoelectric. T waves diffusely flattened. U waves present. Normal R wave progression.

STEP 6. Miscellaneous ECG Changes

Diffuse T wave changes and presence of U waves suggestive of hypokalemia.

EXERCISE 38

STEP 1. Rhythm Determination

- Ventricular rate *38*
- QRS shape *Normal*
- R-R rhythm *Slightly irregular*
- QRS interval *0.08*
- QT interval *0.44*

- Atrial rate *=*
- P wave shape *=*
- P-P rhythm *=*

- P-R interval *=*
- P:R conduction ratio *=*

- Dominant pacemaker site *AV junctional*
- Interpretation *Slow junctional rhythm*

STEP 2. Axis Determination

Normal axis

STEP 3. Chamber Enlargement Determination

LVH

STEP 4. Intraventricular Conduction Blocks Determination

Normal conduction

STEP 5. Ischemia, Injury, and Infarction Determination

ST segments depressed and upwardly coved in leads with tall R waves. T waves inverted in same leads. Normal R wave progression.

STEP 6. Miscellaneous ECG Changes

No significant findings. The ECG changes that are seen with digitalis therapy are being masked in this patient by the ST and T wave changes caused by LVH. The slow junctional rhythm is of concern and may be a result of digitalis toxicity.

6

EXERCISE 39

STEP 1. Rhythm Determination

- Ventricular rate *46*
- QRS shape *Small but normal*

- Atrial rate *46*
- P wave shape *Positive except negative in aVR*

- R-R rhythm *Regular*
- QRS interval *0.08*
- QT interval *0.44*

- P-P rhythm *Regular*
- P-R interval *0.15*
- P:R conduction ratio *1:1*

- Dominant pacemaker site *Sinus*
- Interpretation *Marked sinus bradycardia*

STEP 2. Axis Determination

Normal axis

STEP 3. Chamber Enlargement Determination

None

STEP 4. Intraventricular Conduction Blocks Determination

Normal conduction

STEP 5. Ischemia, Injury, and Infarction Determination

ST segments isoelectric. T waves positive in all leads except negative in aVR and V1. Normal R wave progression.

STEP 6. Miscellaneous ECG Changes

Measured QT interval is 0.44 seconds. The corrected QT interval for this heart rate is 0.53 seconds. The portion of the QT that appears shortened is the ST segment. These changes may be significant for hypercalcemia.

EXERCISE 40

STEP 1. Rhythm Determination

- Ventricular rate *120*
- QRS shape *Normal*

- Atrial rate *120*
- P wave shape *Positive except negative in aVR and flattened in aVL*

- R-R rhythm *Regular*
- QRS interval *0.09*
- QT interval *0.34*

- P-P rhythm *Regular*
- P-R interval *0.12*
- P:R conduction ratio *1:1*

- Dominant pacemaker site *Sinus*
- Interpretation *Sinus tachycardia*

STEP 2. Axis Determination

Left axis

STEP 3. Chamber Enlargement Determination

None

STEP 4. Intraventricular Conduction Blocks Determination

LAH

STEP 5. Ischemia, Injury, and Infarction Determination

ST segments isoelectric. T waves tall, pointed, and pinched in chest leads. Tall R waves in V1–V3.

STEP 6. Miscellaneous ECG Changes

Peaked T waves significant for hyperkalemia

EXERCISE 41

STEP 1. Rhythm Determination

- Ventricular rate *88*
- QRS shape *Normal*

- Atrial rate *88*
- P wave shape *Positive except negative in aVR and aVL*

- R-R rhythm *Regular*
- QRS interval *0.06*
- QT interval *0.34*

- P-P rhythm *Regular*
- P-R interval *0.16*
- P:R conduction ratio *1:1*

- Dominant pacemaker site *Sinus*
- Interpretation *NSR*

STEP 2. Axis Determination

Normal axis

STEP 3. Chamber Enlargement Determination

LVH no strain pattern

STEP 4. Intraventricular Conduction Blocks Determination

Normal conduction

STEP 5. Ischemia, Injury, and Infarction Determination

ST segments concave shaped and diffusely elevated. T waves positive in all leads except negative in leads I, aVR, and aVL. Normal R wave progression.

STEP 6. Miscellaneous ECG Changes

ST segments diffusely elevated and concave in shape. P-R segment elevated in lead aVR with a depressed ST segment in that same lead. Changes significant for pericarditis.

EXERCISE 42

STEP 1. Rhythm Determination

- Ventricular rate *115*
- QRS shape *Normal*

- Atrial rate *115*
- P wave shape *Positive except negative in aVR and flattened in aVL*

- R-R rhythm *Regular*
- QRS interval *0.08*
- QT interval *0.34*

- P-P rhythm *Regular*
- P-R interval *0.13*
- P:R conduction ratio *1:1*

- Dominant pacemaker site *Sinus*
- Interpretation *Sinus tachycardia*

STEP 2. Axis Determination

Left axis

STEP 3. Chamber Enlargement Determination

None

STEP 4. Intraventricular Conduction Blocks Determination

LAH

STEP 5. Ischemia, Injury, and Infarction Determination

ST segments isoelectric. T waves tall, pointed, and pinched in leads V1–V4. Tall R waves in leads V1–V3.

STEP 6. Miscellaneous ECG Changes

Tall peaked T waves indicative of hyperkalemia

8

Final Interpretation

$$\boxed{\text{STEP 7}}$$

Final interpretation is the *seventh* and last *step* in the recommended systematic process. It incorporates the analysis and interpretation of the data you have collected. The analysis will be based on the patient's clinical and drug history. It will identify what treatment if any may be needed.

This chapter will describe the final interpretation step and review the steps of the systematic process. It will also provide sufficient ECG exercises to practice utilizing the systematic process, steps 1–7.

FINAL INTERPRETATION

In this final step, you will restate the rhythm diagnosis and establish a 12-lead ECG interpretation. You will base the interpretation on the data you have collected at each step. The data will be correlated to the patient's clinical and drug history, such that if the patient has had an old anterior wall myocardial infarction (MI), you would look for old ECG changes confirming this. Or if the patient were on digoxin, you would look for digoxin effects on the ECG. The data should also be compared with the patient's baseline or previous ECG, if available. A final interpretation diagnosis could be atrial fibrillation and acute inferior wall MI.

This step is important because you must decide whether the changes are new and significant. You must determine whether the changes should be reported, how soon, and to whom. You must determine whether the changes are affecting the patient's cardiac output. Thus you should take the patient's vital signs, listen to his/her lungs, and assess him/her for chest pain and other signs of ischemia.

The interpretation will determine what treatment is needed. Treatment might include drawing cardiac enzymes, giving drugs to control dysrhythmias or chest pain, preparing for pacemaker insertion, preparing for thrombolytic therapy, switching monitoring leads, or just observing for other changes in the ECG configurations.

REVIEW OF STEPS

Table 8.1 provides an overview of the seven steps and identifies some essential points to consider at each step. If still unsure, reread appropriate chapters. For more detailed explanations on any of the information written and discussed in this book, see any of the excellent textbooks listed in the bibliography.

Step 1. In this step, you will determine the rhythm diagnosis. Is it normal sinus rhythm, atrial fibrillation, or some other dysrhythmia? It is recommended you use leads II, V1, and V6 in this step. Treat all dysrhythmias that are affecting the patient's cardiac output. Study the QRS, QT interval, and the P wave for possible clues to other abnormalities in the 12-lead ECG.

Step 2. In this step, you will determine whether the axis is normal, deviated to the right, left, or indeterminate. Axis provides a clue to other ECG changes present. It is recommended you use leads I and aVF to determine the axis. Remember this provides an estimate of the axis, not the specific degrees.

Step 3. In this step, you will determine chamber enlargement. Chamber enlargements interpreted on an ECG are either right or left atrial abnormalities, or right or left ventricular hypertrophy. It is recommended that you look at the P waves in leads II and V1 for atrial abnormalities, and look at the QRS configuration in leads V1 or V2 and V5 or V6 for ventricular hypertrophy.

7

Table 8.1.
Systematic Approach Flow Chart[a]

Systematic Approach

Step 1   Rhythm Determination

> If symptoms of low CO, treat first.
> If wide QRS and not ventricular dysrhythmias, look for BBB.
> If abnormal QT interval, look for miscellaneous causes.
> If notched or widened P wave, look for atrial abnormalities.

Step 2   Axis Determination

> If RAD, look for LPH, RVH, or lateral MI.
> If LAD, look for LAH, LVH, or inferior MI.

Step 3   Chamber Enlargement Determination

> Examine height and width of P waves in leads II and V1 for atrial abnormalities.
> Examine chest leads V1 or V2 and V5 or V6, comparing height of R and S waves for ventricular hypertrophy.

Step 4   IVCB Determination

> Examine leads I and III for hemiblocks.
> Examine width and configuration of QRS in leads V1 and V6 for bundle branch blocks.

Step 5   Ischemia, Injury, Infarction Determination

> Analyze ST segment, T wave, and Q wave findings.
> Look for normal R wave progression in V leads.
> Note in which leads changes found.
> Determine age of changes.
> Determine differential diagnosis.

Step 6   Miscellaneous ECG Changes

> Analyze ST segment, T wave, and QT intervals.
> Monitor drug and serum electrolyte levels.

Step 7   Final Interpretation

> Compare changes with previous ECG.
> Correlate with clinical and drug history.
> Report any new significant findings.
> Treat as necessary.

[a] **Abbreviations: CO = cardiac output; BBB = bundle branch block; RAD = right axis deviation; LPH = left posterior hemiblock; RVH = right ventricular hypertrophy; LAD = left axis deviation; LAH = left anterior hemiblock; LVH = left ventricular hypertrophy; IVCB = intraventricular conduction block.**

Step 4. In this step, you will determine the presence of intraventricular conduction blocks. It is recommended you look at the limb leads, especially leads I and III for hemiblocks. For the presence of bundle branch blocks (BBBs), look at the chest leads, especially V1 and V6, for QRS configurations that are widened and different in shape.

Step 5. In this step, you will determine the presence of myocardial ischemia, injury, or infarction. Look for specific ST segment and T wave changes, and for the presence of significant Q waves. Then determine in which leads these changes are occurring and their age.

Step 6. In this step, you will determine whether selected miscellaneous ECG changes are present, such as electrolyte imbalances, drug effects, and other conditions. Look for changes in the ST segment and T wave, and for changes in the QT interval.

Step 7. In the final step, you will establish a 12-lead ECG interpretation and combine it with a rhythm diagnosis. Then be prepared to act on the information you have collected.

CLINICAL SIGNIFICANCE

The ability to interpret a 12-lead ECG is clinically a very useful skill for health care practitioners. It assists in determining what monitoring lead to use for a patient with a certain diagnosis, and it identifies signs, symptoms, and problems requiring assessment and enables you to prepare for appropriate treatment. It also assists in helping you to decide when to notify the physician.

Applying a systematic approach to interpreting a 12-lead ECG makes it easier for you to analyze and hopefully utilize in your clinical practice. Also, practicing this skill will assist you in learning.

Key questions to ask at this step are:

What is the clinical and drug history of this patient?
- Assess for history of an MI, hypertension, or angina.
- Monitor serum drug and electrolyte levels.
- Assess drug history.

How does this ECG compare with the patient's baseline and previous ECG?
- Report significant changes to the physician.
- Look for widening QRS intervals or P-R intervals.
- Look for new ST segment and T wave changes.
- Look for dysrhythmias.
- Assess for axis changes.

Are these changes new or old?
- If new, report.

Should I report these changes?
- All new significant changes should be reported.

What is the significance of the interpretation in terms of the patient's condition?
- Assess vital signs, lung, and heart sounds.
- Assess for angina and signs and symptoms of decreased cardiac output.

What treatment should I prepare to administer?
- Provide oxygen.
- Establish an IV.
- Initiate Rx as ordered.
- Be prepared for electrical, thrombolytic, or drug therapy.
- Order appropriate laboratory work such as cardiac enzymes or electrolytes.

SELF-ASSESSMENT EXERCISES 43–67

In the following 25 ECG examples, apply the complete systematic process. Use the self-assessment form and the study guide found in the Appendix to assist you in interpreting these 12-lead ECG examples. Remember to consider the clinical situation provided with each example. Also try to consider what treatment, if any, you think might be indicated.

Check your answers with the suggested interpretations found at the end of this chapter.

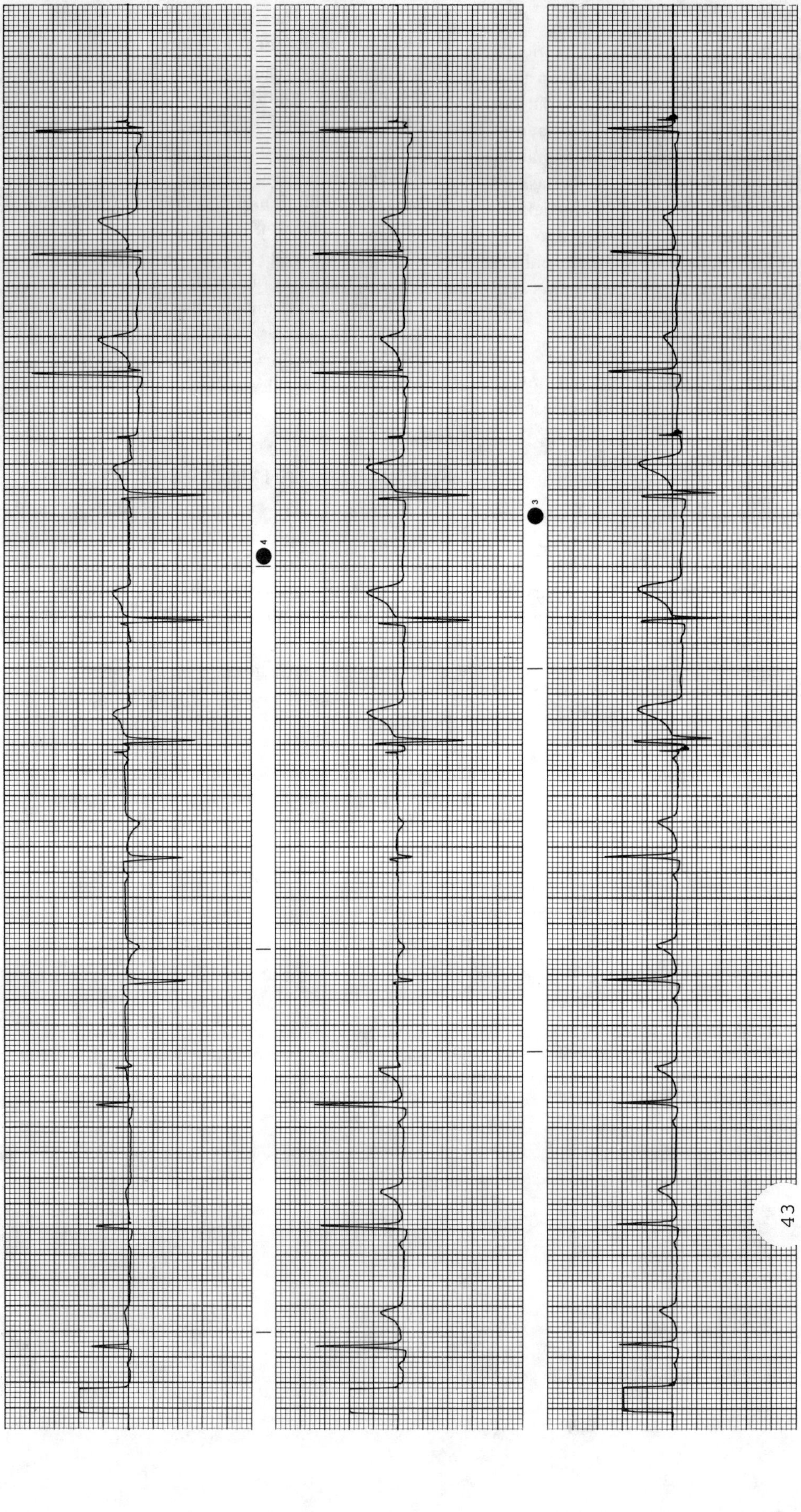

Exercise 43. A 45-year-old man admitted to CCU with unstable angina. He is now complaining of midsternal chest pain, which is aggravated by taking a deep breath.

43

SELF-ASSESSMENT ANSWERS TO EXERCISES 43–67

EXERCISE 43

STEP 1. Rhythm Determination

- Ventricular rate *64*
- QRS shape *Normal*

- Atrial rate *64*
- P wave shape
  *Positive except
  negative in aVR,
  flattened in aVL, and
  diphasic in V1*

- R-R rhythm *Regular*
- QRS interval *0.08*
- QT interval *0.40*

- P-P rhythm *Regular*
- P-R interval *0.16*
- P:R conduction ratio
  1:1

- Dominant pacemaker site *Sinus*
- Interpretation *NSR*

STEP 2. Axis Determination

Normal axis

STEP 3. Chamber Enlargement Determination

None

STEP 4. Intraventricular Conduction Blocks Determination

Normal conduction

STEP 5. Ischemia, Injury, and Infarction Determination

Diffuse concave-shaped ST segment elevations. T waves positive in all leads except negative in aVR and aVL. Normal R wave progression.

STEP 6. Miscellaneous ECG Changes

Diffuse concave-shaped ST segment elevations with P-R interval elevations and ST depressions in aVR significant for pericarditis.

STEP 7. Final Interpretation

Abnormal 12-lead ECG. Normal sinus rhythm with diffuse ST changes indicative of pericarditis. Assess difference in the quality of chest pain from that on admission. Teach patient to be able to differentiate between the two types of pain. Medicate chest pain with antiinflammatory agents rather than nitrates. Monitor for increased frequency of atrial dysrhythmias.

7

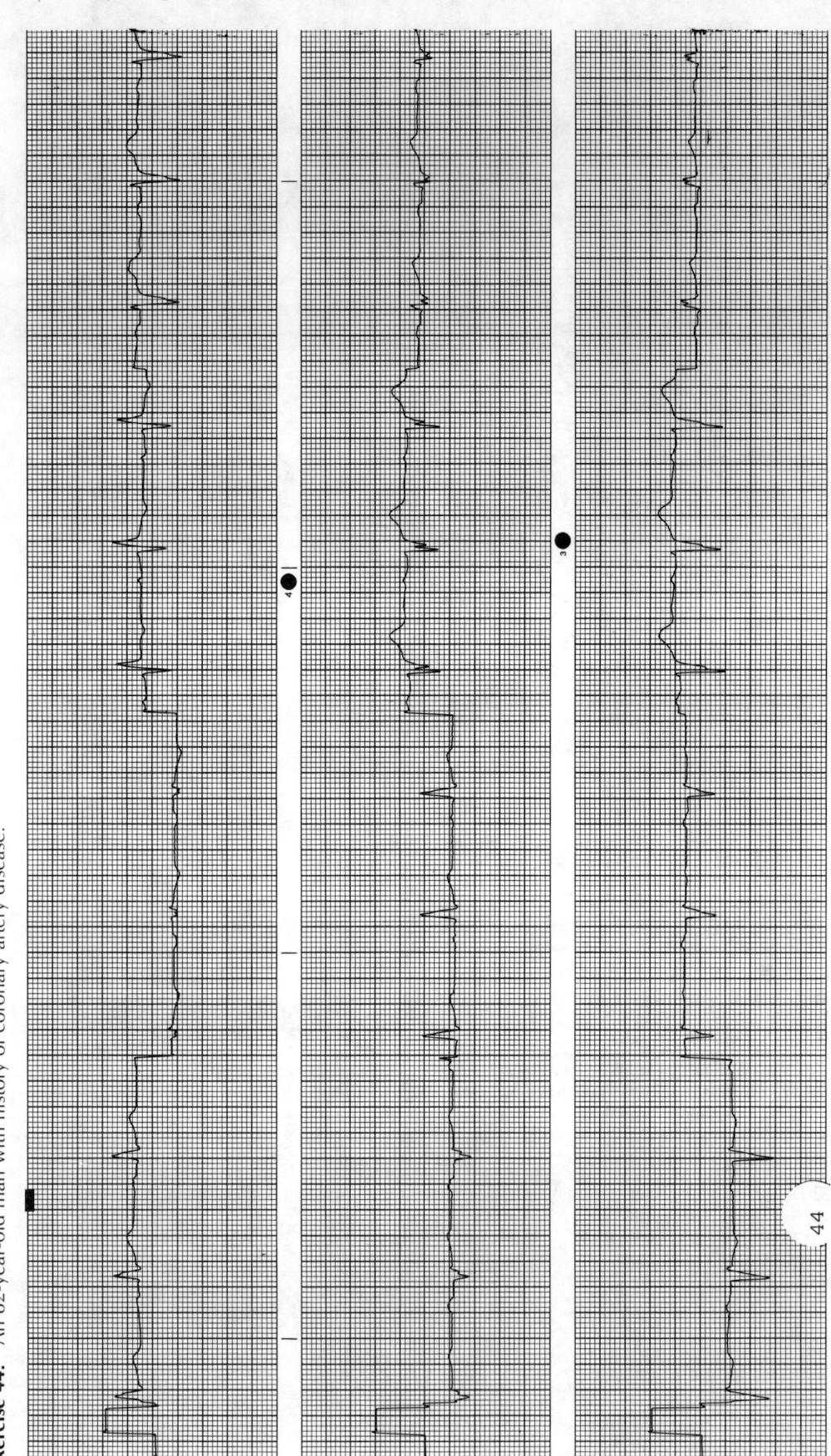

Exercise 44.   An 82-year-old man with history of coronary artery disease.

EXERCISE 44

STEP 1. Rhythm Determination

- Ventricular rate 65
- QRS shape *Widened*

- Atrial rate 65
- P wave shape *Widened, positive and notched except negative in aVR and diphasic in V1, flat in aVL*

- R-R rhythm *Regular*
- QRS interval *0.13*
- QT interval *0.40*

- P-P rhythm *Regular*
- P-R interval *0.24*
- P:R conduction ratio *1:1*

- Dominant pacemaker site *Sinus*
- Interpretation *NSR with 1st degree AV block*

STEP 2. Axis Determination

Left axis

STEP 3. Chamber Enlargement Determination

Left atrial abnormality

STEP 4. Intraventricular Conduction Blocks Determination

RBBB

STEP 5. Ischemia, Injury, and Infarction Determination

ST segments isoelectric. T waves positive in all leads except negative in leads III, aVR, and V1. Normal R wave progression. Significant Q waves in leads II, III, and aVF.

STEP 6. Miscellaneous ECG Changes

No significant findings

STEP 7. Final Interpretation

Abnormal 12-lead ECG. Normal sinus rhythm with 1st degree AV block and RBBB. LAD. Left atrial abnormality also present. Q waves in inferior leads represent an old inferior MI. Assess age of RBBB. If present on previous ECGs, no further treatment necessary. If new finding, may be indicative of ischemia. If new, monitor serial ECGs and cardiac enzymes. Monitor on limb lead for progression of block.

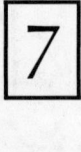

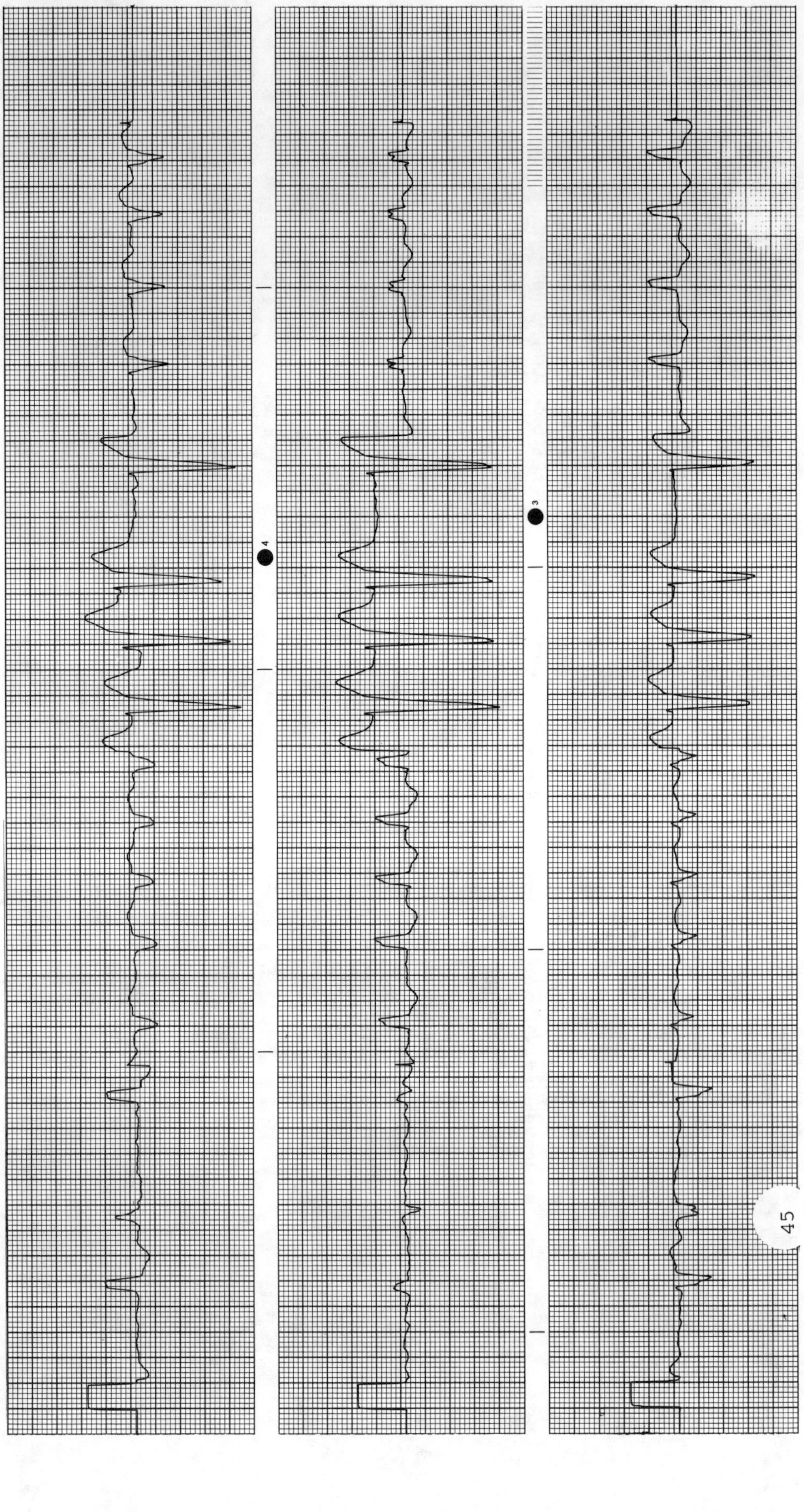

Exercise 45. A 79-year-old woman admitted in CHF.

7

EXERCISE 45

STEP 1. Rhythm Determination

- Ventricular rate 105
- QRS shape Widened
- R-R rhythm Irregular
- QRS interval 0.14
- QT interval 0.40

- Atrial rate =
- P wave shape f waves
- P-P rhythm =
- P-R interval =
- P:R conduction ratio =

- Dominant pacemaker site Atrial
- Interpretation Uncontrolled atrial fibrillation

STEP 2. Axis Determination

Left axis

STEP 3. Chamber Enlargement Determination

None

STEP 4. Intraventricular Conduction Blocks Determination

LBBB

STEP 5. Ischemia, Injury, and Infarction Determination

Cannot be determined in presence of LBBB

STEP 6. Miscellaneous ECG Changes

No significant findings

STEP 7. Final Interpretation

Abnormal 12-lead ECG. Uncontrolled atrial fibrillation with LBBB. LAD. Assess age of LBBB; if chronic, no further treatment necessary. If new, draw serial cardiac enzymes to see whether intraventricular conduction block due to acute MI and be prepared to apply external pacemaker and/or assist in insertion of temporary transvenous pacemaker. Prepare to medicate with digoxin to control ventricular rate. Assess heart and lung sounds to follow response of CHF to diuretic and rate control therapy.

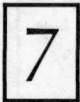

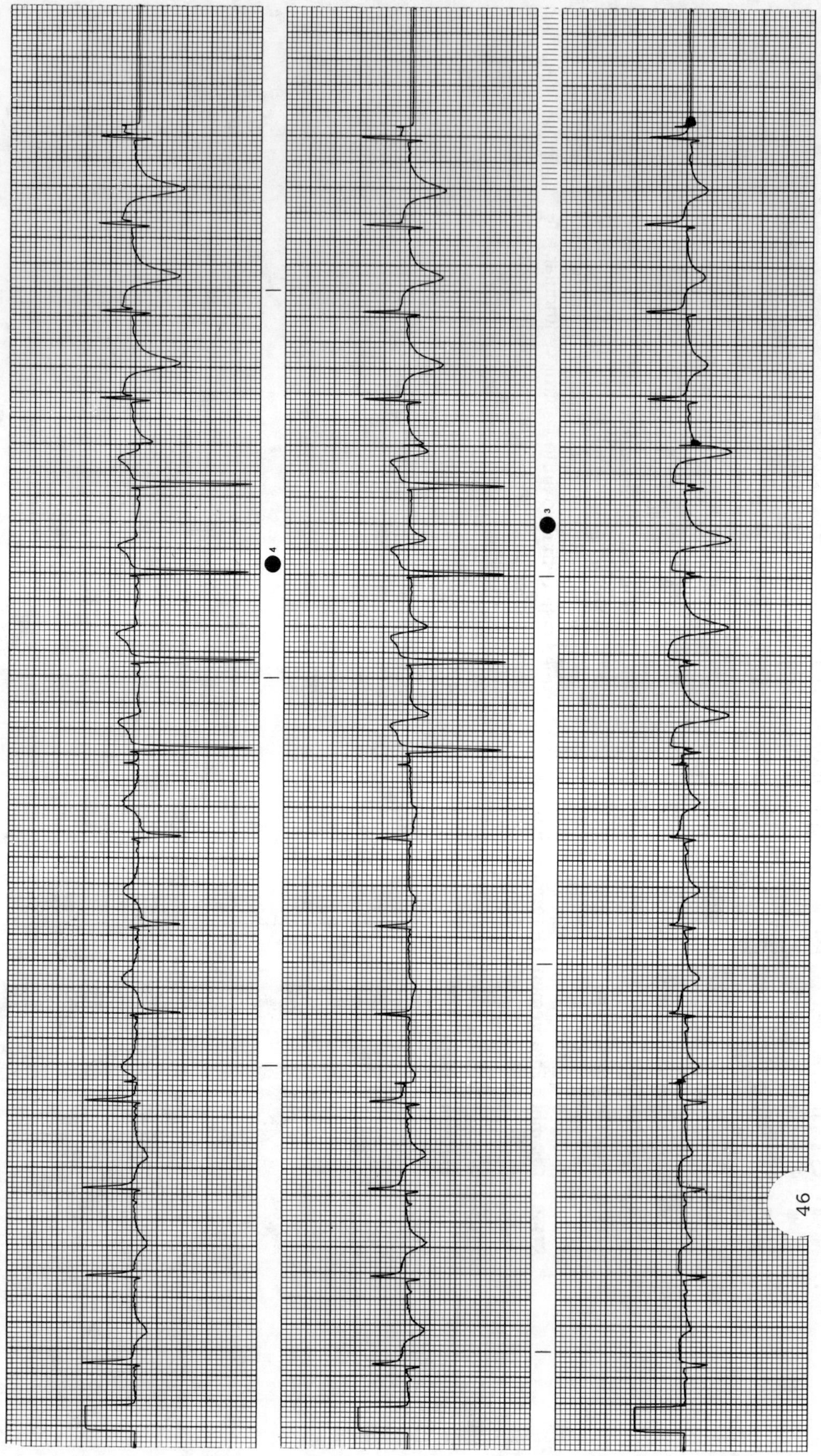

Exercise 46.   A 94-year-old woman admitted to CCU with chest pain. History of hypertension.

46

EXERCISE 46

STEP 1. Rhythm Determination

- Ventricular rate *90*
- QRS shape *Normal*

- Atrial rate *90*
- P wave shape
  Negative except positive in aVR, V1, and V2

- R-R rhythm *Regular*
- QRS interval *0.08*
- QT interval *0.44*

- P-P rhythm *Regular*
- P-R interval *0.10*
- P:R conduction ratio *1:1*

- Dominant pacemaker site *Junctional*
- Interpretation *Accelerated junctional rhythm*

STEP 2. Axis Determination

Normal axis. Use null plane method.

STEP 3. Chamber Enlargement Determination

None

STEP 4. Intraventricular Conduction Blocks Determination

Normal conduction

STEP 5. Ischemia, Injury, and Infarction Determination

ST segment elevations in leads II, III, aVF, V2–V6 with reciprocal depression in leads I and aVL. T waves negative in all leads except positive in lead aVR and V1 and diphasic in V2. Poor R wave progression. Significant Q waves in leads II, III, aVF, V3–V6.

STEP 6. Miscellaneous ECG Changes

No significant findings

STEP 7. Final Interpretation

Abnormal 12-lead ECG. Accelerated junctional rhythm with inferior and anterolateral injury current. Monitor serial ECGs and cardiac enzymes. Assess for evolving inferior and anterolateral infarction. Assess quality and type of chest pain; medicate appropriately. Assess vital signs. Monitor for ventricular dysrhythmias; if present, medicate cautiously with lidocaine IV. Assess heart and lung sounds for signs and symptoms of CHF. Monitor on V1 for development of BBB.

7

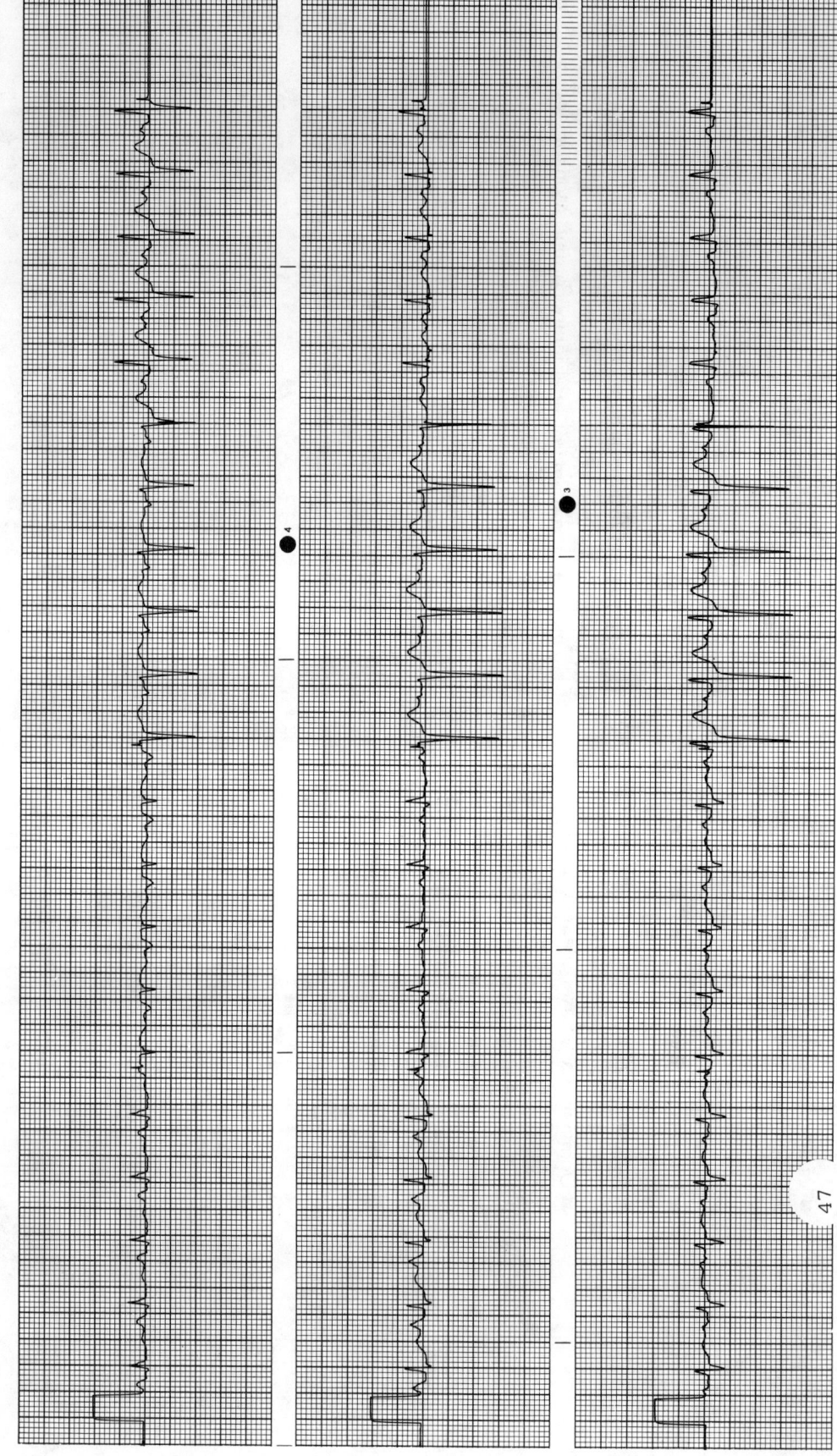

Exercise 47. A 66-year-old man with known heart disease and history of COPD admitted for evaluation and treatment of severe anterior chest pain of 1-hour duration with radiation to left arm and shortness of breath.

47

EXERCISE 47

STEP 1. Rhythm Determination

- Ventricular rate *125*
- QRS shape *Normal, small*

- R-R rhythm *Regular*
- QRS interval *0.06*
- QT interval *0.31*

- Dominant pacemaker site *Sinus*
- Interpretation *Sinus tachycardia*

- Atrial rate *125*
- P wave shape *Positive except negative in aVR and diphasic in V1; tall and wide in II*

- P-P rhythm *Regular*
- P-R interval *0.16*
- P:R conduction ratio *1:1*

STEP 2. Axis Determination

Normal axis

STEP 3. Chamber Enlargement Determination

Left atrial abnormality

STEP 4. Intraventricular Conduction Blocks Determination

Normal conduction

STEP 5. Ischemia, Injury, and Infarction Determination

ST segments isoelectric all leads except nonspecific ST depressions in leads V2–V4. T waves positive in all leads except negative in leads aVR and aVL. Normal R wave progression.

STEP 6. Miscellaneous ECG Changes

No significant findings

STEP 7. Final Interpretation

Abnormal 12-lead ECG. Sinus tachycardia with left atrial abnormality. Monitor serial ECGs and cardiac enzymes. If enzymes positive, consider non-Q wave infarction. Assess quality and type of chest pain; medicate appropriately. This patient would not be a candidate for thrombolytic therapy because ST segments are not elevated. He would be a candidate for heparin therapy if his chest pain is cardiac. Because of his history of COPD, arterial blood gases would probably be clinically of value to assess for hypoxia. Monitor for atrial dysrhythmias.

7

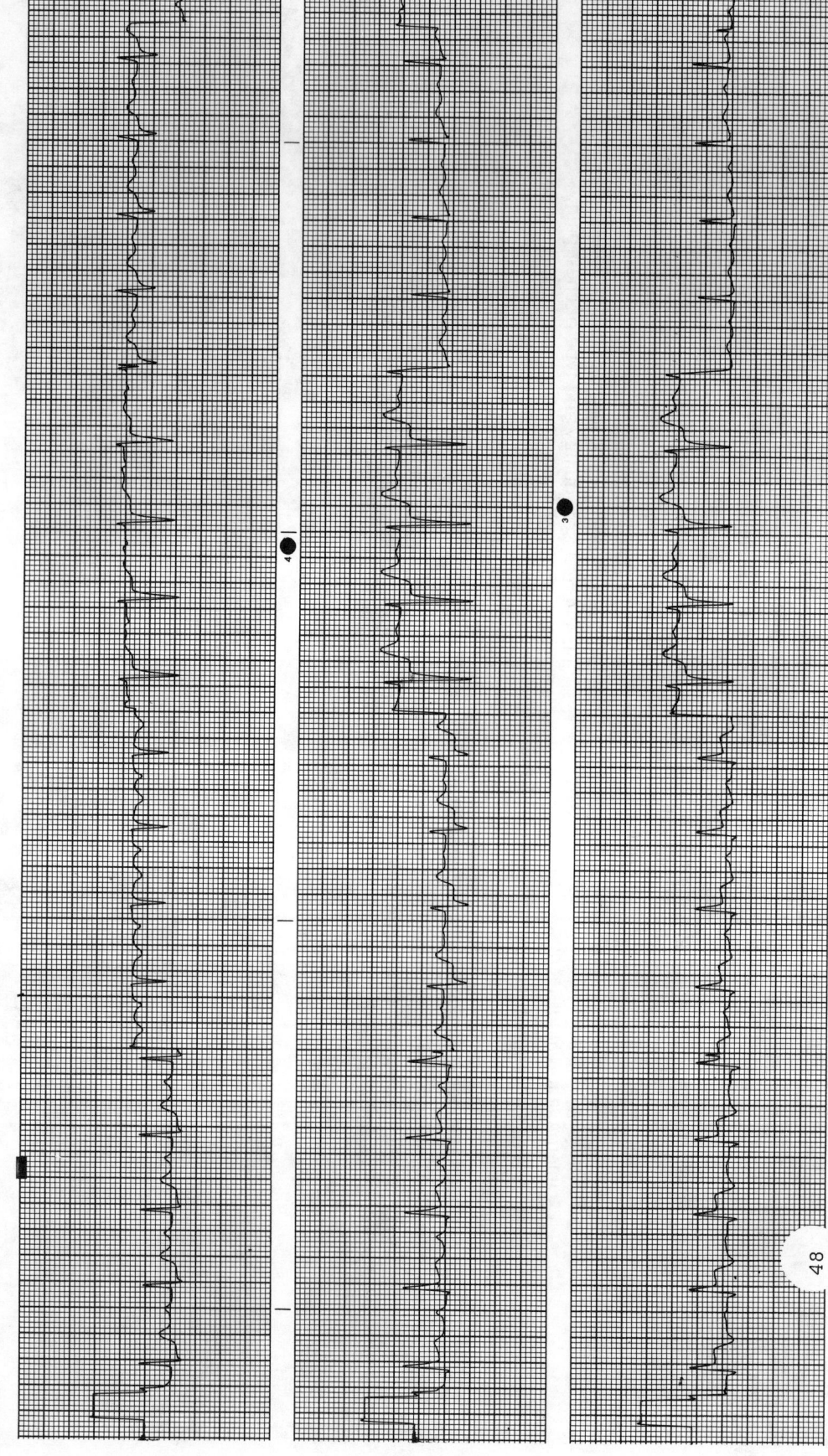

Exercise 48. A 54-year-old woman who has come into the emergency department complaining of chest pain of 6-hour duration. No history of heart disease.

48

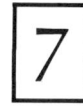

EXERCISE 48

STEP 1. Rhythm Determination

- Ventricular rate *100*
- QRS shape *Slightly widened*

- R-R rhythm *Regular*
- QRS interval *0.11*
- QT interval *0.33*

- Atrial rate *100*
- P wave shape *Positive except negative in aVR and diphasic in V1*
- P-P rhythm *Regular*
- P-R interval *0.22*
- P:R conduction ratio *1:1*

- Dominant pacemaker site *Sinus*
- Interpretation *Sinus tachycardia with borderline 1st degree AV block*

STEP 2. Axis Determination

Normal axis

STEP 3. Chamber Enlargement Determination

None

STEP 4. Intraventricular Conduction Blocks Determination

IVCD

STEP 5. Ischemia, Injury, and Infarction Determination

ST segments elevated and convex in shape in leads II, III, and aVF with reciprocal depressions in leads I and aVL. ST depression also seen in leads V1–V3. T waves positive in all leads except negative in leads III, aVR, and aVF. R waves in V2 taller than those in V3. Q waves appearing in inferior leads.

STEP 6. Miscellaneous ECG Changes

No significant findings

STEP 7. Final Interpretation

Abnormal 12-lead ECG. Sinus tachycardia with borderline 1st degree AV block. IVCD. Inferoposterior MI in evolution. ST segment depressions in septal leads may be indicative of ischemia. Monitor serial ECGs and cardiac enzymes. Assess intensity of chest pain; medicate with morphine unless contraindicated. Monitor vital signs. Thrombolytic therapy would probably not be an option for this patient because she has had chest pain for 6 hours. Monitor for bradycardia and AV blocks.

7

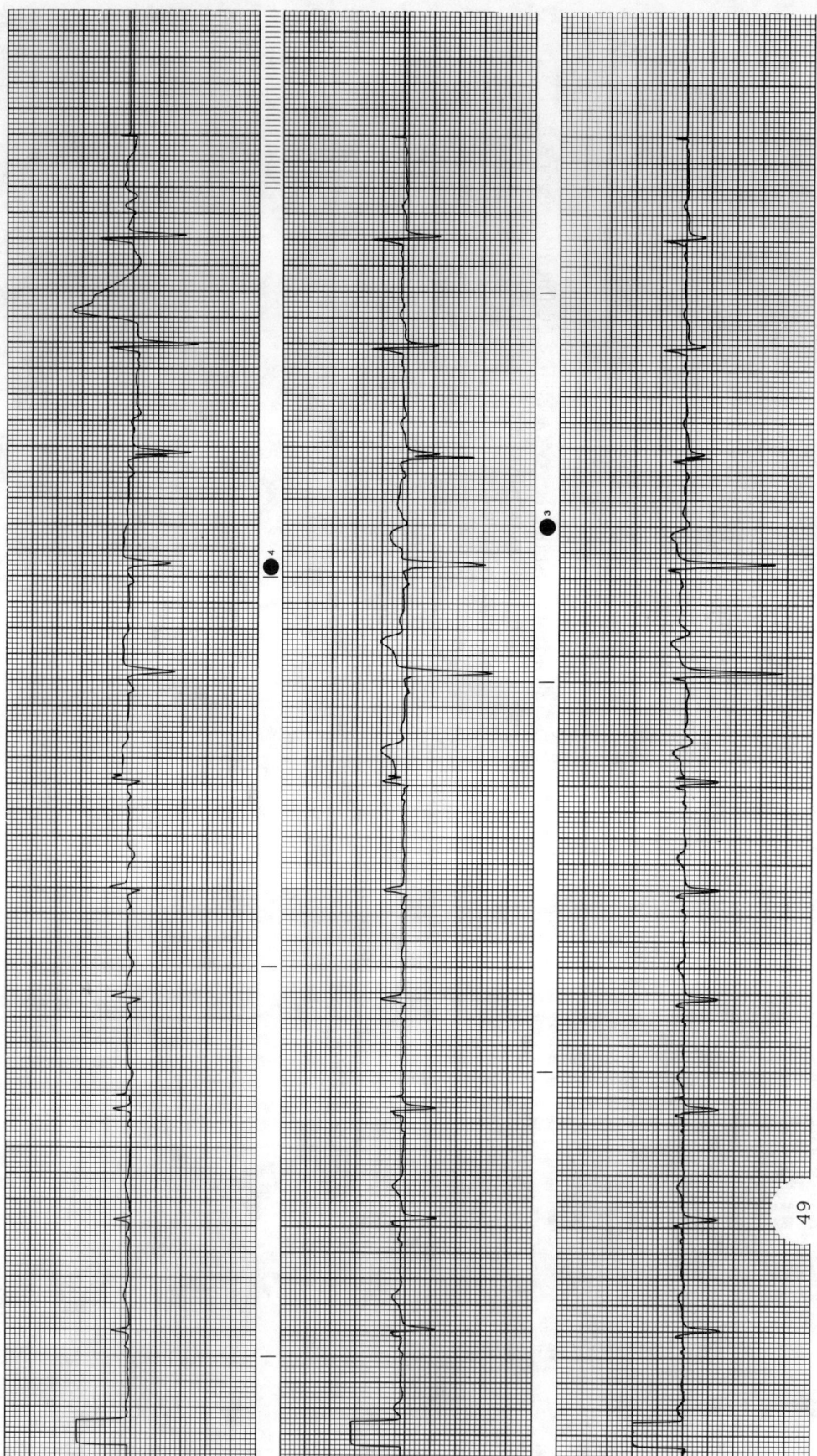

Exercise 49. A 58-year-old man experiencing increasing chest pain over the last week admitted to CCU. Positive smoking history.

49

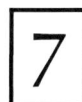

EXERCISE 49

STEP 1. Rhythm Determination

- Ventricular rate *70*
- QRS shape *Normal*

- Atrial rate *70*
- P wave shape *Positive except negative in aVR, V1, V2, and V3*
- P-P rhythm *Regular*
- P-R interval *0.12*
- P:R conduction ratio *1:1*

- R-R rhythm *Regular*
- QRS interval *0.09*
- QT interval *0.39*

- Dominant pacemaker site *Sinus*
- Interpretation *NSR*

STEP 2. Axis Determination

Left axis

STEP 3. Chamber Enlargement Determination

None

STEP 4. Intraventricular Conduction Blocks Determination

Normal conduction

STEP 5. Ischemia, Injury, and Infarction Determination

ST segments elevated in leads V1 and V2. T waves positive in all leads except negative in leads aVR, flattened in aVL, and diphasic in V2–V4. Poor R wave progression V3–V6. Significant Q waves leads V1–V2.

STEP 6. Miscellaneous ECG Changes

No significant findings

STEP 7. Final Interpretation

Abnormal 12-lead ECG. Normal sinus rhythm with LAD. Anteroseptal infarction in evolution. Monitor serial ECGs and cardiac enzymes. Monitor for ventricular dysrhythmias. Counsel about smoking cessation to decrease risk of cardiac disease.

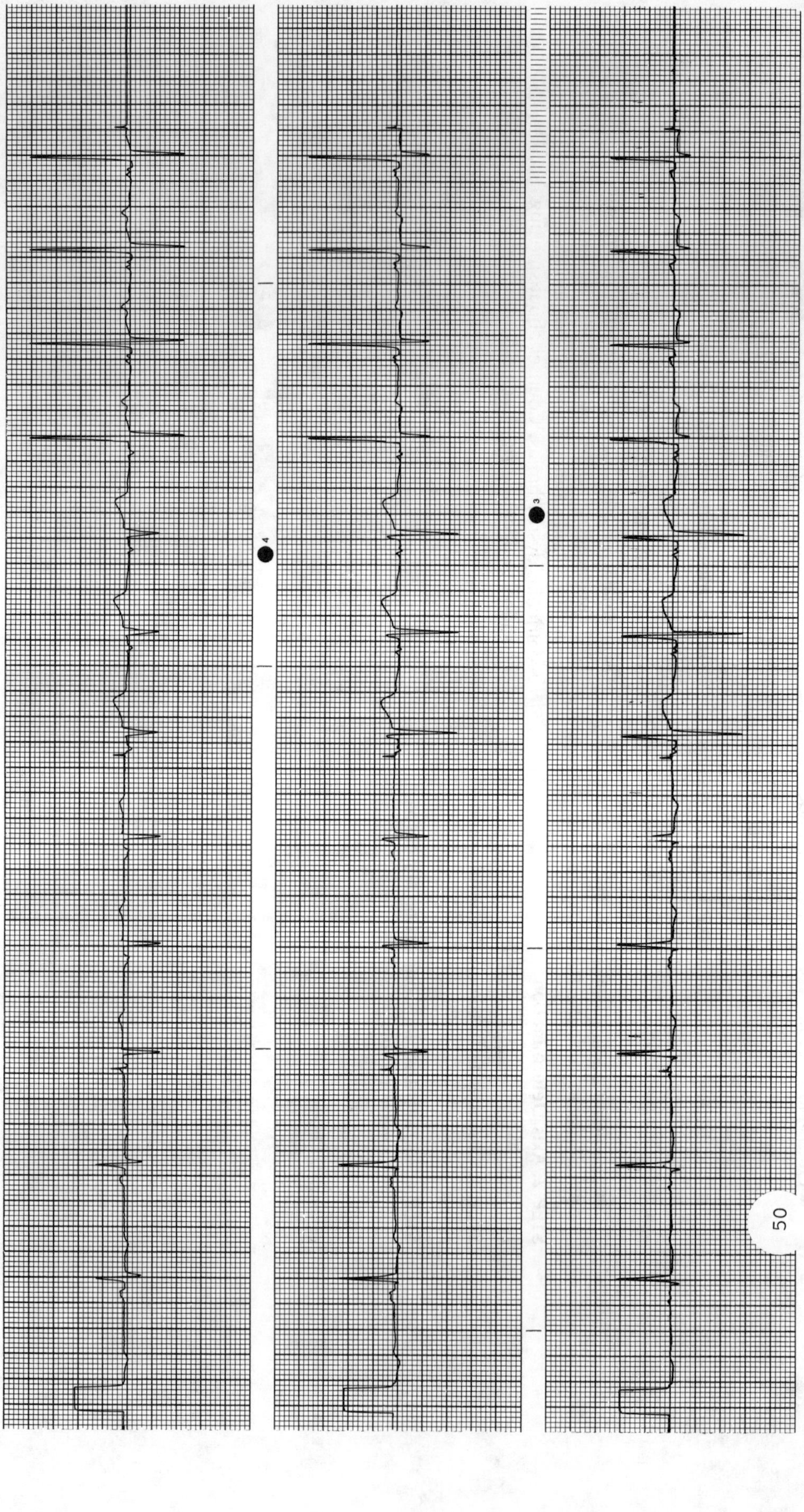

Exercise 50.   A 52-year-old man with a 2-week history of increasing chest pain.

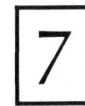

EXERCISE 50

STEP 1. Rhythm Determination

- Ventricular rate *73*
- QRS shape *Normal*

- Atrial rate *73*
- P wave shape *Notched, positive except negative in aVR and diphasic in V1–V2*

- R-R rhythm *Regular*
- QRS interval *0.09*
- QT interval *0.38*

- P-P rhythm *Regular*
- P-R interval *0.16*
- P:R conduction ratio *1:1*

- Dominant pacemaker site *Sinus*
- Interpretation *NSR*

STEP 2. Axis Determination

Normal axis

STEP 3. Chamber Enlargement Determination

Left atrial abnormality

STEP 4. Intraventricular Conduction Blocks Determination

Normal conduction

STEP 5. Ischemia, Injury, and Infarction Determination

ST segments depressed in V6. T waves positive in all leads except negative in leads I, aVF, and V6, flattened in aVL, and diphasic in II, V4, and V5. Normal R wave progression.

STEP 6. Miscellaneous ECG Changes

No significant findings

STEP 7. Final Interpretation

Abnormal 12-lead ECG. Normal sinus rhythm with left atrial abnormality. ST and T wave changes in inferolateral leads appear ischemic. Monitor serial ECGs and cardiac enzymes. If negative, patient will need further workup of coronary artery disease. Counsel patient about risk factor modification.

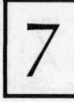

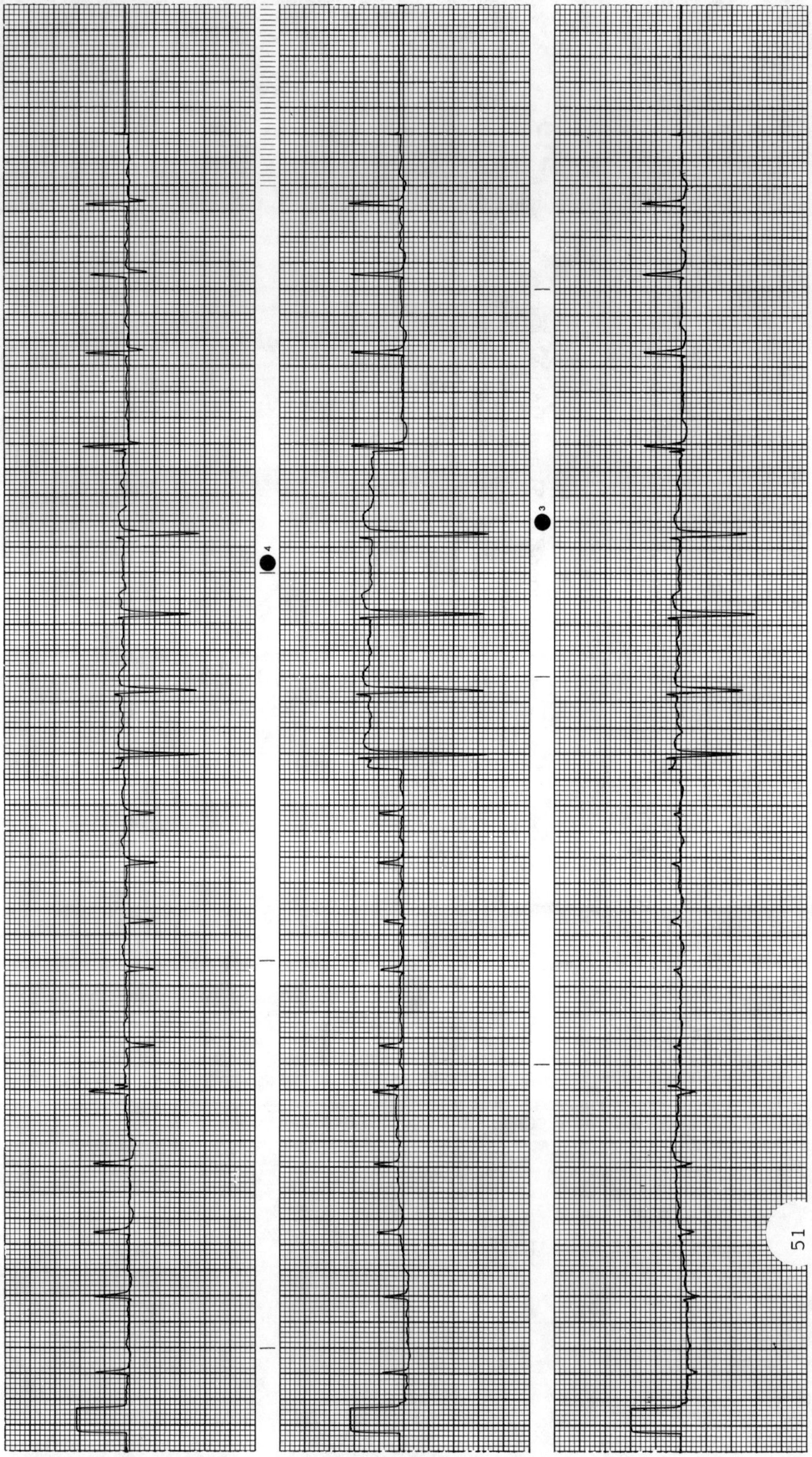

Exercise 51.   A 68-year-old woman with history of coronary artery disease.

7

EXERCISE 51

STEP 1. Rhythm Determination

- Ventricular rate *110*
- QRS shape *Normal, small*
- R-R rhythm *Irregular*
- QRS interval *0.09*
- QT interval *0.32*

- Atrial rate *=*
- P wave shape *f waves*

- P-P rhythm *=*
- P-R interval *=*
- P:R conduction ratio *=*

- Dominant pacemaker site *Atrial*
- Interpretation *Uncontrolled atrial fibrillation*

STEP 2. Axis Determination

Normal axis

STEP 3. Chamber Enlargement Determination

None

STEP 4. Intraventricular Conduction Blocks Determination

Normal conduction

STEP 5. Ischemia, Injury, and Infarction Determination

ST segments sagging in all leads with tall R waves. T waves diffusely flattened. Normal R wave progression.

STEP 6. Miscellaneous ECG Changes

Digitalis effect

STEP 7. Final Interpretation

Abnormal 12-lead ECG. Atrial fibrillation with an uncontrolled ventricular response. ST and T wave changes consistent with digitalis effect. A higher dose of digoxin or the addition of a calcium channel blocker (Verapamil) may be of help to slow the heart rate. No other treatment is necessary.

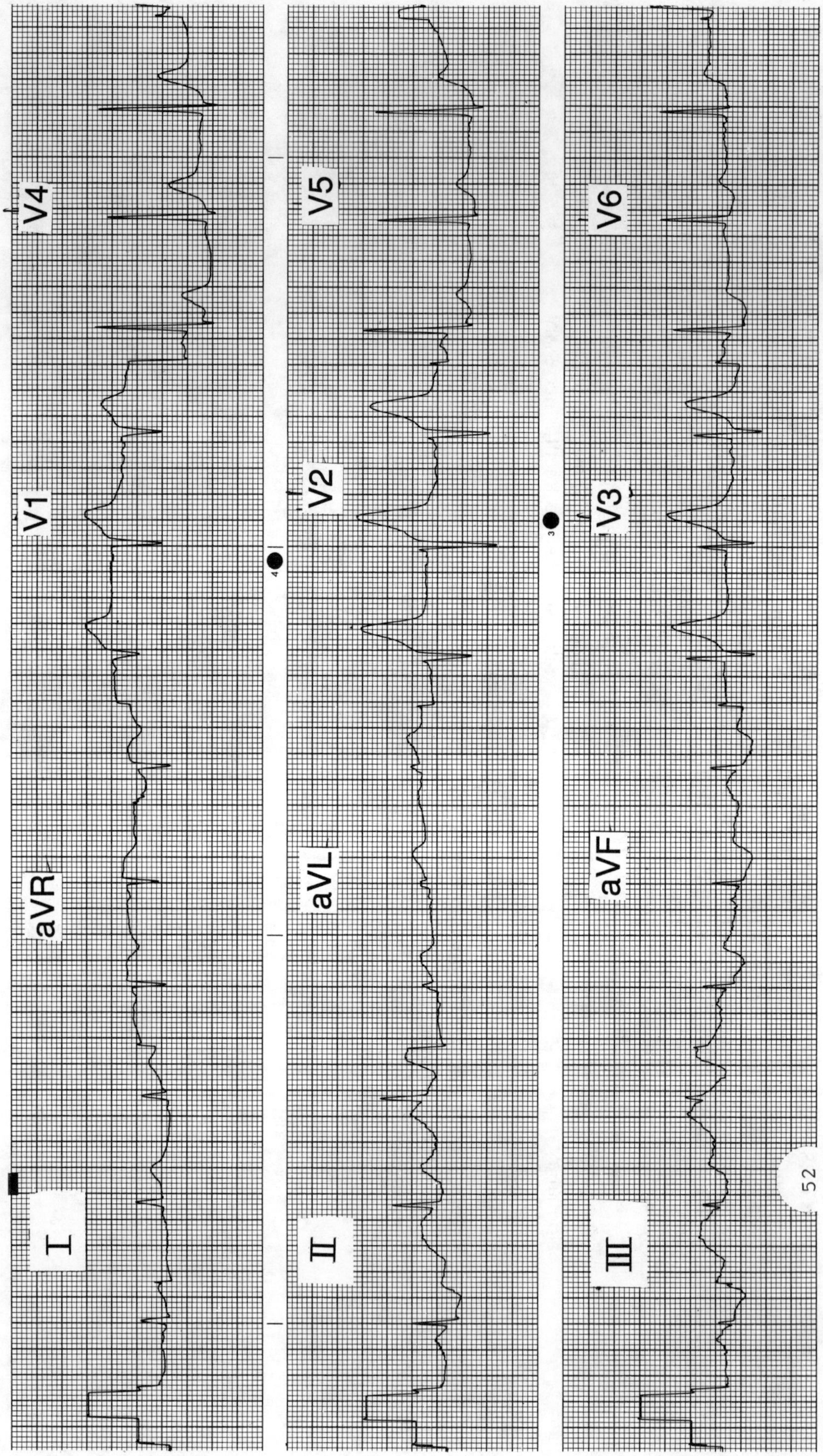

Exercise 52. A 53-year-old man who entered emergency department with chest pain described as indigestion and shortness of breath.

I

aVR

V1

V4

II

aVL

V2

V5

III

aVF

V3

V6

52

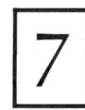

EXERCISE 52

STEP 1. Rhythm Determination

- Ventricular rate *70*
- QRS shape *Normal*

- R-R rhythm *Irregular*
- QRS interval *0.08*
- QT interval *0.37*

- Atrial rate *70*
- P wave shape *Positive except negative aVR, and diphasic V1–V2*

- P-P rhythm *Irregular*
- P-R interval *0.16*
- P:R conduction ratio *1:1*

- Dominant pacemaker site *Sinus*
- Interpretation *Sinus arrhythmia*

STEP 2. Axis Determination

Normal axis

STEP 3. Chamber Enlargement Determination

None

STEP 4. Intraventricular Conduction Blocks Determination

Normal conduction

STEP 5. Ischemia, Injury, and Infarction Determination

ST segments elevated in leads aVL, V1, V2, and V3 with reciprocal depressions in leads II, III, and aVF, V5–V6. T waves positive in all leads except diphasic in leads III, aVF, and aVR with hyperacute T waves in leads V2–V4. Normal R wave progression.

STEP 6. Miscellaneous ECG Changes

No significant findings

STEP 7. Final Interpretation

Abnormal 12-lead ECG. Sinus arrhythmia with acute anteroseptal injury current (infarction). Prepare to administer thrombolytic therapy. Monitor serial ECGs and cardiac enzymes. Monitor for ventricular dysrhythmias. Administer oxygen. Monitor vital signs. Treat indigestion-type anginal pain with nitrates and/or morphine as indicated. Monitor on lead V1 for the development of BBB.

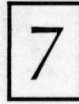

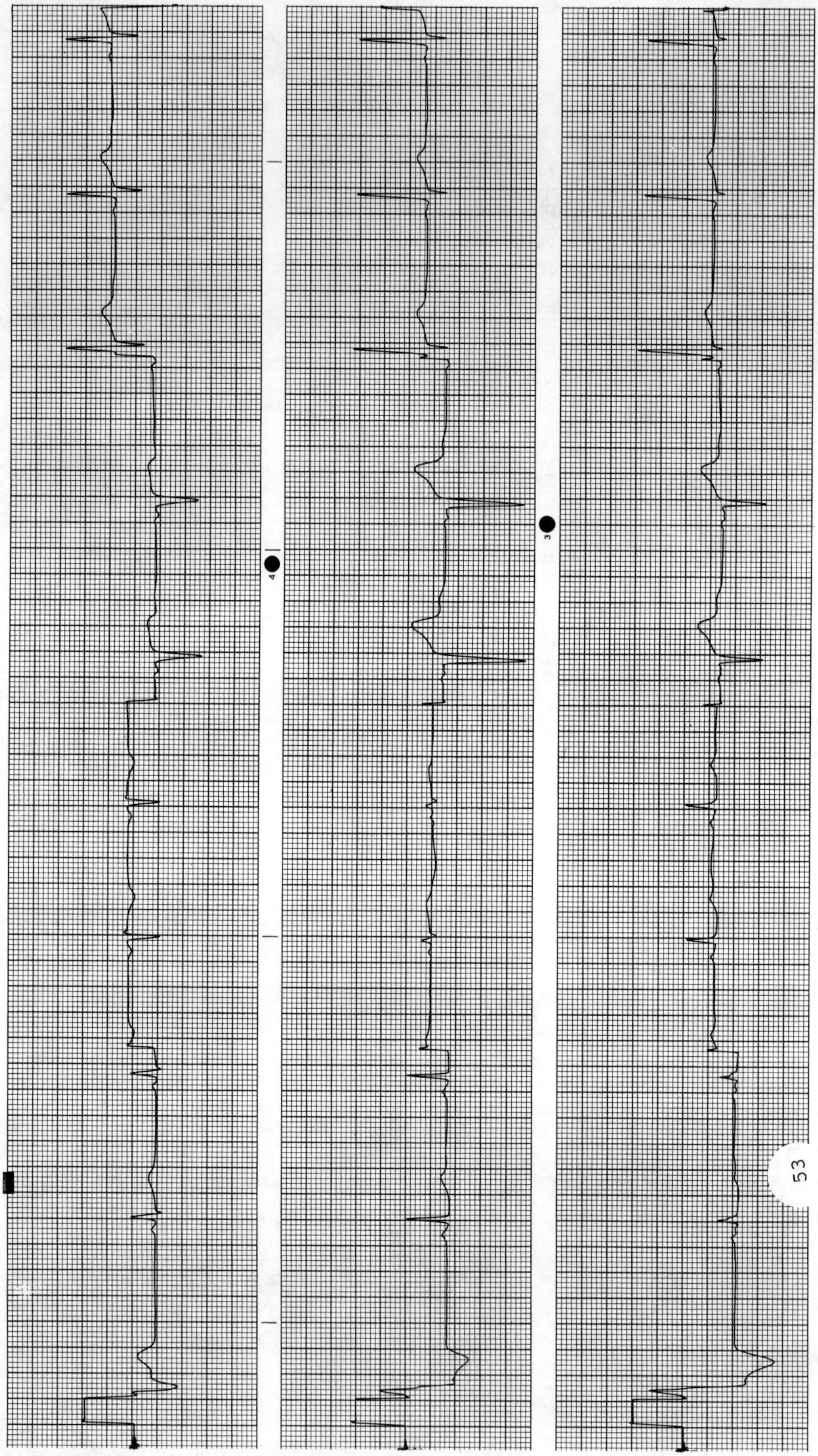

Exercise 53. ECG from the person in Exercise 52, 4 hours after treatment with tissue-plasminogen activator.

EXERCISE 53

STEP 1. Rhythm Determination

- Ventricular rate *50*
- QRS shape *Normal*

- R-R rhythm *Regular*
- QRS interval *0.08*
- QT interval *0.40*

- Dominant pacemaker site *Sinus*
- Interpretation *Sinus bradycardia*

STEP 2. Axis Determination

Normal axis

STEP 3. Chamber Enlargement Determination

None

STEP 4. Intraventricular Conduction Blocks Determination

Normal conduction

- Atrial rate *50*
- P wave shape *Positive except negative in aVR and diphasic in V1–V2*
- P-P rhythm *Regular*
- P-R interval *0.15*
- P:R conduction ratio *1:1*

STEP 5. Ischemia, Injury, and Infarction Determination

ST segments returning to baseline in leads V1–V3. T waves positive in all leads except negative in aVR. Loss of R wave in leads V1–V3. Significant Q wave in leads V1–V3.

STEP 6. Miscellaneous ECG Changes

No significant findings

STEP 7. Final Interpretation

Abnormal 12-lead ECG. Sinus bradycardia with evolutionary changes of anteroseptal MI. Monitor serial ECGs and cardiac enzymes. Follow thrombolytic therapy protocol for further anticoagulation. Because of the rapid return to baseline of the ST segments, the TPA appears to have been effective. Monitor for ventricular dysrhythmias.

7

Exercise 54. A 33-year-old man admitted with 3-day history of weakness, vomiting, and tachycardia.

54

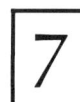

EXERCISE 54

STEP 1. Rhythm Determination

- Ventricular rate *100*
- QRS shape *Normal*

- Atrial rate *100*
- P wave shape
  Positive except negative aVR and aVL, and diphasic in V1 and V2

- R-R rhythm *Regular*
- QRS interval *0.08*
- QT interval *0.34*

- P-P rhythm *Regular*
- P-R interval *0.16*
- P:R conduction ratio *1:1*

- Dominant pacemaker site *Sinus*
- Interpretation *Sinus tachycardia*

STEP 2. Axis Determination

Normal axis

STEP 3. Chamber Enlargement Determination

None

STEP 4. Intraventricular Conduction Blocks Determination

Normal conduction

STEP 5. Ischemia, Injury, and Infarction Determination

ST segments isoelectric. T waves tall and pinched and positive except negative in III and aVR. Small r waves in leads V3 and V4.

STEP 6. Miscellaneous ECG Changes

Diffuse tall, pinched T waves

STEP 7. Final Interpretation

Abnormal 12-lead ECG. Sinus tachycardia with tall pinched T waves, this may be caused by hyperkalemia. Patient found to have a potassium level of 7.1 mEq/L. Monitor for ventricular dysrhythmias. Monitor serum potassium level.

7

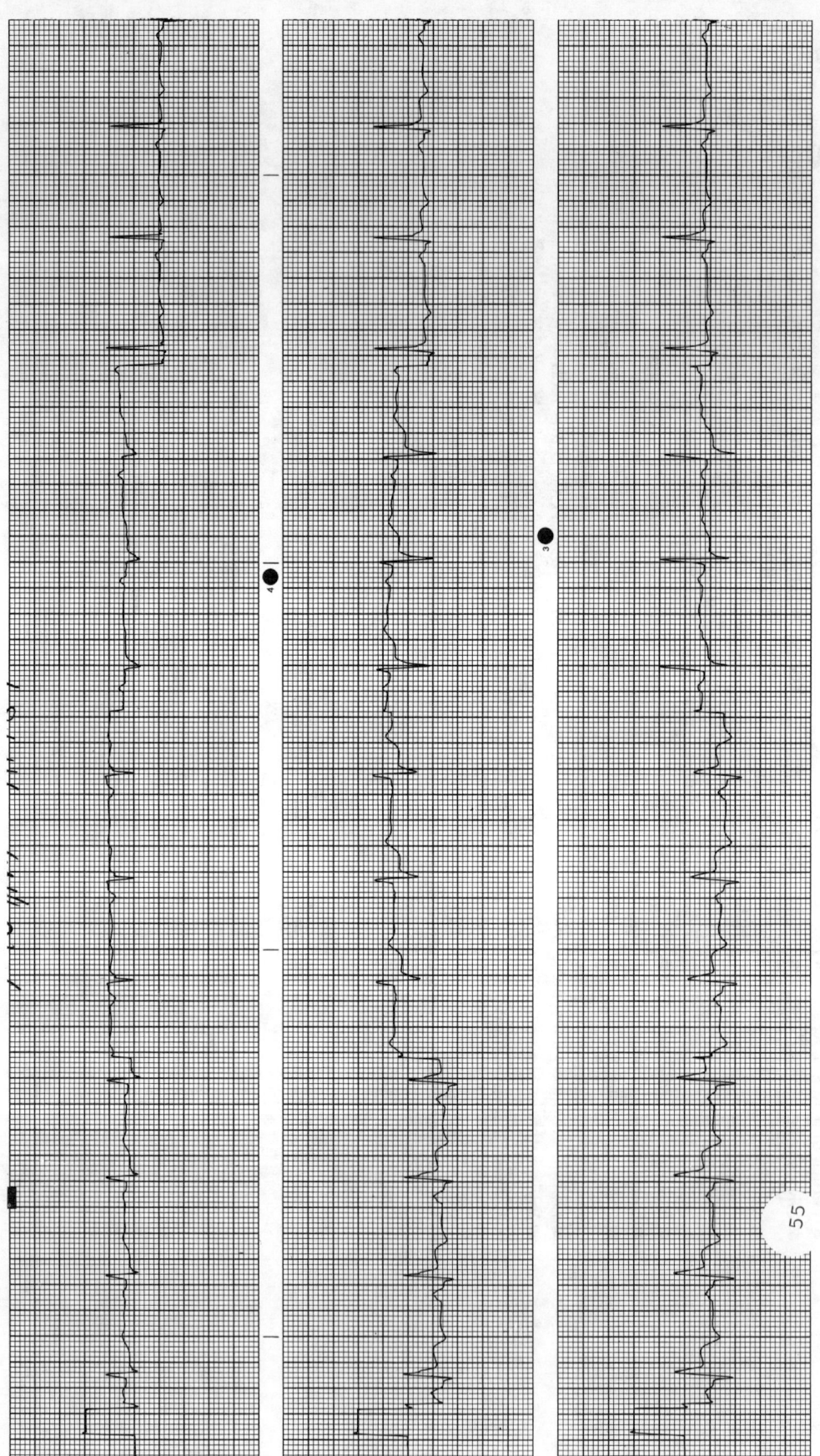

Exercise 55. A 61-year-old woman was admitted to CCU with midsternal chest pain. History of unstable angina.

55

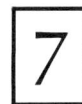

EXERCISE 55

STEP 1. Rhythm Determination

- Ventricular rate *78*
- QRS shape *Slightly widened*

- Atrial rate *78*
- P wave shape *Positive except negative in aVR and aVL*

- R-R rhythm *Regular*
- QRS interval *0.10*
- QT interval *0.40*

- P-P rhythm *Regular*
- P-R interval *0.16*
- P:R conduction ratio *1:1*

- Dominant pacemaker site *Sinus*
- Interpretation *NSR*

STEP 2. Axis Determination

Normal axis

STEP 3. Chamber Enlargement Determination

None

STEP 4. Intraventricular Conduction Blocks Determination

IVCD

STEP 5. Ischemia, Injury, and Infarction Determination

ST segments elevated in leads II, III, aVF, V5, and V6 with reciprocal depressions in leads I, aVL, V2–V3. T waves positive in all leads except negative in leads II, III, aVR, aVF,V1, V4–V6. Significant Q waves in leads II, III, and aVF.

STEP 6. Miscellaneous ECG Changes

No significant findings

STEP 7. Final Interpretation

Abnormal 12-lead ECG. Normal sinus rhythm with IVCD. Evolutionary changes of inferolateral MI. Monitor serial ECGs and cardiac enzymes. Assess quality and type of chest pain; medicate appropriately. Monitor for brady dysrhythmias and 2nd degree heart blocks.

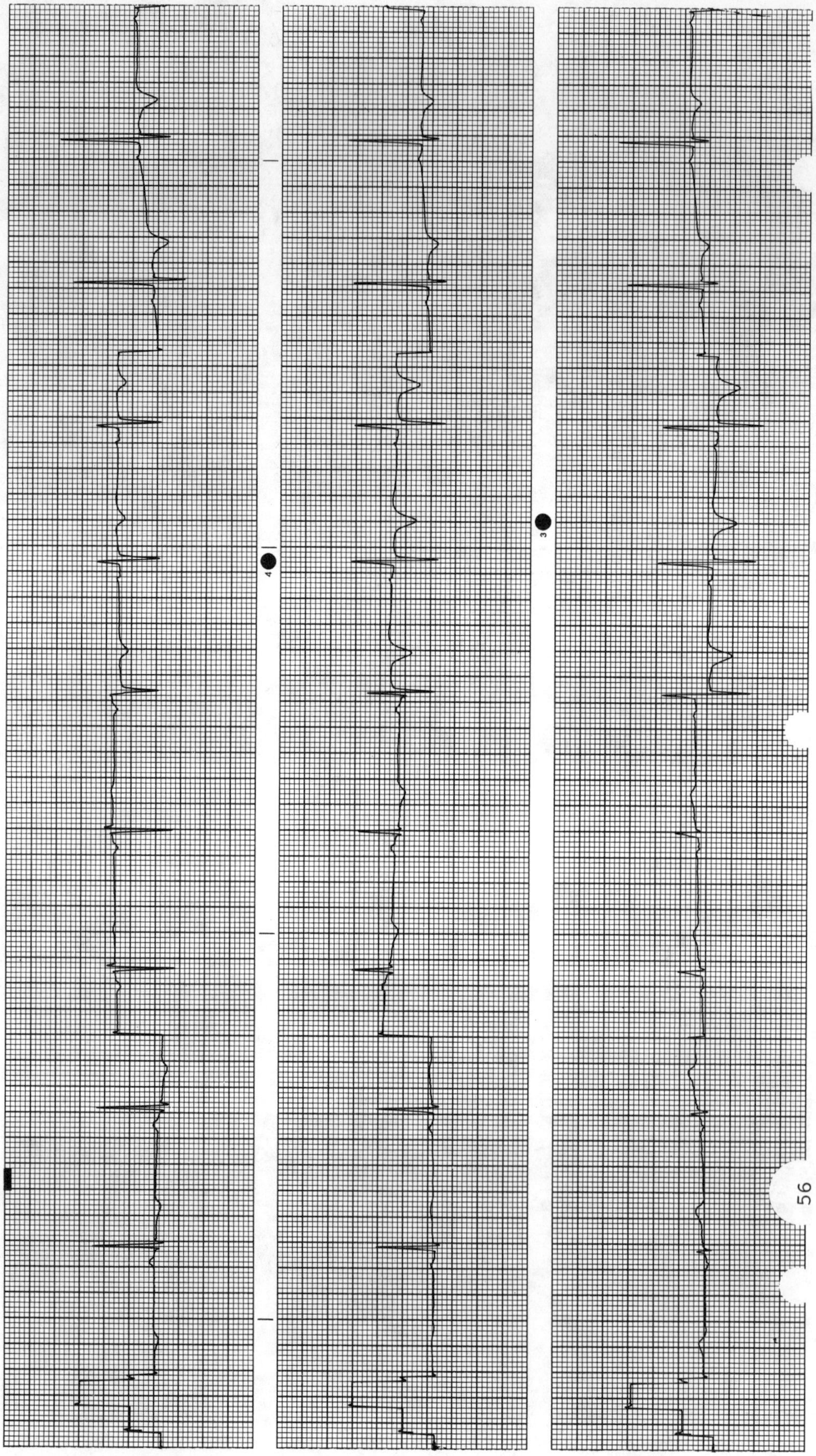

Exercise 56. A 54-year-old woman admitted with chest pain described as pressure. Pain relieved with one nitrogycerin.

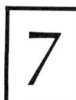

EXERCISE 56

STEP 1. Rhythm Determination

- Ventricular rate *58*
- QRS shape *Normal*

- Atrial rate *58*
- P wave shape
  *Positive except
  negative in III and
  aVR*

- R-R rhythm *Regular*
- QRS interval *0.07*
- QT interval *0.40*

- P-P rhythm *Regular*
- P-R interval *0.16*
- P:R conduction ratio
  1:1

- Dominant pacemaker site *Sinus*
- Interpretation *Sinus bradycardia*

STEP 2. Axis Determination

Normal axis

STEP 3. Chamber Enlargement Determination

None

STEP 4. Intraventricular Conduction Blocks Determination

Normal conduction

STEP 5. Ischemia, Injury, and Infarction Determination

ST segments isoelectric. T waves negative in all leads except positive in leads II, III, aVF, and aVR. Normal R wave progression. R waves appear abnormally tall in leads V1 and V2.

STEP 6. Miscellaneous ECG Changes

No significant findings

STEP 7. Final Interpretation

Abnormal 12-lead ECG. Sinus bradycardia with anterolateral ischemic T wave changes. Because this patient's chest pain was relieved with nitroglycerin, these changes are consistent with classic angina. She should have a further workup to diagnose the extent of her coronary artery disease.

7

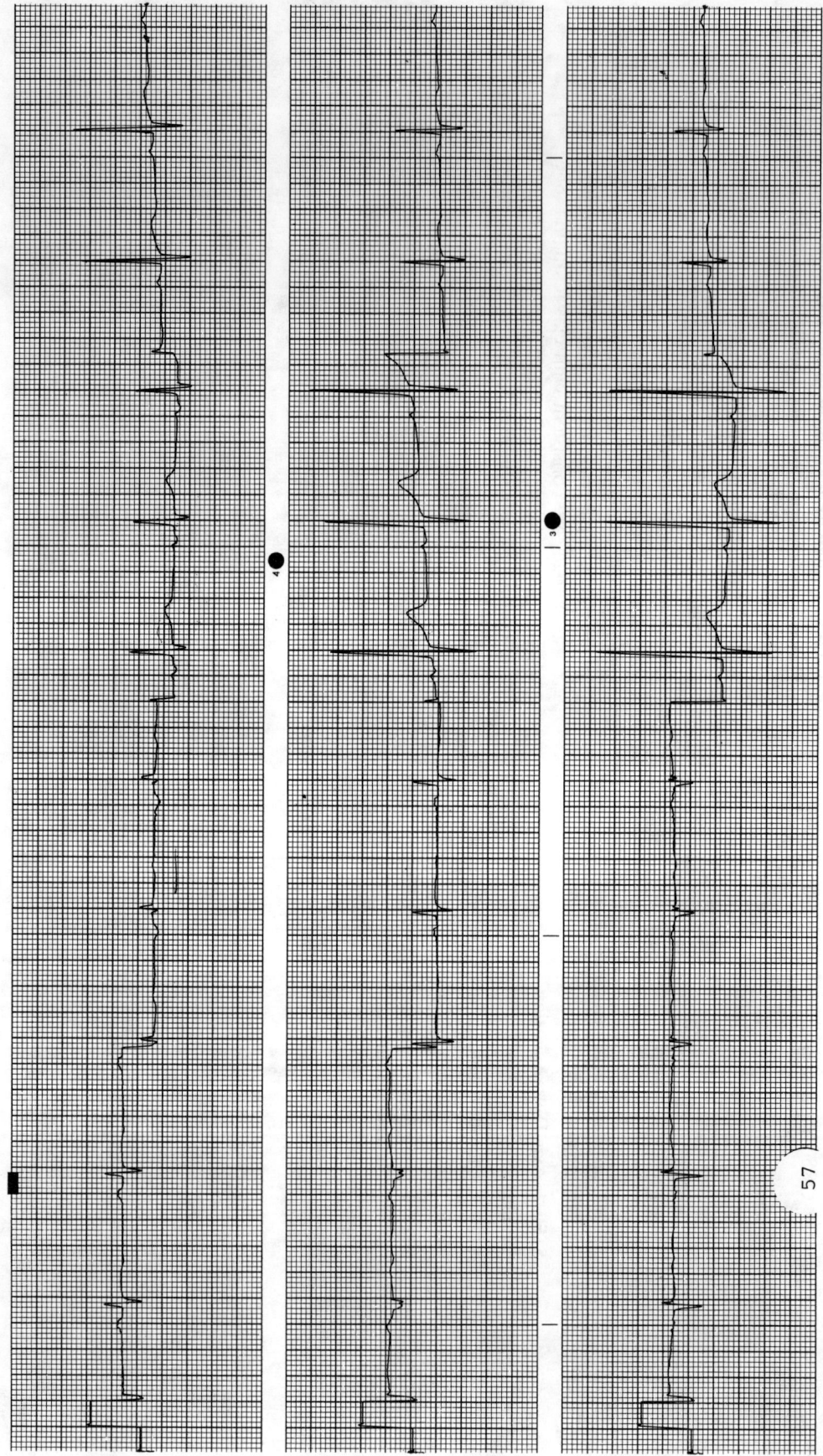

Exercise 57. A 53-year-old man admitted to CCU complaining of chest pain. History of MI 6 years ago. Positive cardiac enzymes.

57

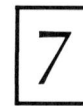

EXERCISE 57

STEP 1. Rhythm Determination

- Ventricular rate *60*
- QRS shape *Normal*

- Atrial rate *60*
- P wave shape *Widened, notched, and positive except negative in aVR and diphasic in V1–V2*
- P-P rhythm *Regular*
- P-R interval *0.16*
- P:R conduction ratio *1:1*

- R-R rhythm *Regular*
- QRS interval *0.08*
- QT interval *0.44*

- Dominant pacemaker site *Sinus*
- Interpretation *Sinus bradycardia*

STEP 2. Axis Determination

Left axis

STEP 3. Chamber Enlargement Determination

Left atrial abnormality

STEP 4. Intraventricular Conduction Blocks Determination

Normal conduction

STEP 5. Ischemia, Injury, and Infarction Determination

ST segments isoelectric. T waves positive in all leads except negative in aVR, flattened in I and aVL, and diphasic in II, III, and aVF. R waves abnormally tall in leads V1–V3. Significant Q waves in leads II, III, and aVF.

STEP 6. Miscellaneous ECG Changes

No significant findings

STEP 7. Final Interpretation

Abnormal 12-lead ECG. Normal sinus rhythm with left atrial abnormality. LAD. Old inferoposterior MI. Because cardiac enzymes were positive without acute ECG changes, this patient had a non-Q wave MI. It is not possible to determine from this ECG the site of the infarct. Further studies such as an echocardiogram would be indicated to determine the exact site. Monitor serial ECGs (Changes consistent with an infarct are not always present on the initial ECG) and cardiac enzymes. Assess quality and type of chest pain; medicate appropriately.

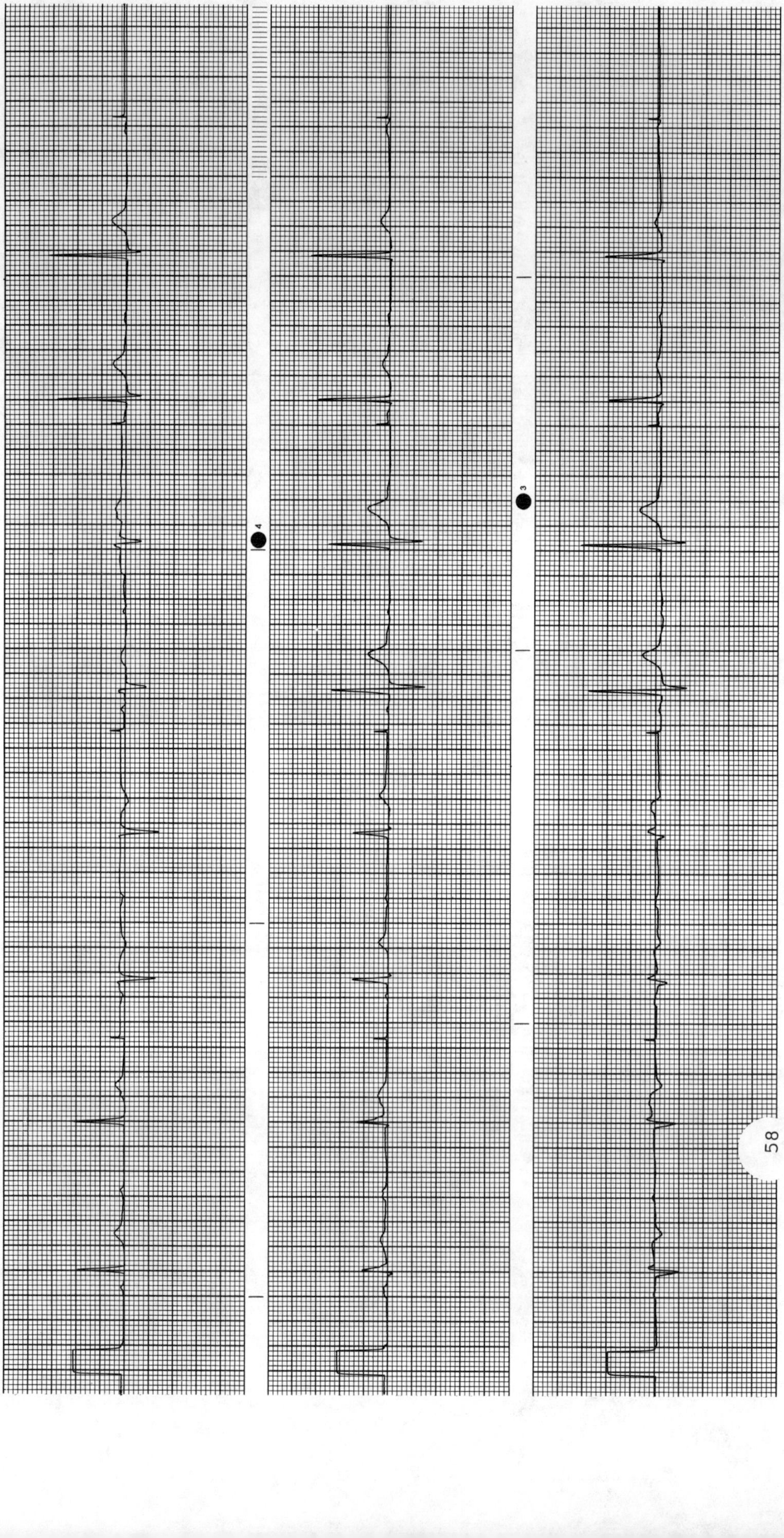

Exercise 58. A 63-year-old admitted with chest pain. History of MI 2 years ago.

58

EXERCISE 58

STEP 1. Rhythm Determination

- Ventricular rate *50*
- QRS shape *Normal*

- Atrial rate *77*
- P wave shape *Widened, notched, and positive except negative in aVR*

- R-R rhythm *Regular*
- QRS interval *0.08*
- QT interval *0.43*

- P-P rhythm *Regular*
- P-R interval *Varies*
- P:R conduction ratio = __

- Dominant pacemaker site *Sinus and AV junctional*
- Interpretation *Complete heart block with junctional escape rhythm*

STEP 2. Axis Determination

Normal axis

STEP 3. Chamber Enlargement Determination

Left atrial abnormality

STEP 4. Intraventricular Conduction Blocks Determination

Normal conduction

STEP 5. Ischemia, Injury, and Infarction Determination

ST segments isoelectric. T waves positive in all leads except negative in aVR and diphasic in leads III and aVF. Abnormally tall R waves in lead V2. Significant Q waves in leads III and aVF.

STEP 6. Miscellaneous ECG Changes

No significant findings

STEP 7. Final Interpretation

Abnormal 12-lead ECG. Complete heart block with junctional escape rhythm. Left atrial abnormality. Evolutionary changes of inferoposterior MI. Assess patient's vital signs to assess tolerance of complete heart block. Prepare to administer atropine IV. Be prepared to apply external pacemaker and to assist with insertion of temporary transvenous pacemaker. Monitor serial ECGs and cardiac enzymes. Assess quality and type of chest pain; medicate appropriately.

7

Exercise 59.   A 54-year-old man admitted with prolonged angina. This is the same patient as in Exercise 34. This ECG was taken after he was given three NTGs.

59

7

EXERCISE 59

STEP 1. Rhythm Determination

- Ventricular rate *81*
- QRS shape *Slightly widened*

- Atrial rate *81*
- P wave shape *Positive except negative in III and aVR*

- R-R rhythm *Regular*
- QRS interval *0.10*
- QT interval *0.35*

- P-P rhythm *Regular*
- P-R interval *0.20*
- P:R conduction ratio *1:1*

- Dominant pacemaker site *Sinus*
- Interpretation *NSR*

STEP 2. Axis Determination

Normal axis. Use null plane method.

STEP 3. Chamber Enlargement Determination

None

STEP 4. Intraventricular Conduction Blocks Determination

IVCD

STEP 5. Ischemia, Injury, and Infarction Determination

ST segments isoelectric. T waves positive in all leads except negative in aVR and flattened in aVL. Normal R wave progression. Q waves in leads I, aVL, V5, and V6 appear slightly more pronounced in this tracing.

STEP 6. Miscellaneous ECG Changes

No significant findings

STEP 7. Final Interpretation

Abnormal 12-lead ECG. Normal sinus rhythm with IVCD. Anterolateral T wave changes seen on previous tracing have improved. Continue to follow serial ECGs and cardiac enzymes. Because ischemic changes seen on previous tracing have improved after sublingual nitroglycerin, previous changes were consistent with classic angina. Monitor on lead V1 to assess for development of BBB.

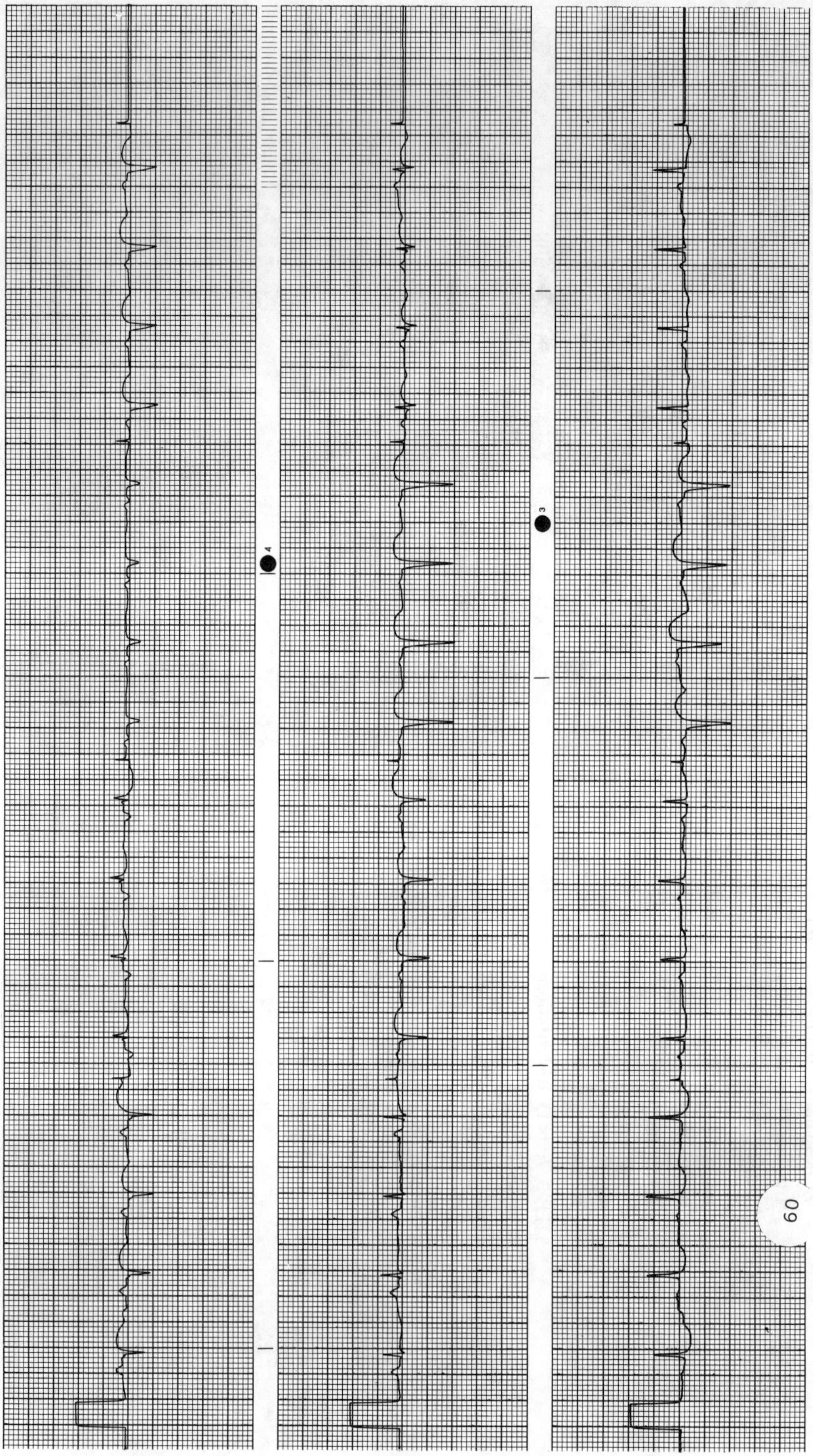

Exercise 60. A 79-year-old man admitted with severe dyspnea.

60

EXERCISE 60

STEP 1. Rhythm Determination

- Ventricular rate 98
- QRS shape *Small, normal*

- Atrial rate 98
- P wave shape *Positive except negative in aVR and diphasic in V1*
- P-P rhythm *Regular*
- P-R interval *0.16*
- P:R conduction ratio *1:1*

- R-R rhythm *Regular*
- QRS interval *0.07*
- QT interval *0.32*

- Dominant pacemaker site *Sinus*
- Interpretation *NSR*

STEP 2. Axis Determination

Right axis

STEP 3. Chamber Enlargement Determination

None

STEP 4. Intraventricular Conduction Blocks Determination

Normal conduction

STEP 5. Ischemia, Injury, and Infarction Determination

ST segments elevated I, aVL, V2–V4. T waves positive all leads except negative in leads II, III, and aVF (reciprocal changes), V5–V6. Loss of R waves in leads V1–V4. Significant Q waves in leads I, aVL, V1–V4.

STEP 6. Miscellaneous ECG Changes

No significant findings

STEP 7. Final Interpretation

Abnormal 12-lead ECG. Normal sinus rhythm with RAD. Evolutionary changes of anterolateral MI. Low voltage suggestive of pulmonary disease. Monitor patient's vital signs. Draw arterial blood gases to assess whether dyspnea secondary to cardiac or pulmonary problem and to determine O_2 requirements. Assess patient's lung sounds for presence of wheezes. Assess patient's heart sounds for signs of CHF. This patient may need both bronchodilators and diuretics to treat his dyspnea. Monitor serial ECGs and cardiac enzymes to determine age of infarction. Monitor on lead V1 for development of BBB.

Exercise 61. A 52-year-old man admitted with chest pain. No previous history of cardiac disease. History of hypertension and smoking.

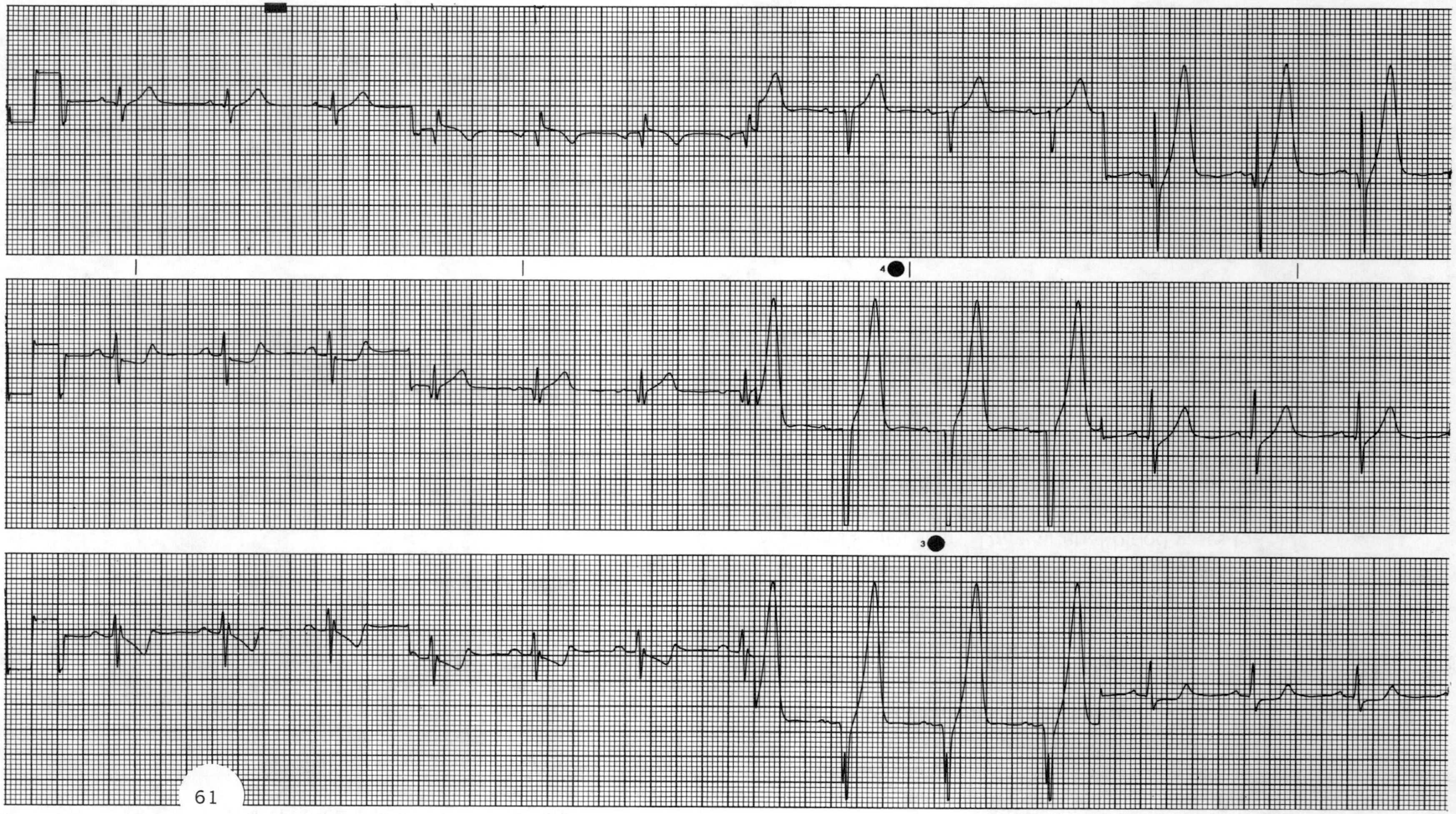

EXERCISE 61

STEP 1. Rhythm Determination

- Ventricular rate *74*
- QRS shape *Normal*

- Atrial rate *74*
- P wave shape
  Positive except negative in aVR and aVL

- R-R rhythm *Regular*
- QRS interval *0.08*
- QT interval *0.34*

- P-P rhythm *Regular*
- P-R interval *0.17*
- P:R conduction ratio *1:1*

- Dominant pacemaker site *Sinus*
- Interpretation *NSR*

STEP 2. Axis Determination

Indeterminate axis

STEP 3. Chamber Enlargement Determination

None

STEP 4. Intraventricular Conduction Blocks Determination

Normal conduction

STEP 5. Ischemia, Injury, and Infarction Determination

ST segments elevated in leads V2–V4 with hyperacute T wave changes in same leads and reciprocal depressions in leads II, III, and aVF. Poor R wave progression. Significant Q waves in leads V1–V4.

STEP 6. Miscellaneous ECG Changes

No significant findings

STEP 7. Final Interpretation

Abnormal 12-lead ECG. Normal sinus rhythm with indeterminate axis. Acute anteroseptal MI. Prepare to administer thrombolytic therapy. Assess patient's vital signs. Administer oxygen. Monitor for ventricular dysrhythmias. Treat chest pain with nitrates and/or intravenous morphine. Monitor serial ECGs and cardiac enzymes for effectiveness of thrombolytic therapy. Assess patient for signs and symptoms of congestive heart failure.

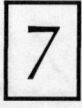

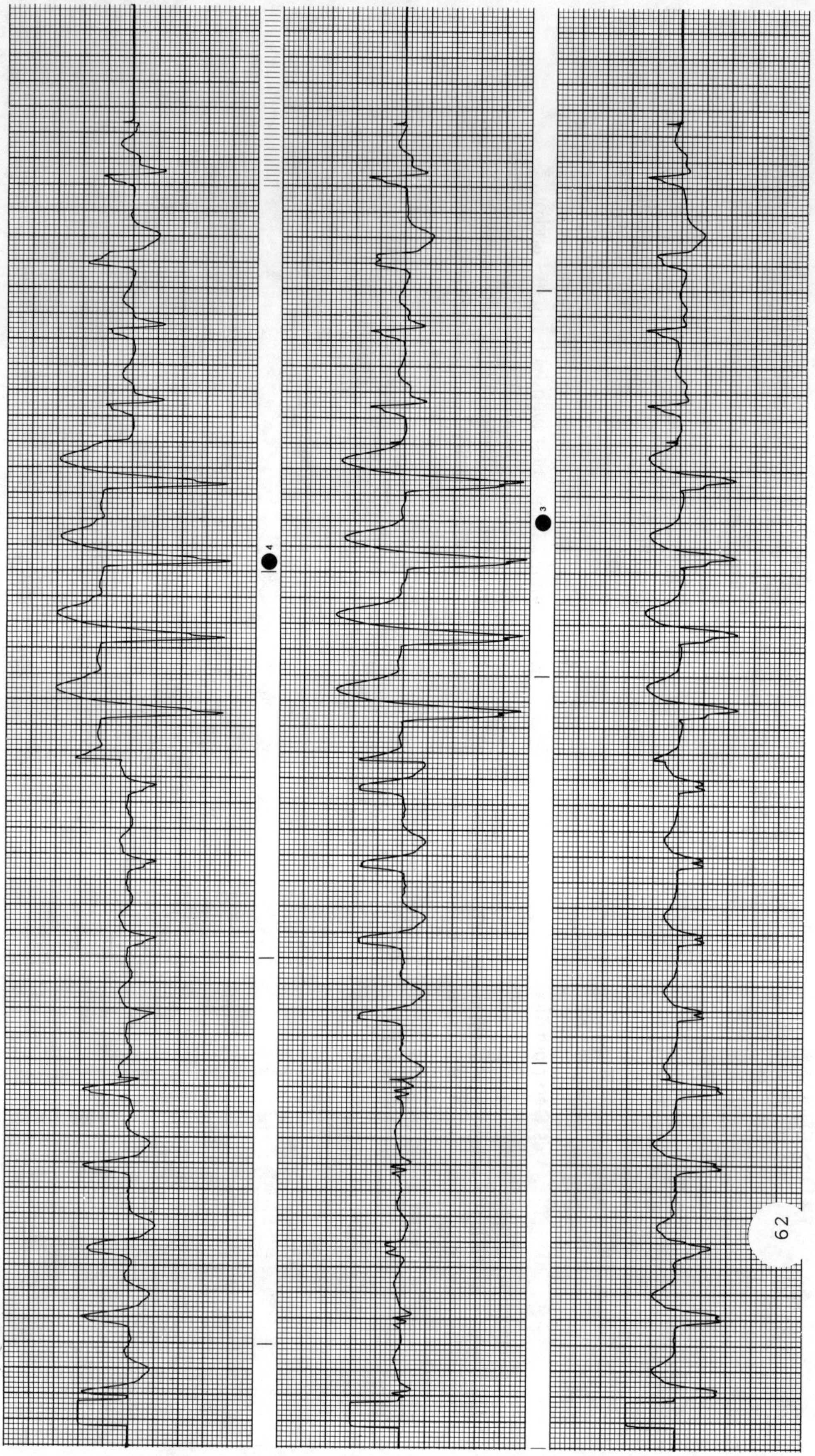

Exercise 62. A 62-year-old man with history of MI 2 years ago.

62

7

EXERCISE 62

STEP 1. Rhythm Determination

- Ventricular rate *100*
- QRS shape *Widened*

- R-R rhythm *Mostly Regular*
- QRS interval *0.17*
- QT interval *0.45*

- Atrial rate *100*
- P wave shape *Buried in T wave*
- P-P rhythm *Regular*

- P-R interval *0.26*
- P:R conduction ratio *1:1*

- Dominant pacemaker site *Sinus*
- Interpretation *Sinus tachycardia with 1st degree AV block and PVCs*

STEP 2. Axis Determination

Left axis

STEP 3. Chamber Enlargement Determination

None

STEP 4. Intraventricular Conduction Blocks Determination

LBBB

STEP 5. Ischemia, Injury, and Infarction Determination

Cannot be determined in the presence of LBBB

STEP 6. Miscellaneous ECG Changes

No significant findings

STEP 7. Final Interpretation

Abnormal 12-lead ECG. Sinus tachycardia with 1st degree AV block and PVCs. LBBB. LAD. Assess age of LBBB; if old, no further treatment necessary. If acute, assess patient for signs and symptoms of myocardial ischemia. If new, monitor serial cardiac enzymes for acute MI. Monitor on rhythm lead for progression to complete heart block. Apply external pacemaker and set heart rate; initiate pacing if rhythm progresses to complete heart block.

7

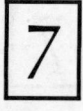

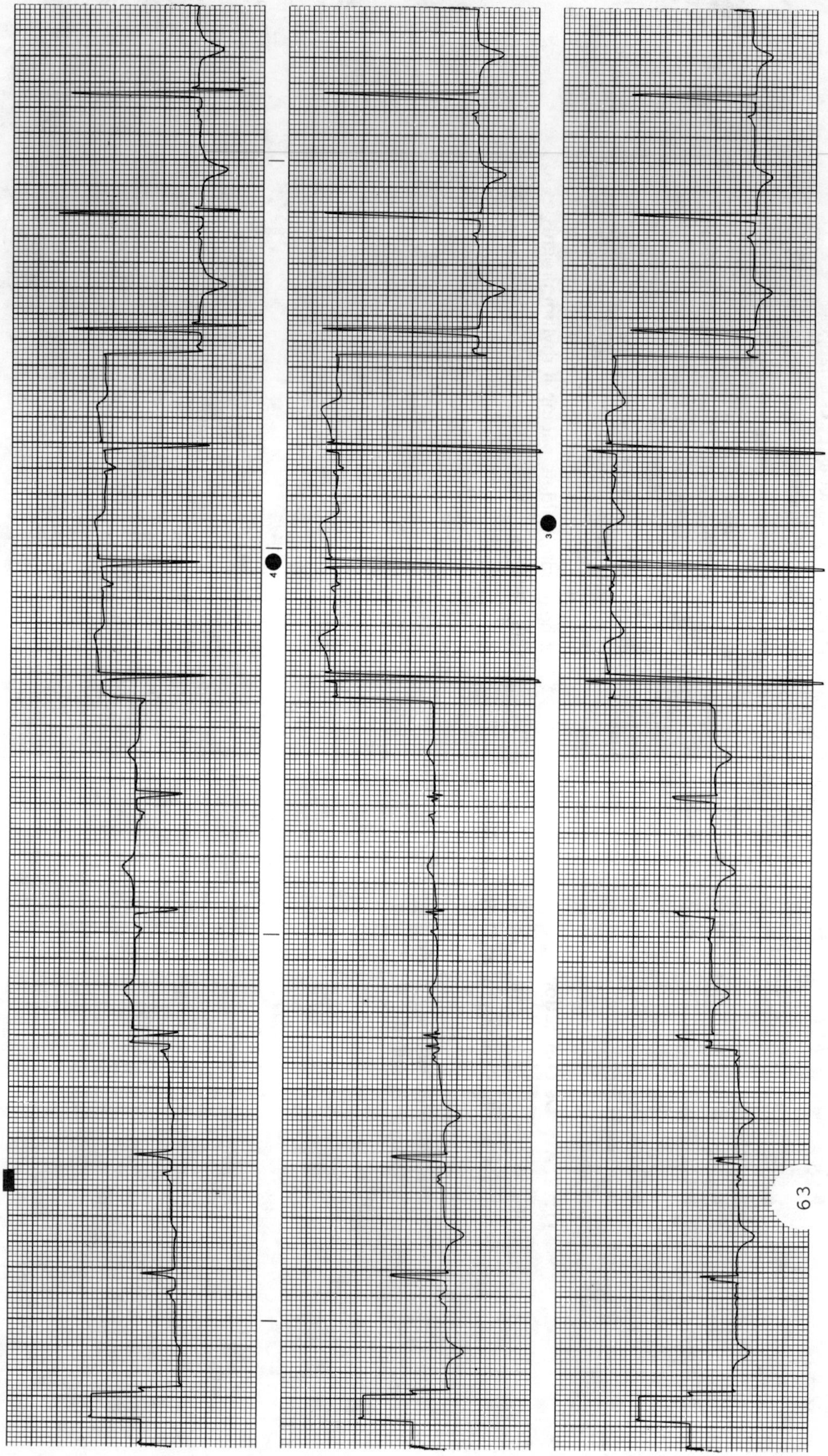

Exercise 63. A 50-year-old woman with longstanding history of hypertension.

63

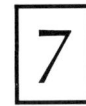

EXERCISE 63

STEP 1. Rhythm Determination

- Ventricular rate 66
- QRS shape *Large, normal*

- R-R rhythm *Regular*
- QRS interval *0.08*
- QT interval *0.44*

- Dominant pacemaker site *Sinus*
- Interpretation *NSR*

- Atrial rate 66
- P wave shape *Notched, wide, positive except negative in aVR and diphasic in V1 and V2*

- P-P rhythm *Regular*
- P-R interval *0.18*
- P:R conduction ratio *1:1*

STEP 2. Axis Determination

Normal axis

STEP 3. Chamber Enlargement Determination

Left atrial abnormality with LVH

STEP 4. Intraventricular Conduction Blocks Determination

Normal conduction

STEP 5. Ischemia, Injury, and Infarction Determination

ST segments upwardly coved with T wave inversions in all leads with tall R waves. Normal R wave progression.

STEP 6. Miscellaneous ECG Changes

No significant findings

STEP 7. Final Interpretation

Abnormal 12-lead ECG. Normal sinus rhythm with left atrial abnormality. LVH with strain. No treatment necessary for this ECG. These findings are consistent with hypertensive heart disease. This patient should be on antihypertensive medication.

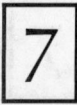

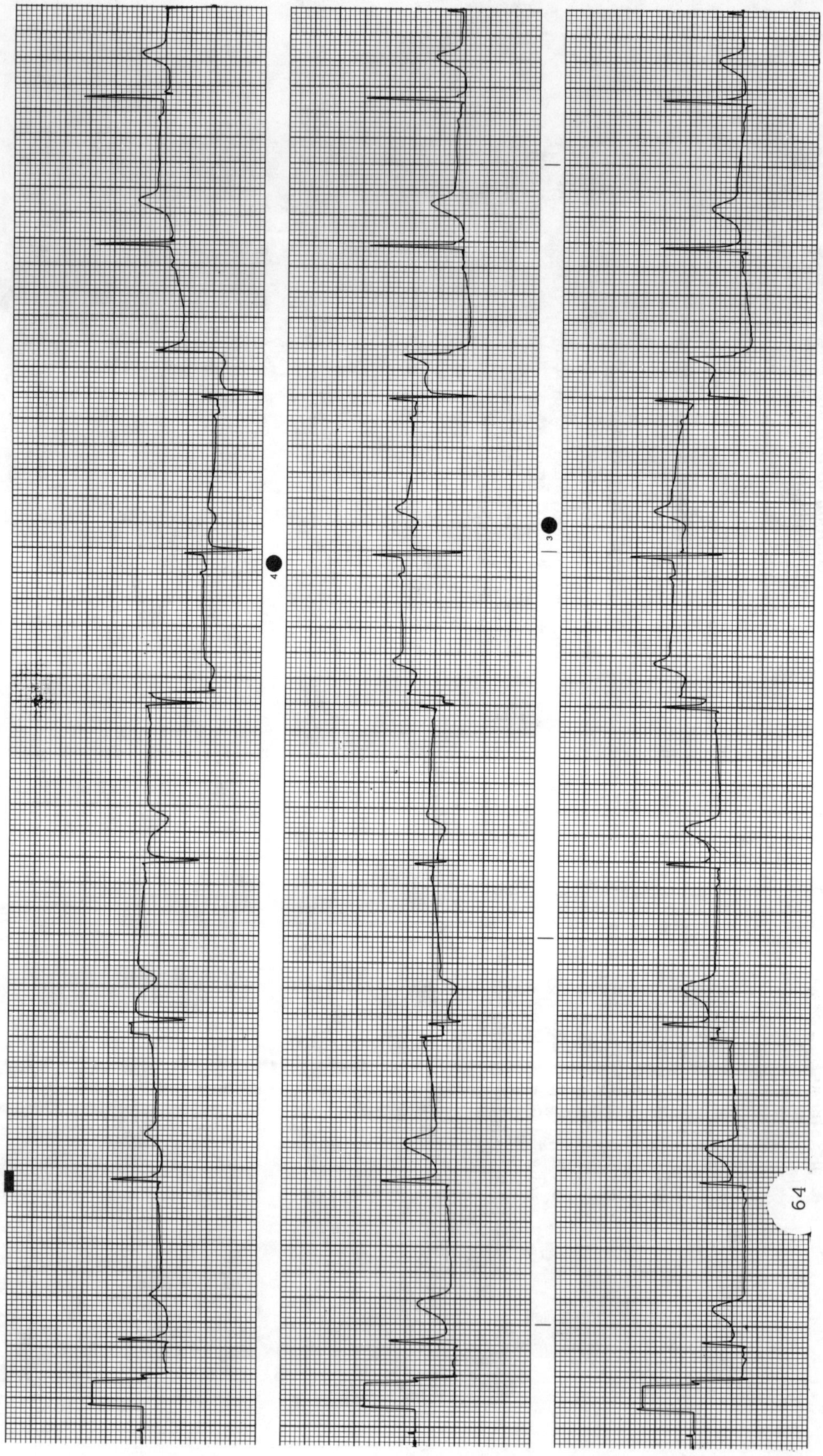

Exercise 64. A 77-year-old woman admitted with substernal left-sided chest pain.

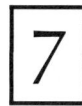

EXERCISE 64

STEP 1. Rhythm Determination

- Ventricular rate *50*
- QRS shape *Normal*

- Atrial rate *50*
- P wave shape
  *Positive except
  negative in III, aVR,
  and aVF*

- R-R rhythm *Regular*
- QRS interval *0.08*
- QT interval *0.43*

- P-P rhythm *Regular*
- P-R interval *0.16*
- P:R conduction ratio
  1:1

- Dominant pacemaker site *Sinus*
- Interpretation *Sinus bradycardia*

STEP 2. Axis Determination

Normal axis

STEP 3. Chamber Enlargement Determination

None

STEP 4. Intraventricular Conduction Blocks Determination

Normal conduction

STEP 5. Ischemia, Injury, and Infarction Determination

ST segments elevated in leads II, III, and aVF with reciprocal depressions in lead aVL. ST segments depressed in leads V1–V3. T waves positive in all leads except negative in leads aVR, aVL, and V1. Abnormally tall R waves in leads V1–V2. The rest of R wave progression is normal.

STEP 6. Miscellaneous ECG Changes

No significant findings

STEP 7. Final Interpretation

Abnormal 12-lead ECG. Sinus bradycardia with inferoposterior injury current. Assess quality and type of pain; medicate appropriately. Patient received sublingual nitroglycerin with relief of chest pain within 3 minutes. She was being monitored at the time. The nurse noted that ST-T wave changes returned to normal with relief of pain. These ECG changes were caused by variant angina. Monitor serial ECGs and cardiac enzymes; if they remain negative, patient will need further workup of coronary artery disease. She should be placed on a calcium channel blocker to prevent further spasm.

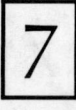

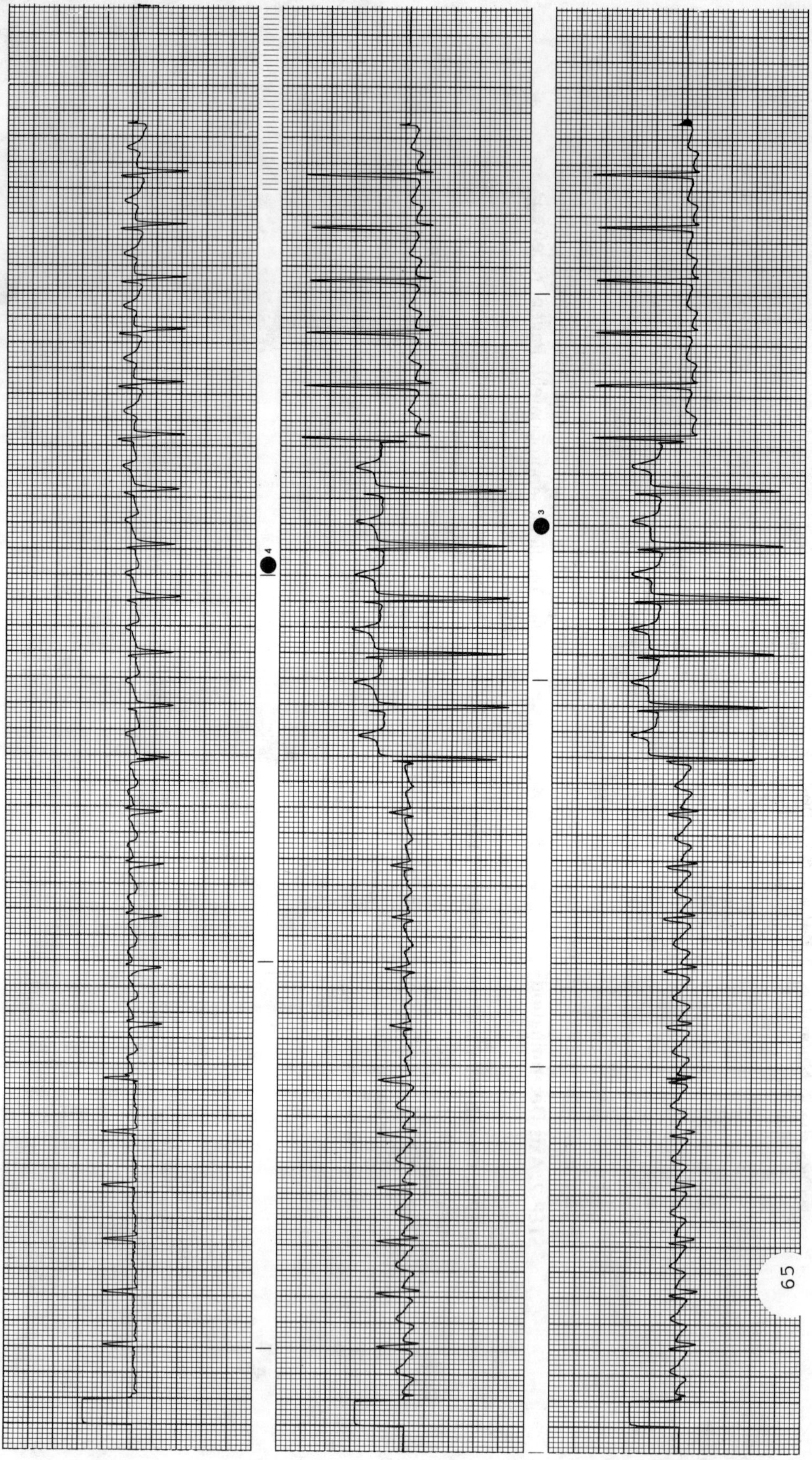

Exercise 65.   A 58-year-old man with history of cardiomyopathy.

65

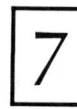

EXERCISE 65

STEP 1. Rhythm Determination

- Ventricular rate *150*
- QRS shape *Normal*

- R-R rhythm *Regular*
- QRS interval *0.09*
- QT interval *0.28*

- Atrial rate *300*
- P wave shape *Saw-toothed*
- P-P rhythm *Regular*
- P-R interval *=*
- P:R conduction ratio *2:1*

- Dominant pacemaker site *Atrial*
- Interpretation *Atrial flutter*

STEP 2. Axis Determination

Normal axis

STEP 3. Chamber Enlargement Determination

None

STEP 4. Intraventricular Conduction Blocks Determination

Normal conduction

STEP 5. Ischemia, Injury, and Infarction Determination

ST segments and T waves difficult to assess because obscured by flutter waves but they appear to be within normal limits. Normal R wave progression.

STEP 6. Miscellaneous ECG Changes

No significant findings

STEP 7. Final Interpretation

Abnormal 12-lead ECG. Atrial flutter. Monitor patient's vital signs to assess for tolerance of this rapid rhythm. If hypotensive or has other signs and symptoms of low cardiac output, prepare for electrical cardioversion. If otherwise stable, prepare to cardiovert chemically with digoxin and quinidine. If the patient has a low ejection fraction secondary to his cardiomyopathy, a calcium channel blocker that decreases contractility, i.e., verapamil, should be used with caution and may be contraindicated. Monitor serial ECGs and cardiac enzymes to determine whether rhythm change caused by an ischemic process. Monitor on lead II and note rhythm changes.

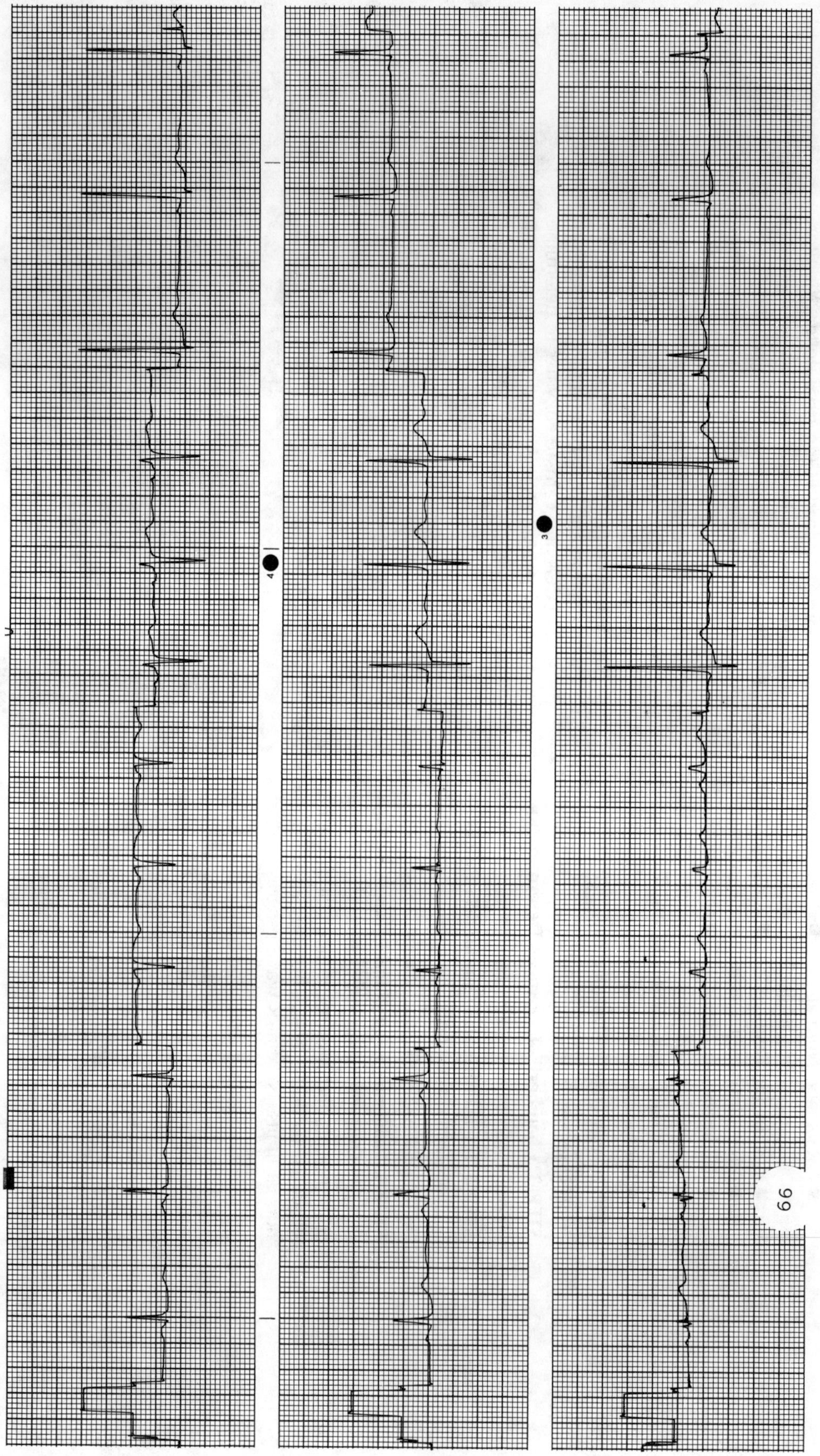

Exercise 66. A 59-year-old man admitted with severe chest pain. History of smoking.

7

EXERCISE 66

STEP 1. Rhythm Determination

- Ventricular rate 65
- QRS shape *Normal*

- Atrial rate 65
- P wave shape
  Positive except negative in aVR

- R-R rhythm *Irregular*
- QRS interval *0.08*
- QT interval *0.40*

- P-P rhythm *Irregular*
- P-R interval *0.16*
- P:R conduction ratio *1:1*

- Dominant pacemaker site *Sinus*
- Interpretation *Sinus arrhythmia*

STEP 2. Axis Determination

Normal axis

STEP 3. Chamber Enlargement Determination

None

STEP 4. Intraventricular Conduction Blocks Determination

Normal conduction

STEP 5. Ischemia, Injury, and Infarction Determination

ST segments isoelectric. T waves positive in all leads except negative in aVR and flattened in aVL. R wave progression normal.

STEP 6. Miscellaneous ECG Changes

No significant findings

STEP 7. Final Interpretation

Normal 12-lead ECG with sinus arrhythmia. Assess type and quality of chest pain. This patient's chest pain was diagnosed as cardiac. He was admitted to the CCU where he had serial ECGs and cardiac enzymes. His ECG did not change but his cardiac enzymes did become positive. These findings are consistent with a non-Q wave infarction and illustrate the point that the ECG is only one tool used to diagnose cardiac disease. When diagnosing angina and/or myocardial injury, the patient's symptoms are critical to making a treatment decision and must always be considered.

7

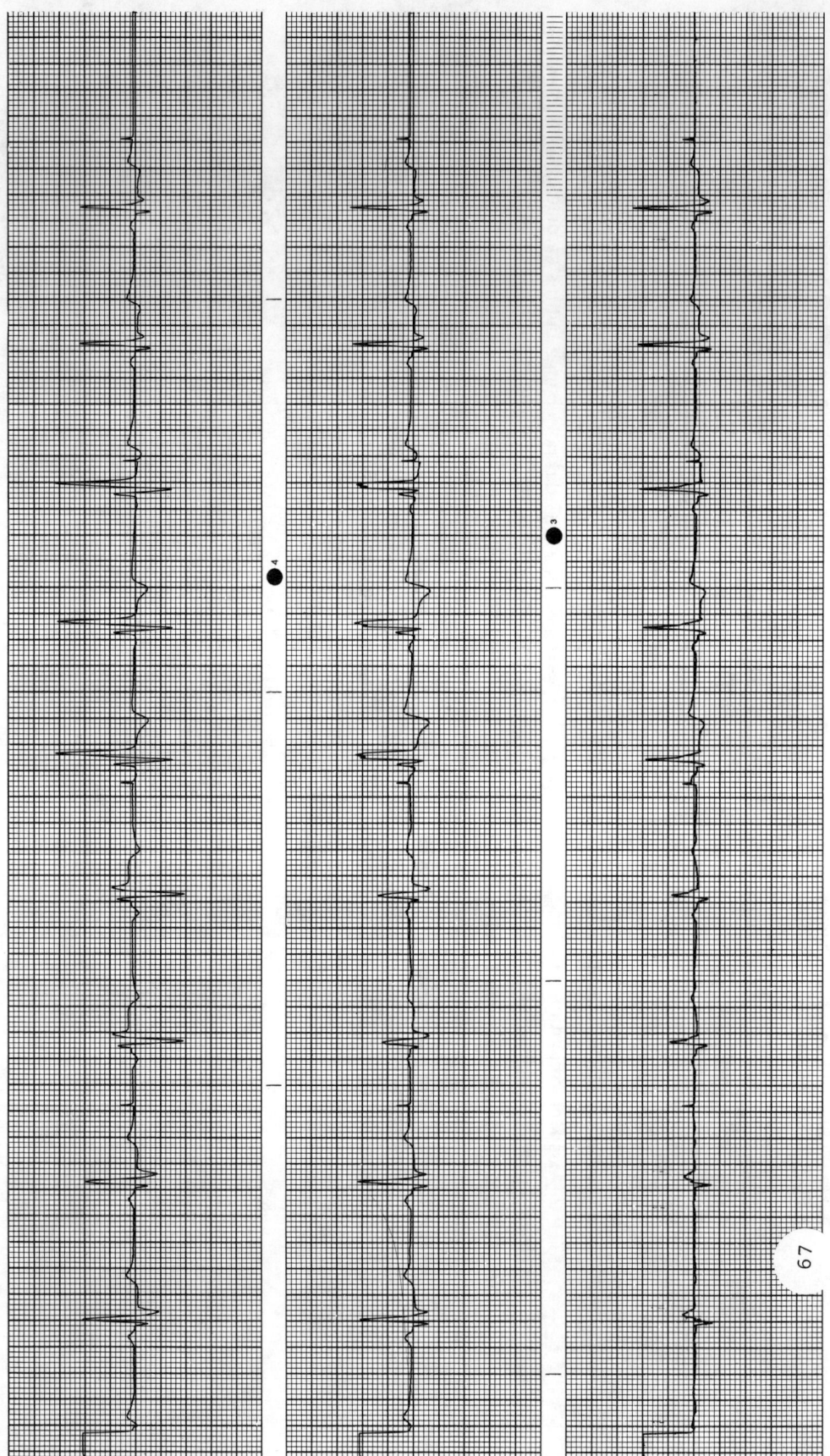

Exercise 67. A 50-year-old man with history of an MI at the age of 32. Past month has been complaining of increasing chest pain.

67

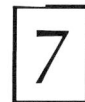

EXERCISE 67

STEP 1. Rhythm Determination

- Ventricular rate 58
- QRS shape Widened, notched

- Atrial rate 58
- P wave shape Positive except negative in aVR and flattened in V1

- R-R rhythm Regular
- QRS interval 0.16
- QT interval 0.48

- P-P rhythm Regular
- P-R interval 0.16
- P:R conduction ratio 1:1

- Dominant pacemaker site Sinus
- Interpretation Sinus bradycardia

STEP 2. Axis Determination

Normal axis

STEP 3. Chamber Enlargement Determination

None

STEP 4. Intraventricular Conduction Blocks Determination

RBBB

STEP 5. Ischemia, Injury, and Infarction Determination

ST segments isoelectric. T waves positive in all leads except negative in aVR, V1 and V2, and diphasic in V3–V5 (primary changes). R wave progression cannot be assessed. Significant Q waves in leads I, aVL, II, III, aVF, V3–V6.

STEP 6. Miscellaneous ECG Changes

No significant findings. Although the measured QT interval is 0.48 seconds, it is within normal limits because the corrected QT interval for this heart rate is 0.45 seconds.

STEP 7. Final Interpretation

Abnormal 12-lead ECG. Sinus bradycardia with RBBB. Old inferior MI. Evolutionary changes of anterolateral MI. Monitor serial ECGs and cardiac enzymes. Monitor on limb lead to assess for progression of intraventricular block. Determine age of RBBB; if old, of no clinical significance; if new, may be ischemic change.

APPENDIX A
Answers to Chapters 1–7

SELF-ASSESSMENT ANSWERS TO CHAPTER 1

EXERCISE 1

STEP 1: Rhythm Determination
- Ventricular rate *68*
- QRS shape *Normal*
- Atrial rate *68*
- P wave shape *Positive except negative in aVR*

- R-R rhythm *Regular*
- QRS interval *0.08*
- QT interval *0.38*
- P-P rhythm *Regular*
- P-R interval *0.16*
- P:R conduction ratio *1:1*

- Dominant pacemaker site *Sinus*
- Interpretation *NSR*

STEP 2: Axis Determination
Normal

STEP 3: Chamber Enlargement Determination
None

STEP 4: Intraventricular Conduction Blocks Determination
Normal conduction

STEP 5: Ischemia, Injury, and Infarction Determination
ST segments isoelectric. T wave positive in all leads except negative aVR. R wave progression normal.

STEP 6: Miscellaneous ECG Changes
No significant findings

STEP 7: Final Interpretation
Normal 12-lead ECG with normal sinus rhythm

EXERCISE 2

STEP 1: Rhythm Determination
- Ventricular rate *57*
- QRS shape *Normal*
- Atrial rate *57*
- P wave shape *Positive except negative in aVR and flat in aVL*

- R-R rhythm *Regular*
- P-P rhythm *Regular*

- QRS interval *0.08*
- QT interval *0.38*
- P-R interval *0.16*
- P:R conduction ratio *1:1*

- Dominant pacemaker site *Sinus*
- Interpretation *Sinus Bradycardia*

STEP 2: Axis Determination
Normal

STEP 3: Chamber Enlargement Determination
None

STEP 4: Intraventricular Conduction Blocks Determination
Normal conduction

STEP 5: Ischemia, Injury, and Infarction Determination
ST segments isoelectric. T waves positive in all leads except negative in aVR and V1. Normal R wave progression.

STEP 6: Miscellaneous ECG Changes
No significant findings

STEP 7: Final Interpretation
Normal 12-lead ECG with sinus bradycardia. Positive smoking history, counsel regarding cardiac risk factor modification.

EXERCISE 3

STEP 1: Rhythm Determination
- Ventricular rate *88*
- QRS shape *Normal*
- Atrial rate *88*
- P wave shape *Positive except negative in aVR and flat in aVL*

- R-R rhythm *Regular*
- QRS interval *0.08*
- QT interval *0.32*
- P-P rhythm *Regular*
- P-R interval *0.14*
- P:R conduction ratio *1:1*

- Dominant pacemaker site *Sinus*
- Interpretation *NSR*

STEP 2: Axis Determination
Normal

STEP 3: Chamber Enlargement Determination
None

STEP 4: Intraventricular Conduction Blocks Determination
Normal conduction

STEP 5: Ischemia, Injury, and Infarction Determination
ST segments isoelectric. T waves positive in all leads except negative in aVR and flat in aVL. Normal R wave progression.

STEP 6: Miscellaneous ECG Changes
No significant findings

STEP 7: Final Interpretation
Normal 12-lead ECG with normal sinus rhythm. Further assess nature of pain. Medicate for pain as necessary. Follow serial ECGs and cardiac enzymes for any changes.

EXERCISE 4

STEP 1: Rhythm Determination
- Ventricular rate *71*
- QRS shape *Normal*
- Atrial rate *71*
- P wave shape *Positive except negative in aVR and diphasic in V1*

- R-R rhythm *Regular*
- QRS interval *0.08*
- QT interval *0.36*
- P-P rhythm *Regular*
- P-R interval *0.12*
- P:R conduction ratio *1:1*

- Dominant pacemaker site *Sinus*
- Interpretation *NSR*

STEP 2: Axis Determination
Normal

STEP 3: Chamber Enlargement Determination
None

STEP 4: Intraventricular Conduction Block Determination
Normal conduction

STEP 5: Ischemia, Injury, and Infarction Determination
ST segments isoelectric. T waves positive in all leads except negative in aVR and III. Normal R wave progression.

STEP 6: Miscellaneous ECG Changes
No significant findings

STEP 7: Final Interpretation
Normal 12-lead ECG with normal sinus rhythm.

Continue observing for further pain, ECG, and/or cardiac enzyme changes. Positive smoking history, counsel regarding cardiac risk factor modification.

EXERCISE 5

STEP 1: Rhythm Determination
- Ventricular rate *58*
- QRS shape *Normal*
- Atrial rate *58*
- P wave shape *Positive except negative in aVR, diphasic in V1, and flattened in aVL*

- R-R rhythm *Regular*
- QRS interval *0.08*
- QT interval *0.36*
- P-P rhythm *Regular*
- P-R interval *0.16*
- P:R conduction ratio *1:1*

- Dominant pacemaker site *Sinus*
- Interpretation *Sinus bradycardia*

STEP 2: Axis Determination
Normal

STEP 3: Chamber Enlargement Determination
None

STEP 4: Intraventricular Conduction Blocks Determination
Normal conduction

STEP 5: Ischemia, Injury, and Infarction Determination
ST segments isoelectric but sagging in all leads with tall R wave. T waves positive in all leads except negative in aVR. Normal R wave progression.

STEP 6: Miscellaneous ECG Determination
Sagging ST segments in leads with tall R wave—digoxin effect

STEP 7: Final Interpretation
Normal 12-lead ECG with sinus bradycardia. Digoxin effect. Assess and monitor for further chest pain, ECG, and/or cardiac enzyme changes. Counsel regarding smoking to reduce risk of cardiac disease. Difficult to assess for ischemia because ST depressions may all be related to digoxin use. If cardiac enzymes do not elevate, may need to follow up with a thallium stress test to assess for ischemic areas of myocardium.

EXERCISE 6

STEP 1: Rhythm Determination
- Ventricular rate *81*
- QRS shape *Normal*
- Atrial rate *81*
- P wave shape *Positive except negative in aVR and aVL*

- R-R rhythm *Regular*
- QRS interval *0.08*
- QT interval *0.36*
- P-R rhythm *Regular*
- P-R interval *0.16*
- P:R conduction ratio *1:1*
- Dominant pacemaker site *Sinus*
- Interpretation *NSR*

STEP 2: Axis Determination
Normal

STEP 3: Chamber Enlargement Determination
None

STEP 4: Intraventricular Conduction Blocks Determination
Normal conduction

STEP 5: Ischemia, Injury, and Infarction Determination
ST segments isoelectric. T waves positive in all leads except negative in aVR and negative and flat in aVL. Normal R wave progression.

STEP 6: Miscellaneous ECG Changes
No significant findings

STEP 7: Final Interpretation
Normal 12-lead ECG with normal sinus rhythm. Assess nature of pain and other associated signs and symptoms to try to establish cause of pain. If cardiac source suspected by history, admit and observe for ECG and/or cardiac enzyme changes.

SELF-ASSESSMENT ANSWERS TO CHAPTER 2

EXERCISE 7
STEP 1: Rhythm Determination
- Ventricular rate *90*
- QRS shape *Normal*

- Atrial rate *90*
- P wave shape *Positive except negative in aVR and aVL, and diphasic in V1, V2*

- R-R rhythm *Mostly regular*
- QRS interval *0.08*
- QT interval *0.32*
- P-P rhythm *Mostly regular*
- P-R interval *0.14*
- P:R conduction ratio *1:1*
- Dominant pacemaker site *Sinus*
- Interpretation *NSR with occasional APBs*

STEP 2: Axis Determination
Normal

STEP 3: Chamber Enlargement Determination
None

STEP 4: Intraventricular Conduction Blocks Determination
Normal conduction

STEP 5: Ischemia, Injury, and Infarction Determination
ST segments isoelectric. T waves positive in all leads except flattened in aVR and negative in I, aVL, V5, and V6. R wave progression normal.

STEP 6: Miscellaneous ECG Changes
No significant findings

STEP 7: Final Interpretation
Abnormal 12-lead ECG. Normal sinus rhythm with occasional APBs. Inverted T waves in lateral leads may

indicate lateral ischemia. Further assess and treat chest pain. Fever and hypoxemia increase myocardial demand, so observe for further ischemic ECG and vital sign changes. Once fever and hypoxemia corrected, assess ECG for continued presence of lateral changes. Assess cardiac enzymes to R/O non-Q wave infarction.

Observe monitor for increased APBs or the development of atrial dysrhythmias, such as atrial tachycardia, atrial fibrillation, or atrial flutter.

EXERCISE 8
STEP 1: Rhythm Determination
- Ventricular rate *78*
- QRS shape *Normal*

- Atrial rate *320*
- P wave shape *Saw-toothed*

- R-R interval *Regular*
- QRS interval *0.10*
- QT interval *cannot measure*
- P-P rhythm *Regular*
- P-R interval *Absent*
- P:R conduction ratio *4:1*
- Dominant pacemaker site *Atrial*
- Interpretation *Atrial flutter with a controlled ventricular response*

STEP 2: Axis Determination
Normal

STEP 3: Chamber Enlargement Determination
None

STEP 4: Intraventricular Conduction Blocks Determination
Incomplete LBBB

STEP 5: Ischemia, Injury, and Infarction Determination
ST and T waves buried in flutter waves. Normal R wave progression.

STEP 6: Miscellaneous ECG Changes
No significant findings

STEP 7: Final Interpretation
Abnormal 12-lead ECG. Atrial flutter with a controlled ventricular response. Incomplete LBBB. No sign of any pacemaker activity. Assess for further chest pain and treat as necessary.

Assess whether atrial flutter new or chronic. Prepare for possible treatment of intravenous digoxin and verapamil or electrical cardioversion.

EXERCISE 9

STEP 1: Rhythm Determination
- Ventricular rate 58
- QRS shape *Normal wih occasional wide beats*
- R-R rhythm *Irregular due to premature beats*
- QRS interval 0.08
- QT interval 0.42
- Atrial rate 58
- P wave shape *Positive except aVR negative*
- P-P rhythm *Regular except occasional absent P wave*
- P-R interval 0.16
- P:R conduction ratio 1:1
- Dominant pacemaker site *Sinus*
- Interpretation *Sinus bradycardia with ventricular trigeminy*

STEP 2: Axis Determination
Normal

STEP 3: Chamber Enlargement Determination
None

STEP 4: Intraventricular Conduction Blocks Determination
Normal conduction

STEP 5: Ischemia, Injury, and Infarction Determination
ST segments elevated in V1, V2, V3. T waves positive in all leads except flat to inverted in aVR, aVL and V4. Significant Q waves in V2, V3, and V4.

STEP 6: Miscellaneous ECG Changes
No significant findings

STEP 7: Final Interpretation
Abnormal ECG. Sinus bradycardia with ventricular trigeminy. Anteroseptal MI, age indeterminate. Assess further ECGs and cardiac enzymes for further changes. If remain negative, ischemic admission

symptoms will need further workup. Assess heart and lung sound—R/O signs and symptoms of heart failure.

Treat PVCs with lidocaine; be alert for development of heart block or significant bradycardia in the setting of lidocaine treatment in a patient with bradycardia. Monitor for change in rhythm either control of PVCs or deterioration to VT or VF.

Monitor patient for development of axis change and/or a BBB. Suggested monitor lead to use is V1.

EXERCISE 10

STEP 1: Rhythm Determination
- Ventricular rate 190
- QRS shape *Normal*
- R-R rhythm *Regular*
- QRS interval 0.06
- QT interval 0.22
- Atrial rate *Unable to measure*
- P wave shape *Buried*
- P-P rhythm ==
- P-R interval ==
- P:R conduction ratio ==
- Dominant pacemaker site *Atrial*
- Interpretation *Supraventricular tachycardia (SVT)*

STEP 2: Axis Determination
Normal

STEP 3: Chamber Enlargement Determination
None

STEP 4: Intraventricular Conduction Blocks Determination
Normal conduction

STEP 5: Ischemia, Injury, and Infarction Determination
ST segment sagging in leads II, III, aVF, V2–V6. T waves difficult to assess but appear normal. Normal R wave progression.

STEP 6: Miscellaneous Changes
Sagging ST segments in leads with tall R wave—probable digoxin effect

STEP 7: Final Interpretation
Abnormal 12-lead ECG. SVT with probable digoxin effect. Ischemic changes due to tachycardia or myocardial disease cannot be ruled out. Further assess patient for signs and symptoms of ischemia—chest pain, shortness of breath, sweating, nausea and vomiting, and hypotension. Assess serial cardiac enzymes for elevations indicative of MI.
Prepare for treatment of SVT with intravenous digoxin, verapamil, or electric cardioversion.
Provide O_2 and assess vital signs for deterioration of condition.
Monitor for change in rhythm, either conversion to sinus rhythm or deterioration to a ventricular rhythm.

EXERCISE '11

STEP 1: Rhythm Determination
- Ventricular rate *46*
- QRS shape *Normal*
- Atrial rate *92*
- P wave shape *Positive except negative in aVR and diphasic in V1 and V2*
- R-R rhythm *Regular*
- QRS interval *0.08*
- QT interval *0.48*
- P-P rhythm *Regular*
- P-R interval *0.36*
- P:R conduction ratio *2:1*
- Dominant pacemaker site *Sinus*
- Interpretation *Second degree AV block with 2:1 conduction*

STEP 2: Axis Determination
Left axis

STEP 3: Chamber Enlargement Determination
None

STEP 4: Intraventricular Conduction Blocks Determination
Normal conduction

STEP 5: Ischemia, Injury, and Infarction Determination
ST segments isoelectric. T waves positive in all leads except negative in aVR and III. R wave progression normal.

STEP 6: Miscellaneous ECG Changes
No significant findings, measured QT interval is long (0.48), but the corrected QT for this heart rate is 0.50. Therefore, this QT interval is not prolonged for this slow heart rate.

STEP 7: Final Interpretation
Abnormal 12-lead ECG. Second degree AV block with 2:1 conduction. Take vital signs. Administer atropine to increase heart rate and, hopefully, relieve chest pain. Be prepared to use external pacemaker and for insertion of temporary invasive pacemaker. Monitor cardiac enzymes. Assess drug history for digoxin or diltiazem (calcium channel blocker). If pain not relieved, treat.

EXERCISE 12

STEP 1: Rhythm Determination
- Ventricular rate *240*
- QRS shape *Wide & Bizarre*
- R-R rhythm *Regular*
- QRS interval *0.22*
- QT interval *==*
- Atrial rate *Cannot measure*
- P wave shape *==*
- P-P rhythm *==*
- P-R interval *==*
- P:R conduction ratio *==*
- Dominant pacemaker site *Ventricular*
- Interpretation *Ventricular tachycardia*

STEP 2: Axis Determination
Right axis

STEP 3: Chamber Enlargement Determination
None

STEP 4: Intraventricular Conduction Blocks Determination
No conduction problem, wide QRS due to ventricular dysrythmia.

STEP 5: Ischemia, Injury, and Infarction Determination
Cannot be determined due to ventricular dysrhythmia.

STEP 6: Miscellaneous ECG Changes
No significant findings

STEP 7: Final Interpretation
Abnormal 12-lead ECG. Ventricular tachycardia. Take vital signs and assess for presence of pulse. Prepare for emergency cardioversion. Prepare lidocaine bolus and maintenance drip.

SELF-ASSESSMENT ANSWERS TO CHAPTER 3

EXERCISE 13
STEP 1: Rhythm Determination
- Ventricular rate *47*
- QRS shape *Normal*
- R-R rhythm *Regular*
- QRS interval *0.11*
- Atrial rate *47*
- P wave shape *Positive except negative aVR and flat in III*
- P-P rhythm *Regular*
- P-R interval *0.28*
- QT interval *0.48*
- P:R conduction ratio *1:1*
- Dominant pacemaker site *Sinus*
- Interpretation *Sinus bradycardia with 1st degree AV block*

STEP 2: Axis Determination
Left axis

STEP 3: Chamber Enlargement Determination
None

STEP 4: Intraventricular Conduction Blocks Determination

IVCD, LAH

STEP 5: Ischemia, Injury, and Infarction Determination

ST segments isoelectric. T waves positive in all leads except negative in I, aVR, and aVL. Poor R wave progression.

STEP 6: Miscellaneous ECG Changes

No significant findings. Measured QT interval is long (0.48), but corrected QT is 0.49. Therefore, QT interval is not prolonged.

STEP 7: Final Interpretation

Abnormal 12-lead ECG. Sinus bradycardia with 1st degree AV block and IVCD with LAH. Poor R wave progression in chest leads. Compare with previous ECG to determine age and/or significance of poor R wave progression. Possible anteroseptal MI, age indeterminate. Assess vital signs and observe for symptoms of low cardiac output. Assess type and level of chest pain; medicate appropriately. Monitor ECG for further T wave inversion in lateral leads and cardiac enzymes.

EXERCISE 14

STEP 1: Rhythm Determination

- Ventricular rate *90*
- Atrial rate *90*
- QRS shape *Small and widened*
- P wave shape *Positive except negative aVR, V1 and flattened in aVL*
- R-R rhythm *Regular*
- P-P rhythm *Regular*
- QRS interval *0.10*
- P-R interval *0.16*
- QT interval *0.32*
- P:R conduction ratio *1:1*
- Dominant pacemaker site *Sinus*
- Interpretation *NSR*

STEP 2: Axis Determination

Right axis deviation

STEP 3: Chamber Enlargement Determination

None

STEP 4: Intraventricular Conduction Blocks Determination

IVCD

STEP 5: Ischemia, Injury, and Infarction Determination

1-mm ST segment elevations in leads II, III, aVF. T waves positive in all leads except flat in leads I and

aVL; negative in aVR. Poor R wave progression in chest leads. No reciprocal changes noted for ST segment elevations.

STEP 6: Miscellaneous ECG Changes

No significant findings

STEP 7: Final Interpretation

Abnormal 12-lead ECG. Normal sinus rhythm with RAD and IVCD. Possible old anteroseptal infarction. Injury current in inferior leads. Possible inferior infarction versus variant angina. Assess vital signs, quality, and location of chest pain and cardiac enyzmes. Medicate with nitroglycerin. If pain relieved with nitroglycerin and ST segments return to baseline and cardiac enzymes negative, diagnosis of variant angina.

EXERCISE 15

STEP 1: Rhythm Determination

- Ventricular rate *100*
- Atrial rate *100*
- QRS shape *Normal*
- P wave shape *Positive except negative in aVR and flat in aVL and V1–V3*
- R-R rhythm *Regular*
- P-P rhythm *Regular*
- QRS interval *0.09*
- P-R interval *0.16*
- QT interval *0.36*
- P:R conduction ratio *1:1*
- Dominant pacemaker site *Sinus*
- Interpretation *Sinus tachycardia*

STEP 2: Axis Determination

Normal

STEP 3: Chamber Enlargement Determination

None

Step 4: Intraventricular Conduction Blocks Determination

Normal conduction

STEP 5: Ischemia, Injury, and Infarction Determination

1-mm ST elevations in leads II, III, and aVF with reciprocal ST segment depressions in leads V3 and V4. T waves positive in all leads except negative in II, III, and aVF; flat in aVR. Normal R wave progression. Q waves evolving in leads II, III, and aVF.

STEP 6: Miscellaneous ECG Changes

No significant findings

STEP 7: Final Interpretation

Abnormal 12-lead ECG. Sinus tachycardia. Evolving

inferior MI. Monitor for dysrhythmias. Monitor for signs and symptoms of decreased cardiac output.

EXERCISE 16

STEP 1: Rhythm Determination
- Ventricular rate *64*
- QRS shape *Normal*
- Atrial rate *64*
- P wave shape *Positive except negative in aVR, aVL, and diphasic in V1*

- R-R rhythm *Regular*
- QRS interval *0.08*
- QT interval *0.40*
- P-P rhythm *Regular*
- P-R interval *0.16*
- P:R conduction ratio *1:1*

- Dominant pacemaker site *Sinus*
- Interpretation *NSR*

STEP 2: Axis Determination
Normal. Because QRS complex equiphasic in lead I, cannot use easy quadrant method. Must use null plane method (axis 90°).

STEP 3: Chamber Enlargement Determination
None

STEP 4: Intraventricular Conduction Blocks Determination
Normal conduction

STEP 5: Ischemia, Injury, and Infarction Determination
ST segments isoelectric. T waves positive in all leads except negative in aVR, aVL, and V1. Poor R wave in leads V2 and V3.

STEP 6: Miscellaneous ECG Changes
No significant findings

STEP 7: Final Interpretation
Normal ECG with normal sinus rhythm. Assess vital signs. Assess type and quality of chest pain; medicate as appropriate. If chest pain assessed as cardiac, monitor serial ECGs and cardiac enzymes. Compare ECG with previous one if available.

EXERCISE 17

STEP 1: Rhythm Determination
- Ventricular rate *72*
- QRS shape *Normal*
- Atrial rate *72*
- P wave shape *Positive except negative in aVR and aVL, diphasic in V1 and V2*

- R-R rhythm *Regular*
- QRS interval *0.10*
- QT interval *0.40*
- P-P rhythm *Regular*
- P-R interval *0.16*
- P:R conduction ratio *1:1*

- Dominant pacemaker site *Sinus*
- Interpretation *NSR*

STEP 2: Axis Determination
Normal

STEP 3: Chamber Enlargement Determination
None

STEP 4: Intraventricular Conduction Blocks Determination
IVCD

STEP 5: Ischemia, Injury, and Infarction Determination
ST segments depressed and upwardly coved in leads I, II, V5, and V6. T waves positive in all leads except negative in I, aVL, V5, and V6. R wave progression normal.

STEP 6: Miscellaneous ECG Changes
No significant findings

STEP 7: Final Interpretation
Abnormal 12-lead ECG. Normal sinus rhythm with IVCD and nonspecific ST-T wave changes in lateral leads. Monitor serial ECGs and cardiac enzymes. Assess chest pain for quality and type and medicate as appropriate.

EXERCISE 18

STEP 1: Rhythm Determination
- Ventricular rate *72*
- QRS shape *Normal*
- Atrial rate *72*
- P wave shape *Positive except negative aVR, V1*

- R-R rhythm *Regular*
- QRS interval *0.08*
- QT interval *0.44*
- P-P rhythm *Regular*
- P-R interval *0.18*
- P:R conduction ratio *1:1*

- Dominant pacemaker site *Sinus*
- Interpretation *NSR*

STEP 2: Axis Determination
Indeterminate. Because all QRS complexes are diphasic neither the easy quadrant nor the null plane method can be used. It is impossible to determine the direction of the axis, therefore the axis is indeterminate.

STEP 3: Chamber Enlargement Determination
None

STEP 4: Intraventricular Conduction Blocks Determination
Normal conduction

STEP 5: Ischemia, Injury, and Infarction Determination
ST segments isoelectric. T waves positive in all leads except negative in aVR and V1, flattened in leads V2–V4. Normal R wave progression. Significant Q waves in leads III and aVF.

STEP 6: Miscellaneous ECG Changes
No significant findings

STEP 7: Final Interpretation
Abnormal 12-lead ECG. Normal sinus rhythm with indeterminate axis. Inferior MI, age indeterminate. Continue to monitor serial ECGs and cardiac enzymes. If patient should have further chest pain, perform ECG during pain episode.

SELF-ASSESSMENT ANSWERS TO CHAPTER 4

EXERCISE 19
STEP 1: Rhythm Determination
- Ventricular rate *90*
- Atrial rate *90*
- QRS shape *Slightly widened*
- P wave shape *Positive except negative aVR, aVL, V1 and V2*
- R-R rhythm *Regular*
- P-P rhythm *Regular*
- QRS interval *0.10*
- P-R interval *0.18*
- QT interval *0.36*
- P-R conduction ratio *1:1*
- Dominant pacemaker site *Sinus*
- Interpretation *NSR*

STEP 2: Axis Determination
Normal

STEP 3: Chamber Enlargement Determination
Right atrial abnormality. Borderline LVH.

STEP 4: Intraventricular Conduction Blocks Determination
IVCD

STEP 5: Ischemia, Injury, and Infarction Determination
ST segments upwardly coved in leads I, III, aVF, V4–V6. T waves positive all leads except negative in leads aVR, aVL, V4–V6. Poor R wave progression.

STEP 6: Miscellaneous ECG Changes
No significant findings

STEP 7: Final Interpretation
Abnormal 12-lead ECG. Normal sinus rhythm with IVCD, right atrial abnormality, and borderline LVH. Nonspecific ST-T wave changes probably repolarization changes related to LVH. Assess vital signs. Monitor serial ECGs and cardiac enzymes for an infarction. Monitor on lead V1 to assess for completion of intraventricular conduction block. Assess for signs and symptoms of congestive heart failure and atrial dysrhythmias related to right atrial abnormality.

EXERCISE 20
STEP 1: Rhythm Determination
- Ventricular rate *78*
- Atrial rate *78*
- QRS shape *Normal*
- P wave shape *Positive except negative aVR, aVL, diphasic V1 and V2*
- R-R rhythm *Regular*
- P-P rhythm *Regular*
- QRS interval *0.09*
- P-R interval *0.18*
- QT interval *0.36*
- P:R conduction ratio *1:1*
- Dominant pacemaker site *Sinus*
- Interpretation *NSR*

STEP 2: Axis Determination
Left axis

STEP 3: Chamber Enlargement Determination
Left atrial abnormality with LVH

STEP 4: Intraventricular Conduction Blocks Determination
Normal conduction

STEP 5: Ischemia, Injury, and Infarction Determination
ST segments depressed in all leads with tall R waves with upward coving in lead V6. T waves positive in all leads but flattened in limb leads and V5. R wave progression abnormal.

STEP 6: Miscellaneous ECG Changes
No significant findings

STEP 7: Final Interpretation
Abnormal 12-lead ECG. Normal sinus rhythm with left atrial abnormality, LVH, and left axis deviation. Assess vital signs, heart and lung sounds for congestive heart failure. Watch for atrial and ventricular dysrhythmias. Assess drug history.

EXERCISE 21

STEP 1: Rhythm Determination
- Ventricular rate *82*
- QRS shape *Normal*
- R-R rhythm *Regular*
- QRS interval *0.08*
- QT interval *0.36*
- Dominant pacemaker site *Sinus*
- Interpretation *NSR*

- Atrial rate *82*
- P wave shape *Positive except negative aVR, flat in V4–V6*
- P-P rhythm *Regular*
- P-R interval *0.12*
- P:R conduction ratio *1:1*

STEP 2: Axis Determination
Normal axis

STEP 3: Chamber Enlargement Determination
LVH

STEP 4: Intraventricular Conduction Blocks Determination
Normal conduction

STEP 5: Ischemia, Injury, and Infarction Determination
ST segments depressed in all leads with tall R waves and upwardly coved depressions in leads V4–V6. T waves flattened in all leads. R wave progression normal.

STEP 6: Miscellaneous ECG Changes
No significant findings

STEP 7: Final Interpretation
Abnormal 12-lead ECG. Normal sinus rhythm with LVH. Assess vital signs, heart and lung sounds for signs and symptoms of congestive heart failure. Monitor serial ECGs and cardiac enzymes for MI. Assess quality and type of chest pain; medicate appropriately. Assess drug history.

EXERCISE 22

STEP 1: Rhythm Determination
- Ventricular rate *90*
- QRS shape *Normal*
- R-R rhythm *Regular, occasional irregular beat*
- QRS interval *0.09*
- QT interval *0.36*

- Atrial rate *90*
- P wave shape *Tall and pointed II, diphasic V1–V2, negative in aVR and aVL*
- P-P rhythm *Regular*
- P-R interval *0.14*
- P:R conduction ratio *1:1*

- Dominant pacemaker site *Sinus*
- Interpretation *NSR with occasional PVC*

STEP 2: Axis Determination
Left axis

STEP 3: Chamber Enlargement Determination
Biatrial abnormality with LVH

STEP 4: Intraventricular Conduction Blocks Determination
Normal conduction

STEP 5: Ischemia, Injury, and Infarction Determination
ST segments sagging in leads I, aVL, and V6. T waves positive in all leads except negative in aVR, V1, and V2. Poor R wave progression.

STEP 6: Miscellaneous ECG Changes
ST segments sagging in leads with tall R wave

STEP 7: Final Interpretation
Abnormal 12-lead ECG. Normal sinus rhythm with occasional PVCs. Biatrial abnormality with LVH. Question of digitalis effect or strain pattern. Monitor serial ECGs and cardiac enzymes for MI. Assess vital signs, heart, and lung sounds for signs and symptoms of congestive heart failure. Monitor for increase in ventricular dysrhythmias, treat as necessary.

EXERCISE 23

STEP 1: Rhythm Determination
- Ventricular rate *77*
- QRS shape *Normal, tall*
- R-R rhythm *Regular*
- QRS interval *0.08*
- QT interval *0.44*

- Atrial rate *77*
- P wave shape *Notched I, II, aVF, V4–V5, diphasic III, V1 and V2, positive aVL and V3*
- P-P rhythm *Regular*
- P-R interval *0.18*
- P:R conduction ratio *1:1*

- Dominant pacemaker site *Sinus*
- Interpretation *NSR*

STEP 2: Axis Determination
Normal axis

STEP 3: Chamber Enlargement Determination
Left atrial abnormality and LVH

STEP 4: Intraventricular Conduction Blocks Determination
Normal conduction

STEP 5: Ischemia, Injury, and Infarction Determination
ST segments upwardly coved and depressed in leads

V5–V6. T waves inverted in leads II, III, aVF, V1–V6. Poor wave progression.

STEP 6: Miscellaneous ECG Changes
No significant findings

STEP 7: Final Interpretation
Abnormal 12-lead ECG. Normal sinus rhythm with left atrial abnormality and LVH with strain pattern. Monitor serial ECGs and cardiac enzymes for MI. Assess vital signs, heart and lung sounds for congestive heart failure. Assess type and quality of chest pain; medicate appropriately. Already having hypertrophic changes related to systemic hypertension. Counsel regarding blood pressure control.

EXERCISE 24

STEP 1: Rhythm Determination
- Ventricular rate *96*
- QRS shape *Small*

- R-R rhythm *Regular*
- QRS interval *0.09*
- QT interval *0.32*

- Atrial rate *96*
- P wave shape *Positive and flat except negative in aVR and aVF*
- P-P rhythm *Regular*
- P-R interval *0.18*
- P:R conduction ratio *1:1*

- Dominant pacemaker site *Sinus*
- Interpretation *NSR*

STEP 2: Axis Determination
Indeterminate axis

STEP 3: Chamber Enlargement Determination
None

STEP 4: Intraventricular Conduction Blocks Determination
Normal conduction

STEP 5: Ischemia, Injury, and Infarction Determination
ST segments isoelectric. T waves positive in all leads except negative in aVR and V1, and flat in aVL. Abnormal R wave progression due to low voltage. Significant Q waves in leads II, III, and aVF.

STEP 6: Miscellaneous ECG Changes
No significant findings

STEP 7: Final Interpretation
Abnormal 12-lead ECG. Normal sinus rhythm with an indeterminate axis. Inferior MI, age indeterminate. Monitor serial ECGs and cardiac enzymes for MI. Assess vital signs, heart and lung sounds for signs of congestive heart failure versus COPD. Monitor for atrial dysrhythmias.

SELF-ASSESSMENT ANSWERS TO CHAPTER 5

EXERCISE 25
STEP 1: Rhythm Determination
- Ventricular rate *96*
- QRS shape *Widened and notched in V1*

- R-R rhythm *Slightly irregular*
- QRS interval *0.16*
- QT interval *0.40*

- Atrial rate *96*
- P wave shape *Positive except negative in aVR and diphasic in V1*
- P-P rhythm *Slightly irregular*
- P-R interval *0.18*
- P:R conduction ratio *1:1*

- Dominant pacemaker site *Sinus*
- Interpretation *NSR with APB*

STEP 2: Axis Determination
Right axis

STEP 3: Chamber Enlargement Determination
None

STEP 4: Intraventricular Conduction Blocks Determination
RBBB with left posterior hemiblock

STEP 5: Ischemia, Injury, and Infarction Determination
ST segments elevated in leads II, III, aVF. T waves positive in all leads except negative in leads aVR and V1. The T wave changes in leads III and aVF are primary T wave changes (T waves should be negative in these leads with a RBBB). R wave progression normal. Significant Q waves in leads II, III, and aVF.

STEP 6: Miscellaneous ECG Changes
No significant findings

STEP 7: Final Interpretation
Abnormal 12-lead ECG. Normal sinus rhythm with one APB. (Note second complex in leads I, II, and III. Need to examine rhythm strip to confirm.) RAD with bifascicular block. Assess age of conduction blocks; if new may be ischemic changes. Monitor serial ECGs and cardiac enzymes for MI. Assess vital signs. Monitor for progression of heart block. Apply external pacemaker. Be prepared for insertion of transvenous temporary pacemaker. Assess type and quality of chest pain; medicate appropriately.

EXERCISE 26

STEP 1: Rhythm Determination

- Ventricular rate *60*
- QRS shape *Widened*
- Atrial rate *60*
- P wave shape *Positive except negative in aVR, diphasic in V1*
- R-R rhythm *Regular*
- QRS interval *0.14*
- QT interval *0.44*
- P-P rhythm *Regular*
- P-R interval *0.19*
- P:R conduction ratio *1:1*
- Dominant pacemaker site *Sinus*
- Interpretation *Sinus bradycardia*

STEP 2: Axis Determination
Borderline left axis

STEP 3: Chamber Enlargement Determination
None

STEP 4: Intraventricular Conduction Blocks Determination
LBBB

STEP 5: Ischemia, Injury, and Infarction Determination
ST segments depressed and upwardly coved in leads with tall R waves. T waves positive in leads II, III, aVR, aVF, V1–V6 and negative I, aVL. R wave progression normal.

STEP 6: Miscellaneous ECG Changes
No significant findings

STEP 7: Final Interpretation
Abnormal 12-lead ECG. Sinus bradycardia with borderline left axis deviation. LBBB. Primary T wave changes indicative of lateral ischemia. Monitor cardiac enzymes for MI. Monitor on limb lead for progression of heart block. If LBBB old, no treatment required. If LBBB new, apply external pacemaker and be prepared for insertion of temporary transvenous pacemaker. Assess vital signs. Assess type and quality of chest pain; medicate appropriately.

EXERCISE 27

STEP 1: Rhythm Determination

- Ventricular rate *75*
- ORS shape *Normal*
- Atrial rate *75*
- P wave shape *Positive except negative aVR and aVL, diphasic in V1*
- R-R rhythm *Regular*
- QRS interval *0.08*
- QT interval *0.40*
- P-P rhythm *Regular*
- P-R interval *0.19*
- P:R conduction ratio *1:1*

- Dominant pacemaker site *Sinus*
- Interpretation *NSR*

STEP 2: Axis Determination
Left axis

STEP 3: Chamber Enlargement Determination
None

STEP 4: Intraventricular Conduction Blocks Determination
LAH

STEP 5: Ischemia, Injury, and Infarction Determination
ST segments isoelectric. T waves positive in all leads except negative in leads aVR and aVL and flattened in lead I. Poor R wave progression in leads V2–V3.

STEP 6: Miscellaneous ECG Changes
No significant findings

STEP 7: Final Interpretation
Abnormal 12-lead ECG. Normal sinus rhythm with LAD and LAH. Poor R wave progression in anteroseptal leads may be indicative of a previous infarct. Assess vital signs. Assess type and quality of chest pain; if patient's vital signs stable, give sublingual nitroglycerin for chest pain. Monitor serial ECGs and cardiac enzymes.

EXERCISE 28

STEP 1: Rhythm Determination

- Ventricular rate *70*
- QRS shape *Normal*
- Atrial rate *70*
- P wave shape *Positive except negative aVR, diphasic III, V1*
- R-R rhythm *Regular*
- QRS interval *0.08*
- QT interval *0.42*
- P-P rhythm *Regular*
- P-R interval *0.19*
- P:R conduction ratio *1:1*

- Dominant pacemaker site *Sinus*
- Interpretation *NSR*

STEP 2: Axis Determination
Left axis

STEP 3: Chamber Enlargement Determination
None

STEP 4: Intraventricular Conduction Blocks Determination
Normal conduction. Even though there is a LAD, there is no LAH because there is no Q wave in I or an S wave in III.

STEP 5: Ischemia, Injury, and Infarction Determination
ST segments isoelectric. T waves positive in all leads

except negative in aVR, III, and aVF. Abnormally tall R waves V1 and V2. Significant Q waves in leads II, III, and aVF.

STEP 6: Miscellaneous ECG Changes
No significant findings

STEP 7: Final Interpretation
Abnormal 12-lead ECG. Normal sinus rhythm with inferior and posterior MI, age indeterminate. Left axis deviation secondary to inferior MI. Compare with previous ECGs to assess for any acute changes.

EXERCISE 29

STEP 1: Rhythm Determination
- Ventricular rate *51*
- Atrial rate *=*
- QRS shape *Notched V1*
- P wave shape *=*
- R-R rhythm *Regular*
- P-P rhythm *=*
- QRS interval *0.10*
- P-R interval *=*
- QT interval *0.40*
- P:R conduction ratio *=*
- Dominant pacemaker site *Junctional*
- Interpretation *Junctional rhythm*

STEP 2: Axis Determination
Left axis

STEP 3: Chamber Enlargement Determination
None

STEP 4: Intraventricular Conduction Blocks Determination
Incomplete RBBB

STEP 5: Ischemia, Injury, and Infarction Determination
ST segment elevations in leads II, III, aVF with reciprocal ST depressions in lead I, aVL. T waves merged with ST segments leads II, III, and aVF; positive in all leads except negative in aVR and flat in V1. Abnormally tall R waves in leads V1 and V2.

STEP 6: Miscellaneous ECG Changes
No significant findings

STEP 7: Final Interpretation
Abnormal 12-lead ECG. Junctional rhythm. Incomplete RBBB. Acute inferior and posterior MI. Assess serial ECGs and cardiac enzymes. Monitor on limb lead to assess rhythm. If QRS becomes wider, monitor on V1 to assess for completion of RBBB and/

or complete heart block. Prepare for thrombolytic therapy.

EXERCISE 30

STEP 1: Rhythm Determination
- Ventricular rate 38
- Atrial rate 38
- QRS shape *Widened*
- P wave shape *Positive but generally flattened, except negative aVR*
- R-R rhythm *Mostly regular*
- P-P rhythm *Regular*
- QRS interval *0.14*
- P-R interval *0.16*
- QT interval *0.48*
- P:R conduction ratio *1:1*
- Dominant pacemaker site *Sinus*
- Interpretation *Marked sinus bradycardia with PVC*

STEP 2: Axis Determination
Left axis

STEP 3: Chamber Enlargement Determination
None

STEP 4: Intraventricular Conduction Blocks Determination
RBBB with LAH

STEP 5: Ischemia, Injury, and Infarction Determination
ST segments isoelectric. T waves positive in all leads except negative in aVR and V1. Abnormal R wave progression.

STEP 6: Miscellaneous ECG Changes
No significant findings

STEP 7: Final Interpretation
Abnormal 12-lead ECG. Marked sinus bradycardia with PVC. Left axis deviation. Bifascicular block. Monitor ECGs and cardiac enzymes for acute MI. Assess age of bifascicular block. Patient has had bifascicular block on previous ECG, needs no emergency treatment. Observe for progression to complete heart block. Monitor for more frequent PVCs and treat as necessary. Assess vital signs and signs and symptoms of low cardiac output. Treat low heart rate if cardiac output being compromised. Increasing the heart rate may help eliminate PVCs. Assess type and quality of chest pain; medicate appropriately.

SELF-ASSESSMENT ANSWERS TO CHAPTER 6

EXERCISE 31
STEP 1: Rhythm Determination
- Ventricular rate *61*
- QRS shape *Normal*
- Atrial rate *61*
- P wave shape *Positive except negative aVR and aVL*

- R-R rhythm *Regular*
- QRS interval *0.08*
- QT interval *0.38*
- P-P rhythm *Regular*
- P-R interval *0.16*
- P:R conduction ratio *1:1*

- Dominant pacemaker site *Sinus*
- Interpretation *NSR*

STEP 2: Axis Determination
Normal axis

STEP 3: Chamber Enlargement Determination
None

STEP 4: Intraventricular Conduction Blocks Determination
Normal conduction

STEP 5: Ischemia, Injury, and Infarction Determination
ST segment elevations leads II, III, and aVF with reciprocal depressions and T wave inversions in leads I and aVL. ST segments depressed in leads V2–V3. T waves negative in aVR. Normal R wave progression. Q waves evolving in leads II, III, and aVF.

STEP 6: Miscellaneous ECG Changes
No significant findings

STEP 7: Final Interpretation
Abnormal 12-lead ECG. Normal sinus rhythm with inferior MI evolving. Assess quality and type of chest pain; medicate appropriately. Monitor serial ECGs and cardiac enzymes. Monitor for dysrhythmias such as Wenckebach and atrial dysrhythmias. Assess how long patient has been having chest pain. Consider using thrombolytic agent. Will probably need further follow-up to assess patency of angioplasty site. Assess drug history.

EXERCISE 32
STEP 1: Rhythm Determination
- Ventricular rate *67*
- QRS shape *Normal*
- Atrial rate *67*
- P wave shape *Positive except negative III, aVR and flattened in aVF*

- R-R rhythm *Regular*
- QRS interval *0.09*
- QT interval *0.38*
- P-P rhythm *Regular*
- P-R interval *0.14*
- P:R conduction ratio *1:1*

- Dominant pacemaker site *Sinus*
- Interpretation *NSR*

STEP 2: Axis Determination
Normal axis

STEP 3: Chamber Enlargement Determination
None

STEP 4: Intraventricular Conduction Blocks Determination
Normal conduction

STEP 5: Ischemia, Injury, and Infarction Determination
ST segments depressed leads I, aVL, and squared off and depressed in leads V2–V4. T waves positive in all leads except negative in aVR. R wave progression normal.

STEP 6: Miscellaneous ECG Changes
No significant findings

STEP 7: Final Interpretation
Abnormal 12-lead ECG. Normal sinus rhythm with ischemic changes anterolateral leads. Assess serial ECGs and cardiac enzymes for acute non-Q wave MI. If cardiac enzymes positive for non-Q wave MI, observe for postinfarction angina. Monitor for dysrhythmias. Counsel on smoking cessation to reduce risk of heart disease.

EXERCISE 33
STEP 1: Rhythm Determination
- Ventricular rate *92*
- QRS shape *Normal*
- Atrial rate *92*
- P wave shape *Positive except negative III, aVR, and flat in aVF*

- R-R rhythm *Regular*
- QRS interval *0.10*
- QT interval *0.36*
- P-P rhythm *Regular*
- P-R interval *0.28*
- P:R conduction ratio *1:1*

- Dominant pacemaker site *Sinus*
- Interpretation *NSR with 1st degree AV block*

STEP 2: Axis Determination
Normal axis

STEP 3: Chamber Enlargement Determination
None

STEP 4: Intraventricular Conduction Blocks Determination

IVCD

STEP 5: Ischemia, Injury, and Infarction Determination

ST segment elevations in leads II, III, and aVF with reciprocal depressions in leads I, aVL, and V1. T waves positive in all leads except aVR. Normal R wave progression.

STEP 6: Miscellaneous ECG Changes

No significant findings

STEP 7: Final Interpretation

Abnormal 12-lead ECG. Normal sinus rhythm with 1st degree AV block and an IVCD. Inferior injury current. Assess type and quality of chest pain; medicate appropriately. After medicating with two sublingual nitroglycerin, the ST segments all returned to baseline. The patient probably experienced variant angina. Monitor serial ECGs and cardiac enzymes to rule out an MI. Monitor for progression of AV block and development of sinus bradycardia.

EXERCISE 34

STEP 1: Rhythm Determination

- Ventricular rate 65
- QRS shape *Slightly widened*

- Atrial rate 65
- P wave shape *Positive except negative in aVR*

- R-R rhythm *Regular*
- QRS interval *0.10*
- QT interval *0.36*

- P-P rhythm *Regular*
- P-R interval *0.24*
- P:R conduction ratio *1:1*

- Dominant pacemaker site *Sinus*
- Interpretation *NSR with 1st degree AV block*

STEP 2: Axis Determination

Normal axis. Use null plane method.

STEP 3: Chamber Enlargement Determination

None

STEP 4: Intraventricular Conduction Blocks Determination

IVCD

STEP 5: Ischemia, Injury, and Infarction Determination

ST segments isoelectric. T waves positive in all leads except negative in leads I, aVR, V1–V4, and diphasic in V5–V6. Normal R wave progression.

STEP 6: Miscellaneous ECG Changes

No significant findings

STEP 7: Final Interpretation

Abnormal 12-lead ECG. Normal sinus rhythm with 1st degree AV block and IVCD. Anterolateral T wave changes appear ischemic. Monitor serial ECGs and cardiac enzymes. Assess type and quality of chest pain; medicate appropriately. Sublingual nitroglycerin was given with prompt relief of the chest pain. If pain had not been relieved, IV nitroglycerin should have been initiated. The cardiac enzymes remained negative. The ECG changes were those of classic angina. Assess drug history.

EXERCISE 35

STEP 1: Rhythm Determination

- Ventricular rate 49
- QRS shape *Normal*

- Atrial rate 49
- P wave shape *Positive except negative in aVR, and flattened in III and aVL*

- R-R rhythm *Regular*
- QRS interval *0.10*
- QT interval *0.44*

- P-P rhythm *Regular*
- P-R interval *0.16*
- P:R conduction ratio *1:1*

- Dominant pacemaker site *Sinus*
- Interpretation *Sinus bradycardia*

STEP 2: Axis Determination

Normal axis

STEP 3: Chamber Enlargement Determination

None

STEP 4: Intraventricular Conduction Blocks Determination

IVCD

STEP 5: Ischemia, Injury, and Infarction Determination

ST segments isoelectric except J point ST elevations in leads V2–V3. T waves positive in all leads except negative in leads III, aVR, aVF. Tall R waves in leads V1–V2. Significant Q waves in leads II, III, and aVF.

STEP 6: Miscellaneous ECG Changes

No significant findings

STEP 7: Final Interpretation

Abnormal 12-lead ECG. Sinus bradycardia with IVCD. Changes consistent with inferior and true posterior MI. These changes do not appear to be recent. Monitor serial ECGs and cardiac enzymes. Assess quality and type of chest pain; medicate appropriately. Monitor on rhythm lead and watch for Wenckebach, PACs, or slower sinus bradycardia. Treat with atropine if necessary.

EXERCISE 36
STEP 1: Rhythm Determination
- Ventricular rate *68*
- QRS shape *Normal*
- Atrial rate *68*
- P wave shape *Positive except negative in leads III and aVR and diphasic in V1*

- R-R rhythm *Regular*
- QRS interval *0.09*
- QT interval *0.36*
- P-P rhythm *Regular*
- P-R interval *0.14*
- P:R conduction ratio *1:1*

- Dominant pacemaker site *Sinus*
- Interpretation *NSR*

STEP 2: Axis Determination
Left axis. Use null plane method.

STEP 3: Chamber Enlargement Determination
None

STEP 4: Intraventricular Conduction Blocks Determination
Normal conduction

STEP 5: Ischemia, Injury, and Infarction Determination
ST segment elevations in leads I, aVL, V2–V6. T waves positive in all leads except negative in leads III and aVR and flattened in lead aVF. Poor R wave progression. Significant Q waves in leads I and aVL.

STEP 6: Miscellaneous ECG Changes
No significant findings

STEP 7: Final Interpretation
Abnormal 12-lead ECG. Normal sinus rhythm with acute anterolateral MI. Prepare for administration of thrombolytic agent. Monitor serial ECGs and cardiac enzymes. Cardiac enzymes were positive. Assess vital signs. Assess quality and type of chest pain: medicate appropriately. Be prepared to administer intravenous nitroglycerin drip. Observe monitor for ventricular dysrhythmias and BBB development. Assess patient's heart and lung sounds for signs and symptoms of congestive heart failure. Monitor on V1 rhythm lead.

SELF-ASSESSMENT ANSWERS TO CHAPTER 7

EXERCISE 37
STEP 1: Rhythm Determination
- Ventricular rate *90*
- QRS shape *Normal*
- Atrial rate *90*
- P wave shape *Positive except negative in aVR, flattened in aVL, and diphasic in V1*

- R-R rhythm *Regular*
- QRS interval *0.08*
- QT interval *0.36*
- P-P rhythm *Regular*
- P-R interval *0.12*
- P:R conduction ratio *1:1*

- Dominant pacemaker site *Sinus*
- Interpretation *NSR*

STEP 2: Axis Determination
Left axis

STEP 3: Chamber Enlargement Determination
None

STEP 4: Intraventricular Conduction Blocks Determination
LAH

STEP 5: Ischemia, Injury, and Infarction Determination
ST segments isoelectric. T waves diffusely flattened. U waves present. Normal R wave progression.

STEP 6: Miscellaneous ECG Changes
Diffuse T wave changes and presence of U waves suggestive of hypokalemia

STEP 7: Final Interpretation
Abnormal 12-lead ECG. Normal sinus rhythm with LAD and LAH. Diffuse nonspecific T wave changes and presence of U waves suggestive of hypokalemia. Monitor electrolytes, especially potassium level. Potassium level was 2.3 mEq/L. Prepare to replace potassium. Monitor for ventricular dysrhythmias. Observe for hyperkalemia on ECG during repletion of potassium.

EXERCISE 38

STEP 1: Rhythm Determination
- Ventricular rate 38
- QRS shape *Normal*
- R-R rhythm *Slightly irregular*
- QRS interval *0.08*
- QT interval *0.44*

- Atrial rate =
- P wave shape =
- P-P rhythm =
- P-R interval =
- P:R conduction ratio =

- Dominant pacemaker site *Junctional*
- Interpretation *Slow junctional rhythm*

STEP 2: Axis Determination
Normal axis

STEP 3: Chamber Enlargement Determination
LVH

STEP 4: Intraventricular Conduction Blocks Determination
Normal conduction

STEP 5: Ischemia, Injury, and Infarction Determination
ST segments depressed and upwardly coved in leads with tall R waves. T waves inverted in same leads. Normal R wave progression.

STEP 6: Miscellaneous ECG Changes
No significant findings. The ECG changes that are seen with digitalis therapy are being masked in this patient by the ST and T wave changes caused by LVH. The slow junctional rhythm is of concern and may be a result of digitalis toxicity.

STEP 7: Final Interpretation
Abnormal 12-lead ECG. Slow junctional rhythm with LVH. Hold digoxin and draw a digoxin level. Digoxin level was 4.5 (therapeutic range ≤2.0). Measure potassium levels while digoxin level high. Monitor patient for progression to complete heart block and development of ventricular dysrhythmias. Monitor vital signs. Monitor for signs and symptoms of low cardiac output; may need external pacemaker or temporary transvenous pacemaker until digoxin level returns to therapeutic range.

EXERCISE 39

STEP 1: Rhythm Determination
- Ventricular rate 46
- QRS shape *Small but normal*

- R-R rhythm *Regular*
- QRS interval *0.08*
- QT interval *0.44*

- Atrial rate *46*
- P wave shape *Positive except negative in aVR*
- P-P rhythm *Regular*
- P-R interval *0.15*
- P:R conduction ratio *1:1*

- Dominant pacemaker site *Sinus*
- Interpretation *Marked sinus bradycardia*

STEP 2: Axis Determination
Normal axis

STEP 3: Chamber Enlargement Determination
None

STEP 4: Intraventricular Conduction Blocks Determination
Normal conduction

STEP 5: Ischemia, Injury, and Infarction Determination
ST segments isoelectric. T waves positive in all leads except negative in aVR and V1. Normal R wave progression.

STEP 6: Miscellaneous ECG Changes
Measured QT interval is 0.44 seconds. The corrected QT interval for this heart rate is 0.53 seconds. The portion of the QT that appears shortened is the ST segment. These changes may be significant for hypercalcemia.

STEP 7: Final Interpretation
Abnormal 12-lead ECG. Marked sinus bradycardia with shortened QT intervals may be significant for hypercalcemia. Calcium level drawn and was 11.4 mg/dl. Monitor patient for ventricular dysrhythmias. Assess patient for signs and symptoms of myocardial ischemia. Prepare to treat with calcium-lowering drugs. Assess quality and type of abdominal pain; medicate appropriately.

EXERCISE 40

STEP 1: Rhythm Determination
- Ventricular rate *120*
- QRS shape *Normal*

- R-R rhythm *Regular*
- QRS interval *0.09*
- QT interval *0.34*

- Atrial rate *120*
- P wave shape *Positive except negative in aVR and flattened in aVL*
- P-P rhythm *Regular*
- P-R interval *0.12*
- P:R conduction ratio *1:1*

- Dominant pacemaker site *Sinus*
- Interpretation *Sinus tachycardia*

STEP 2: Axis Determination
Left axis

STEP 3: Chamber Enlargement Determination
None

STEP 4: Intraventricular Conduction Blocks Determination
LAH

STEP 5: Ischemia, Injury, and Infarction Determination

ST segments isoelectric. T waves tall, pointed, and pinched in chest leads. Tall R waves in V1–V3.

STEP 6: Miscellaneous ECG Changes

Peaked T waves significant for hyperkalemia

STEP 7: Final Interpretation

Abnormal 12-lead ECG. Sinus tachycardia with LAD and LAH. T wave changes may be significant for hyperkalemia. Tall R waves in anterior chest leads not of significance in this patient because they are secondary in thin-chested young men. Draw electrolytes. Potassium level was 6.7 mEq/L. Monitor for ventricular dysrhythmias. Monitor serum potassium levels as hyperkalemia treated.

EXERCISE 41

STEP 1: Rhythm Determination

- Ventricular rate 88
- QRS shape *Normal*
- Atrial rate 88
- P wave shape *Positive except negative in aVR and aVL*
- R-R rhythm *Regular*
- QRS interval *0.06*
- QT interval *0.34*
- P-P rhythm *Regular*
- P-R interval *0.16*
- P:R conduction ratio *1:1*
- Dominant pacemaker site *Sinus*
- Interpretation *NSR*

STEP 2: Axis Determination

Normal axis

STEP 3: Chamber Enlargement Determination

LVH no strain pattern

STEP 4: Intraventricular Conduction Blocks Determination

Normal conduction

STEP 5: Ischemia, Injury, and Infarction Determination

ST segments concave shaped and diffusely elevated. T waves positive in all leads except negative in leads I, aVR, and aVL. Normal R wave progression.

STEP 6: Miscellaneous ECG Changes

ST segments diffusely elevated and concave in shape. P-R segment elevated in lead aVR with a depressed ST segment in that same lead. Changes significant for pericarditis.

STEP 7: Final Interpretation

Abnormal 12-lead ECG. Normal sinus rhythm. LVH diffuse ST and T wave changes indicative of pericarditis. Assess quality and type of chest pain; medicate appropriately. Assess heart sounds for pericardial friction rub. Monitor for increased frequency of atrial dysrhythmias. Monitor serial ECGs and cardiac enzymes. MI was ruled out in this patient, and his chest pain was attributed to pericarditis. Prepare to medicate patient with anti-inflammatory agents.

EXERCISE 42

STEP 1: Rhythm Determination

- Ventricular rate *115*
- QRS shape *Normal*

- Atrial rate *115*
- P wave shape *Positive except negative in aVR and flattened in aVL*
- R-R rhythm *Regular*
- QRS interval *0.08*
- QT interval *0.34*
- P-P rhythm *Regular*
- P-R interval *0.13*
- P:R conduction ratio *1:1*
- Dominant pacemaker site *Sinus*
- Interpretation *Sinus tachycardia*

STEP 2: Axis Determination

Left axis

STEP 3: Chamber Enlargement Determination

None

STEP 4: Intraventricular Conduction Blocks Determination

LAH

STEP 5: Ischemia, Injury, and Infarction Determination

ST segments isoelectric. T waves tall, pointed, and pinched in leads V1–V4. Tall R waves in leads V1–V3.

STEP 6: Miscellaneous ECG Changes

Tall peaked T waves indicative of hyperkalemia.

STEP 7: Final Interpretation

Abnormal 12-lead ECG. Sinus tachycardia with LAD and LAH. T wave changes may be indicative of hyperkalemia. Tall R waves secondary to a young, thin-chested man and are of no clinical significance. Draw serum electrolytes. Serum potassium was 6.2 mEq/L. Monitor for ventricular dysrhythmias. Prepare to treat hyperkalemia with potassium-lowering agents. Monitor serial serum potassium levels.

APPENDIX B

Self-Assessment Analysis Form

STEP 1: Rhythm Determination
- Ventricular rate _____
- QRS shape _____
- R-R rhythm _____
- QRS interval _____
- QT interval _____

- Atrial rate _____
- P wave shape _____
- P-P rhythm _____
- P-R interval _____
- P:R conduction ratio
_____

- Dominant pacemaker site _____
- Interpretation _____

STEP 2: Axis Determination
Normal __ Right __ Left __ Indeterminate __

STEP 3: Chamber Enlargement Determination
Atrial Abnormality: Right __ Left __
Ventricular Hypertrophy: Right __ Left __

STEP 4: Intraventricular Conduction Blocks Determination
RBBB __ LBBB __
Incomplete RBBB __ Incomplete LBBB __ IVCD __
LAH __ LPH __

STEP 5: Ischemia, Injury, and Infarction Determination
Inferior leads (II, III, aVF): _____
Anterior leads (V1–V6): _____
Lateral leads (I, aVL, V5–V6): _____
Anteroseptal leads (V1–V4): _____
Posterior leads (V1–V2 Reciprocal): _____
Diffuse _____

STEP 6: Miscellaneous ECG Changes
Electrolytes: _____
Drugs: _____
Pericarditis: _____
Other: _____

STEP 7: Final Interpretation

_____
_____
_____

APPENDIX C
Study Guide[a]

STEP	CRITERIA	SIGNIFICANCE

1. Rhythm Determination
Use leads II, V1, V6
	Compare with NSR
	Rate: 60–100 BPM
	  Both atrial and ventricular
	Rhythm: regular
	  Both atrial and ventricular
	QRS Shape: normal
	QT interval: <0.44 seconds
	P Wave Shape: normal
	P-R Interval: 0.12–0.20 seconds
	P:R Conduction ratio: 1:1
		■ Treat rhythms that affect cardiac output.
		■ Look for other etiologies such as MI, drug and electrolyte imbalances.
		■ If wide QRS and not ventricular dysrhythmia, look for BBB.
		■ If abnormal QT interval, look for miscellaneous causes.
		■ If notched or widened P wave, look for atrial abnormalities.

2. Axis Determination
Look at leads I, aVF
Use Easy Quadrant Method
	Normal = Positive I, aVF
	RAD = Negative I; Positive aVF
	LAD = Positive I; Negative aVF
	Indeterminate = Negative I, aVF
		RAD = LPH
		      RVH
		      Lateral MI
		LAD = LAH
		      LVH
		      Inferior MI
		
		■ If equiphasic in leads I or aVF, use Null plane method.
		■ If equiphasic in all leads, axis is indeterminate.

3. Chamber Enlargement Determination Examine height & width of P wave in leads II & V1 for atrial abnormalities.	Rt Atrial = Lead II Tall pointed P wave > 2.5 mm Lead V1 Diphasic P wave Initial positive deflection taller than terminal negative deflection. Lt Atrial = Lead II P wave > 0.12 seconds in width & notched. Looks like an "M." Lead V1 Diphasic P wave with terminal negative deflection deeper and wider than initial positive deflection.	■ Right atrial abnormality due to COPD or pulmonary embolus. ■ Look for atrial dysrhythmias with atrial abnormalities.

[a] ↑ = elevation; ↓ = inversion or depression; ST = ST segment; Ca = calcium; < = less than; > = greater than.

STEP	CRITERIA	SIGNIFICANCE
Examine QRS in chest leads especially V1 or V2 and V5 or V6 for ventricular hypertrophy.	RVH = Lead V1 R > S Strain pattern = ST ↓ & asymmetrical T wave in right heart leads. Lead V6 Deep S wave RAD	■ LVH cannot be identified when LBBB present. ■ Right heart leads = III, aVF, V1, V2.
	LVH = S in lead V1 + R in lead V5 > 35 mm. Strain pattern = ST ↓ & asymmetrical T wave inversion in left heart leads. LAD	■ Left heart leads = I, aVL, V5, V6.
4. Intraventricular Conduction Blocks Determination	RBBB = Lead V1 rSR pattern QRS duration ≥ 0.12 seconds V6 Wide S wave	■ If BBB acute, rule out infarction.
Examine width & configuration of leads V1 & V6 for bundle branch blocks.	LBBB = Lead V1 Wide negative QRS QRS duration ≥ 0.12 second Lead V6 Large R wave	■ If LBBB, cannot determine LVH or MI presence.
Determine axis and examine QRS configuration in leads I & III for hemiblocks.	LAH = Left axis with no evidence of inferior MI Normal QRS duration Lead I qr configuration Lead III rS configuration	■ If other reasons for axis changes such as MI, look for changes in QRS configurations in leads I and III.
	LPH = Rt axis with no evidence of RVH Normal QRS duration Lead I rS configuration Lead III qR configuration	■ LPH is very rare finding.
	Bifascicular = Block in more than one area i.e., RBBB with LAH or LPH. LBBB alone	■ Bifascicular blocks can occur in combination with AV Blocks and can lead to CHB.
	Incomplete Block = Resembles pattern of RBBB or LBBB. QRS duration 0.10–0.11 seconds	■ Treat with pacemaker as needed.
	IVCD = QRS duration between 0.10–0.11 seconds but does not resemble either type of BBB	

STEP	CRITERIA	SIGNIFICANCE
5. Ischemia, Injury, and Infarction Determination	ST segment ↑ > 1 mm convex or coved shape.	■ To make definite differential diagnosis, clinical and drug history must be correlated to ECG findings.
Examine ST segment for ↑ or ↓.	ST segment ↓ > 0.5 mm horizontal, down-sloping or squared off.	■ Assess cardiac enzymes. ■ Cannot diagnose infarction in presence of LBBB.
Examine T wave for ↑ or ↓.	T wave flat, pointed & symmetrical, inverted, or diphasic.	■ *Q wave infarction* = ↑ ST segment, ↓ T waves & path. Q waves. Loss of R wave progression may signify an old MI.
Examine for pathological Q waves.	Pathological Q waves = > 0.04 second wide & depth > ⅓ of R wave.	■ *Non Q wave infarction* = ↓ ST segment and/or ↓ T waves. Squared off ST segment shape. Deeply inverted & symmetrical T waves.
Look for these changes in limb & chest leads.	Reciprocal changes in opposite leads.	■ *Classic angina* = ↓ ST & ↓ T waves. Downsloping or horizontal ST segment shape.
Determine whether localized to specific leads or diffuse leads.	Age of changes: Acute = ↑ ST segment. Evolving = ↑ ST segment isoelectric & inverted T waves.	■ *Variant angina* = ↑ ST segment that return to baseline with rest or NTG.
Anterior leads = V1–V6 Inferior leads = II, III, aVF Anteroseptal leads = V1–V4 Lateral leads = I, aVL, V5, V6 Posterior leads = Reciprocal changes in V1 & V2 and large dominant R waves.	Indeterminate = ST segment & T waves normal with pathological Q waves.	■ Large dominant R in lead V1 without evidence of inferior MI probably caused by RVH or RBBB. ■ Persistent ST ↑, look for ventricular aneurysm.
Determine age of changes Look for R wave progression in chest leads.		■ To diagnosis posterior wall MI, rule out RVH and RBBB, and look for evidence of inferior MI.

6. Miscellaneous ECG Changes
 	
 Examine ST and T waves in all leads.
 	
 Measure QT interval.
	Potassium
	   Low = Flat T wave
	         U wave
	         ST segment ↓
	
	   High = Peak or tented T waves & widened QRS
	
	 Calcium
	   Low = Prolonged QT interval
	
	   High = Shortened QT interval
	
	 Dig. effect = Downward sloping or sagging of ST segment. Asymmetrical ↓ T wave or flat T waves.
	 ST-T wave changes seen in leads with tall R waves.
	
	 Quinidine effect = Prolonged QT interval
		■ To make diagnosis clinical and drug history must be correlated to ECG changes.
		
		 ■ Watch for torsades de pointes with low Ca or quinidine.
		
		 ■ Dig. effect masks ischemic changes.
		
		 ■ With Ca abnormalities, look for changes in the ST segment.
		
		 ■ If QRS lengthens to 1.5 times its original width, stop quinidine.

STEP	CRITERIA	SIGNIFICANCE
	Pericarditis = Diffuse ST ↑, Concave in shape. T wave ↓ only after ST segment returns iso-electric PR interval elevated in aVR while ST segment ↓ in lead aVR.	■ No Q wave formation in pericarditis. ■ In infarction, the T wave usually precedes normalization of ST segment, and the elevations are convex in shape.
7. Final interpretation	Rhythm and 12 lead ECG diagnosis.	■ To make diagnosis clinical and drug history must be correlated to ECG findings.
Combine all information to determine diagnosis.	Compare changes to baseline or serial ECGs.	■ Report new changes. ■ Take vital signs. ■ Assess for angina and other signs & symptoms of ischemia (SOB, dizziness). ■ Assess lung and heart sounds. ■ Prepare for treatment if needed.

BIBLIOGRAPHY

Alspach, J. (1979). Electrical axis: How to recognize deviations on the ECG and interpret them. *American Journal of Nursing, 79,* 1976–1983.

Berne, R. M., & Levy, M. N. (1986). *Cardiovascular Physiology* (5th ed.). St. Louis: C. V. Mosby.

Brown, K., & Jacobson, S. (1988). *Mastering dysrhythmias: A problem-solving guide.* Philadelphia: F. A. Davis Co.

Conover, M. (1980). *Understanding electrocardiography physiological and interpretive concepts* (3rd ed.). St. Louis: C. V. Mosby Co.

Conover, M. (1984). *Exercises in diagnosing ECG tracings* (3rd ed.). St. Louis: C. V. Mosby Co.

Davis, D. (1985). *How to quickly and accurately master ECG interpretation.* Philadelphia: J. B. Lippincott Co.

Dubin, D. (1989). *Rapid interpretation of EKG's* (4th ed.). Tampa: Cover Publishing Co.

Duke, D. (1982). Intraventricular conduction blocks. Part II. *Critical Care Nurse, 2*(4), 58–70.

Frye, S., & Lounsbury, P. (1988). *Cardiac rhythm disorders: An introduction using the nursing process.* Baltimore: Williams & Wilkins.

Goldberger, A. L., & Goldberger, E. (1986). *Clinical electrocardiography. A simplified approach* (3rd ed.). St. Louis: C. V. Mosby Co.

Goldman, M. J. (1982). *Principles of clinical electrocardiography.* Los Altos, CA: Lange Medical Publications.

Hurst, C. (1986). *Dysrhythmia interpretation based on cardiac suppression and irritability.* Philadelphia: J. B. Lippincott.

Karnes, N. (1987). Differentiation of aberrant ventricular conduction from ventricular ectopic beats. *Critical Care Nurse, 4,* 42–55.

Laiken, N., Laiken, S. L., & Karliner, J. S. (1988). *Interpretation of electrocardiograms. A self-instructional approach* (2nd ed.). New York: Raven Press.

Lewis, V. (1987). Monitoring the patient with acute myocardial infarction. *Nursing Clinics of North America, 22*(1)., 15–32.

Marion Laboratories. (1986). *The cardizem ECG ruler.* Kansas City.

Marriott, H. J. L. (1988). *Practical electrocardiography* (8th ed.). Baltimore: Williams & Wilkins.

Meltzer, L., Pinneo, R., & Kitchell, R. (1987). *Intensive coronary care: A manual for nurses* (4th ed.). Bowie, Maryland: Robert J. Brady Co.

Mudge, G. H., Jr. (1986). *Manual of electrocardiography* (2nd ed.). Boston: Little, Brown and Co.

Pecham, M. (1987). *Coronary care modules.* Baltimore: Williams & Wilkins.

Petrie, J. (1988). Distinguishing supraventricular aberrancies from ventricular ectopy. *Focus on Critical Care, 15,* 15–21.

Purcell, J., & Haynes, L. (1984). Using the ECG to detect MI. *American Journal of Nursing, 84,* 627–639.

Searle & Co. (1981). *Norpace cardiac graphics ruler.* Chicago: Medical Communications Department.

Smith-Marker, C. (1982). *12 Lead EKG A practical workbook.* Baltimore: Resource Applications Publishing.

Textbook of advanced cardiac life support. (1987). Dallas: American Heart Association.

Thaler, M. (1988). *The only EKG book you'll ever need.* Philadelphia: J. B. Lippincott Co.

Weeks, L. C. (Ed.). (1986). *Advanced cardiovascular nursing.* Boston: Blackwell Scientific Publications.

INDEX